the shoulder in sport

management, rehabilitation and prevention

Dedication

To my wife Giovanna and my daughters Marianna, Charlotte and Luisamaria for the time stolen from them; to my parents, masters without equal of clinical reasoning and of life

A. F.

Publisher: *Sarena Wolfaard*
Development Editor: *Claire Bonnett*
Commissioning Editor: *Claire Wilson*
Senior Project Manager: *Jess Thompson*
Project Manager: *Tracey Donnelly*
Designer: *Charles Gray*
Illustrator: *David Graham*
Illustration Manager: *Gillian Richards*

Edinburgh ◆ London ◆ New York ◆ Oxford ◆ Philadelphia ◆ St Louis ◆ Sydney ◆ Toronto 2008

Via Val d'Aposa 7 – 40123 Bologna – Italy
seps@alma.unibo.it – www.seps.it

Segretariato Europeo per le Pubblicazioni Scientifiche
The translation of this work has been funded by SEPS

Translated by Helen Wormald

Marco Testa

Frank Musarra

Andrea Foglia

Andrea Fusco

the shoulder in sport
management, rehabilitation and prevention

CHURCHILL LIVINGSTONE

ELSEVIER

An imprint of Elsevier Ltd

© 2008, English Translation
© Masson S.p.A., Milan, 2005

No part of this publication may be reproduced, stored in a retrieval system, or transmitted in any form or by any means, electronic, mechanical, photocopying, recording or otherwise, without the prior permission of the Publishers. Permissions may be sought directly from Elsevier's Health Sciences Rights Department, 1600 John F. Kennedy Boulevard, Suite 1800, Philadelphia, PA 19103-2899, USA: phone: (+1) 215 239 3804; fax: (+1) 215 239 3805; or, e-mail: *healthpermissions@elsevier.com*. You may also complete your request on-line via the Elsevier homepage (http://www.elsevier.com), by selecting 'Support and contact' and then 'Copyright and Permission'.

First edition 2008

ISBN 978-0-443-06874-4

British Library Cataloguing in Publication Data
A catalogue record for this book is available from the British Library

Library of Congress Cataloging in Publication Data
A catalog record for this book is available from the Library of Congress

Note
Neither the Publisher nor the editors and author contributors assume any responsibility for any loss or injury and/or damage to persons or property arising out of or related to any use of the material contained in this book. It is the responsibility of the treating practitioner, relying on independent expertise and knowledge of the patient, to determine the best treatment and method of application for the patient.

The Publisher

ELSEVIER your source for books, journals and multimedia in the health sciences

www.elsevierhealth.com

Working together to grow libraries in developing countries

www.elsevier.com | www.bookaid.org | www.sabre.org

ELSEVIER · BOOK AID International · Sabre Foundation

The Publisher's policy is to use **paper manufactured from sustainable forests**

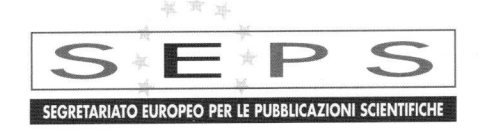

S·E·P·S

SEGRETARIATO EUROPEO PER LE PUBBLICAZIONI SCIENTIFICHE

Via Val d'Aposa 7 – 40123 Bologna – Italy
seps@alma.unibo.it – www.seps.it

Printed in China

Contents

SECTION I
Functional anatomy and recent biomechanical discoveries

SECTION II
Pathology, clinical aspects and diagnostic imaging

Contents

SECTION III
Surgical treatment

Contents

Contents

SECTION V
Current trends in surface electromyography

Contents

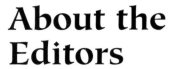

About the Editors

Andrea Fusco

Lecturer in the Theory and Methodology of Manual Therapy on the Master's course in Rehabilitation of Musculoskeletal Disorders at Università degli Studi di Genova and lecturer in Biomechanics on the degree course in Physiotherapy at the same university, with a degree in the Science and Technology of Physical Activities and Sports (STAPS) (Lyon), and in Motor Sciences, and a qualified physiotherapist with credits in sport physiotherapy (Nice) and the Master's course on which he lectures.

He practises independently as a physiotherapist in Genoa, treating athletes, and movement professionals and artists. He is a consultant to many sport and artistic institutions, including the Italian Sailing Federation (FIV), the Associazione Valdostana Maestri di Sci (AVMS) and the Carlo Felice Theatre in Genoa. His experience as a volleyball and beach volleyball player, an accomplished practitioner of winter sports, a physiotherapist and trainer in water polo and sailing, as well as a practitioner of kinomichi and aikido, have helped in his quest for quality in movement as a fusion of efficiency, health and harmony.

Andrea Foglia

A physiotherapist since 1990 after having specialized in Sport Physiotherapy at Nice School of Medicine and Advanced Manual Therapy at Università degli Studi di Genova, he lectured in the Theory and Methodology of Manual Therapy on the Master's course in Rehabilitation of Musculoskeletal Disorders at the same university.

He was an external physiotherapy consultant to professional football teams from 1992 to 2000, and today is a consultant to several sport institutions, including the Italian Football Federation (the National Amateur League) and the Italian Association of Referees, both in the Marche region.

He is currently practising as an independent physiotherapist at L'Officina di Fidia rehabilitation centre in Macerata and at Villa Margherita nursing home in Civitanova Marche, where he is also responsible for training non-medical personnel in physical therapy and rehabilitation.

Frank Musarra

Born in Nijmegen (Netherlands) in 1971, he has a degree in Physiotherapy and in 1996 obtained a specialist qualification with distinction in Sport Rehabilitation and Manual Therapy from Katholieke Universiteit di Leuven (Belgium). His first professional roles were at rehabilitation centres and professional sport associations in Belgium and, after transferring to Italy, he was awarded a Master's degree in Rehabilitation of Musculoskeletal Disorders from the School of Medicine and Surgery of Università degli Studi di Genova; he subsequently lectured on the Theory and Methodology of Manual Therapy.

He has published several papers in national and international scientific journals and, in addition to his role as rapporteur at national and international scientific conventions, currently has an independent physiotherapy practice in Pesaro (PU).

Marco Testa

A physiotherapist and graduate in Motor Sciences with a Diploma in Osteopathy obtained in 1996. He was the Coordinator of advanced training courses in Manual Therapy from 1999 to 2002 and since 2003 has coordinated the Master's course in Rehabilitation of Musculoskeletal Disorders at Università degli Studi di Genova. In this role he has established a series of educational and scientific contacts and cooperation with leading universities in Europe and elsewhere in the field of rehabilitation and sport physiotherapy. Since 2002 he has lectured in Biomechanics on the degree course in Physiotherapy at the same university. Since 1994 he has been head of the Craniocervicomandibular Physiotherapy Laboratory in the Department of Oral Rehabilitation of IRCCS San Rafaele in Milan. He has authored papers published in national and international journals, and has been the Italian editor of several major physiotherapy books for Masson publishing.

He is the only Italian member of the Advisory Board of the Manual Therapy Journal. Since 1988 he has had an independent practice at the 'Centro terapie manuali' in Alassio, of which he is head.

Contributors

Jean Pierre Baeyens
Departments of Experimental Anatomy and Manual Therapy, Vrije Universiteit, Brussels, Belgium

Erik Barbaix
Departments of Human Anatomy and Manual Therapy, Vrije Universiteit, Brussels, Belgium

Roberto Bergamo
Physiotherapist, Turin

Turner A. 'TAB' Blackburn, Jr.
Executive Director, Tulane Institute of Sports Medicine, Adjunct Assistant Professor, Department of Orthopaedics, Tulane School of Medicine, New Orleans, Louisiana, USA

Fabrizio Campi
Shoulder and Elbow Surgery Operating Unit, Ospedale D. Cervesi, Cattolica (RN)

Lorenzo Castellani
School of Specialist Studies II in Orthopaedics and Traumatology, Università degli Studi, Milan

Jan Peter Clarijs
Director of Experimental Anatomy and Manual Therapy Departments, Vrije Universiteit, Brussels, Belgium

Viviana Contardo
Independent professional, Studio Riabilita, Turin

Michel De Maeseneer
Department of Radiology, Vrije Universiteit, Brussels, Belgium

Nicola Gandolfo
Level I Medical Director, Radiology Operating Unit, Azienda Ospedaliera Santa Corona, Pietra Ligure (SV)

Matthew Charles Giordano
'CREA Group' Doctor, Milan

Barbara J. Hoogenboom
Assistant Professor, Physical Therapy, Grand Valley State University, Cook-DeVos Center for Health Sciences, Grand Rapids, Michigan, USA

Veronica Christina Marchione
Università degli Studi di Genova, Master in Rehabilitation of Musculoskeletal Disorders, independent professional, Castelraimondo (MC)

Roberto Merletti
Department of Electronics, Istituto Politecnico di Torino

Andrea Merlo
Electronic Engineer LAM (Movement Analysis Laboratory), AUSL Department of Rehabilitation, Reggio Emilia, Ospedale San Sebastiano, Correggio (RE)

Riccardo Minola
'CREA Group' Doctor, Milan

Ferdinando Odella
Chair of the Italian Society of Shoulder and Elbow Surgery (ICSeG), Consultant II, Division of Orthopaedics and Traumatology, Istituto Ortopedico Gaetano Pini, Milan

Simonetta Odella
Junior Doctor II, Division of Orthopaedics and Traumatology, Istituto Ortopedico Gaetano Pini, Milan

Massimo Paganelli
Orthopaedic Clinic, Università degli Studi, Ferrara

Contributors

Paolo Paladini
Shoulder and Elbow Surgery Operating Unit, Ospedale D. Cervesi, Cattolica (RN)

Luca Pierannunzii
Junior Doctor II Division of Orthopaedics and Traumatology, Istituto Ortopedico Gaetano Pini, Milan

Piergiorgio Pirani
Medical Director, Orthopaedic Operating Unit, Azienda Ospedaliera San Salvatore, Pesaro

Giuseppe Porcellini
Director Shoulder and Elbow Surgery Operating Unit, Ospedale D. Cervesi, Cattolica (RN)

Alberto Rainoldi
Doctor of Research in Physical Medicine and Rehabilitation, Neuromuscular System Engineering Laboratory (LISiN), Politecnico di Torino

Enrico Reggiani
Former Director of the School of Specialist Studies in Sport Medicine, Università degli Studi di Genova

Claudio Scotton
Lecturer in Technique and Teaching Individual Sports, SUISM, Università degli Studi di Torino. Lecturer in the Theory and Methodology of Training, Master in Rehabilitation of Musculoskeletal Disorders, Università degli Studi di Genoa

Giovanni Serafini
Director of Complex, Radiology Operating Unit, Azienda Ospedaliera Santa Corona, Pietra Ligure (SV)

Pierpaolo Summa
'CREA Group' Doctor, Milan

Peter Van Roy
Departments of Experimental Anatomy and Manual Therapy, Vrije Universiteit, Brussels, Belgium

Michael L. Voight
Professor, Belmont University, School of Physical Therapy, Nashville, Tennessee (USA)

Giovanni Villani
Medical Director, Orthopaedic and Traumatology Operating Unit, Santa Rita nursing home, Vercelli

Raul Zini
Director Orthopaedic Operating Unit, Azienda Ospedaliera San Salvatore, Pesaro

Riccardo Zuccarino
Independent professional, Studio Fusco, Genoa

Acknowledgements
Maurizio Marchetti
Medical Director 'Centro Azzarita', Bologna

Abbreviations

ABD abduction

ABER abduction and external rotation position

AC joint acromioclavicular joint

ADD adduction

AIOS acquired instability by overuse syndrome

ALPSA anterior labral periosteal sleeve avulsion

AMBRII atraumatic multidirectional bilateral rehabilitation inferior capsular shift

ANAN National association of swimming and water polo trainers

AP anteroposterior

ARV average rectified value

BFE basic functional examination

BLB bone-ligament-bone

CC correlation coefficient

CC load capacity threshold

CKC closed kinetic chain

CONI Italian national olympic committee

CRaC contract-relax-antagonist-contract

CT Computed tomography

CTF doctor of chemistry and pharmaceutical technology

CV conduction velocity

DOMS delayed onset muscular soreness

EBM evidence based medicine

EMG electromyography

ER external rotation

ERLS external rotation lag sign

ERs external rotators

EXT extension

FE functional evaluation

FI fatigue index

FRA Fédération française d'athlétisme

FTPI functional throwing performance index

GARD glenoid articular rim disruption

GAS general adaptation syndrome

GHL glenohumeral ligament

GIMBE Italian evidence-based medicine group

GLAD glenolabral articular disruption

HAGL humeral avulsion of the glenohumeral ligament

HAMD Hamilton depression rating scale

HR heart rate

IASP International association for the study of pain

ICD International classification of diseases

ICF International classification of functioning

ICFDH International classification of functioning, disability and health

ICIDH-2 International classification of impairments, disabilities and handicaps

ICR instantaneous centre of rotation

IEFCoSTRe European institute of training, systemic consultancy and relational therapy

IGHL inferior glenohumeral ligament

IGHLC inferior glenohumeral ligament complex

IPQ Italian pain questionnaire

IR internal rotation

IRLS internal rotation lag sign

IRRST internal rotation resistance strength test

IRs internal rotators

IZ innervation zone

KEMG kinesiological electromyography

LHB long head of the biceps

LHBB long head of the biceps brachii

LHHB long head of the humeral biceps

MDF median frequency

MDI multidirectional instability

MIP minimal invasive portals

MLCM multidimensional load/carriability model

MMT manual muscle test

MNF mean frequency

Abbreviations

MPQ McGill pain questionnaire
MR magnetic resonance
MRC medical research council
MRI magnetic resonance imaging
MSR muscle strength ratio
MU motor unit
MUAP motor unit action potential
NPV negative predictive value
NWC number of words chosen
OKC open kinetic chain
OT overtraining
OTS overtraining syndrome
PAE passive anterior elevation
PD proton density
PHP prognostic health profile
PL posterolateral portal
PNF proprioceptive neuromuscular facilitation
PPI present pain intensity
PPT pain provocation test
PPV positive predictive value
PRIr pain rating index rank
PRIrc pain rating index rank coefficient
PROM passive range of motion
RC rotator cuff
RHAGL reverse humeral avulsion of the gleno-humeral ligament
RMS root mean square value
ROM range of movement

Rx radiology
SASES Society of American Shoulder and Elbow Surgeons
SC sternoclavicular joint
SDA sedentary daily activities
SENIAM surface electromyography for non-invasive assessment of muscles
SIP sickness impact profile
SLAC superior labrum, anterior cuff lesion
SLAP superior labrum from anterior to posterior
SP scapular plane
SPADI shoulder pain and disability index
SSC stretch-shortening contraction
SSI shoulder severity index
SSP shoulder surgery perception
SSRS subjective shoulder rating scale
SST simple shoulder test
TOS thoracic outlet syndrome
TUBS traumatic unidirectional Bankart-lesion surgery
ULTT upper limb tension test
US ultrasound
VA verbal analogue
VAS visual analogue scale
VUB Vrije Universiteit Brussel
WHO World Health Organization
2D two-dimensional
3D three-dimensional

Preface

Shoulder disorders generally affect athletes involved in certain sports, and their incidence has increased dramatically in recent years owing to the ever-growing demand for extremely high levels of performance throughout long, competitive seasons and with ever-shorter intervals between competitive events.

The growth in the numbers of Italians taking part in sports (12–14 million) has meant that many amateur sportsmen and women are now interested in these problems.

There is additionally a tendency to start youngsters competing early, exposing structures that have not yet matured to acute, repetitive stresses, thus increasing the risk of developing dysfunctional conditions, a prerequisite for subsequent disorders.

The world of sport, therefore, clearly has significant expectations, and eagerly awaits progress in the diagnostics, rehabilitation and surgery of the shoulder.

Owing to recent progress in these fields and to a considerable increase in the scientific literature produced in recent years, it has been possible to abandon terms such as 'scapulohumeral periarthritis' in favour of a more accurate interpretation of shoulder disorders. Such an interpretation is supported by a solid biomechanical and functionalist view of disorders which are primarily multifactorial in origin.

The various causal or risk factors can be correctly identified and excluded only by means of an interdisciplinary approach involving the various professions in an effort to overcome the obstacles to a common, synergic vision.

This book presents the most important advances in the disciplines involved in the prevention and cure of sport injuries with the aim of stimulating a productive interdisciplinary collaboration between physiotherapists, doctors and specialists in motor sciences, while respecting the individual disciplines.

Functional anatomy, surgery, manual therapy, motor rehabilitation, athletic training and technique are dealt with in separate chapters, investigating specific fields such as arthrokinematics, diagnostic imaging, surgical endoscopy, surface electromyography and musculoskeletal therapy.

Acute disorders of the shoulder have been approached from epidemiological, clinical and surgical points of view, while subacute and chronic disorders, which are more widespread and problematic, have been addressed from the point of view of rehabilitation and prevention.

Rehabilitation, with its close links to athletic training, has been examined in particular, along with the prevention of sport injuries, particularly since the latter is sometimes neglected in training programmes. The structure of the book in sections by discipline, supported by an extensive bibliography and some 'unresolved problems', reflects the state of the art thanks to contributions from leading experts in the various fields.

The editors, who are physiotherapists and lecture on the Master's course in the 'Rehabilitation of Musculoskeletal Disorders' at Università degli Studi di Genova, hope that this work will meet the needs not only of health workers and technicians working in the field of sports, but also of lecturers in Physiotherapy and Motor Sciences and students at Specialist Medical Schools who are involved in various roles in the evaluation, treatment and rehabilitation of athletes.

Finally, it is hoped that the work that has been done will help to achieve an interdisciplinary culture with the aim of safeguarding the health of athletes, the fundamental human resource and 'primum movens' of all sport.

A. Fusco, A. Foglia, F. Musarra and M. Testa

FUNCTIONAL ANATOMY AND RECENT BIOMECHANICAL DISCOVERIES

CHAPTER 1

ANATOMICAL VARIANTS OF THE SHOULDER

P. Van Roy
E. Barbaix
J.P. Baeyens
M. De Maeseneer
J.P. Clarijs

Congenital anomalies, like pathological anomalies, of the glenohumeral joint, the acromioclavicular joint (AC joint) and the ligaments surrounding the shoulder may predispose to, or aggravate, impingement of the supraspinatus outlet, for example, an acromial bone, osteophytosis of the inferior surface of the acromioclavicular joint, or calcification and ossification of the coracoclavicular, coracoacromial and glenohumeral ligaments, bursae and tendons.

As well as giving an overview of the bone variants of the glenohumeral joint, the coracoacromial arch, and the acromioclavicular and sternoclavicular joints, this chapter will present a series of clinically significant soft tissue variants. Many anatomical variants can be found concerning the glenoid labrum, the glenohumeral capsule, the glenohumeral ligaments, and the corresponding bursae, as well as the muscles surrounding these structures, and their vascularization and innervation. The possibility of clearly visualizing the soft tissues in magnetic resonance has prompted renewed interest in the various aspects of anatomical variants, owing to their clinical consequences and the need to avoid errors in interpretation.

Glenohumeral joint

Bone structures of the glenohumeral joint

The anatomical variations of the glenoid fossa affect its shape, curvature, orientation and dimensions. Although some glenoid fossae are oval or ovoid, the majority of scapulas have an articular surface that is pear- or comma-shaped at the humeral head (Fig. 1.1). The pear-shape may be the result of the presence, in the upper part of the glenoid cavity, of a smaller anteroposterior diameter, which may be accentuated by the presence of an acetabular notch in the anterior margin. Prescher (1997) reports the presence of a glenoid notch in approximately 55% of cases. This notch causes asymmetry between the anterior and inferior halves of the glenoid cavity (Huber, 1991). As a result of this indentation, a small area of the anterior glenoid labrum does not insert in the rim of the glenoid cavity. A small anterior sublabral hole can be found there (Prescher, 1997). The articulation between the relatively small glenoid cavity and the far larger humeral head predisposes the joint to instability and consequently makes it subject to various types of dislocation. Saha (1971, 1973) points out that to ensure a stable joint configuration, the maximum and minimum diameter of the glenoid cavity should be approximately 75% and 57%, respectively, of the diameter of the humeral head.

A further aspect influences the degree of congruence between the humeral head and the glenoid cavity. Some glenoid cavities are shallow, while others are more sharply concave.

A classification has been devised, based on the size of the radius of curvature of the glenoid fossa in relation to the diameter of the humeral head (greater, equal or smaller), which distinguishes three types of glenoid fossa (A, B and C) (Saha, 1971; Soslowski, 1992; Van der Helm, 1994). In these typologies, the relation between the curvature of the joint surfaces is generally observed in the transverse plane. Iannotti (1992) notes that the humeral head is spherical if

Anatomical variants of the shoulder

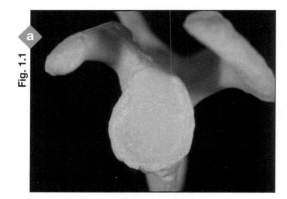

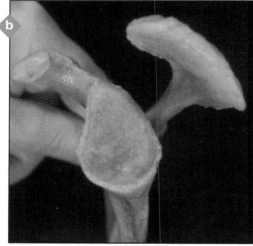

Fig. 1.1

Different glenoid cavity shapes: **(a)** oval-shaped glenoid cavity, **(b)** pear-shaped glenoid cavity showing a smaller anteroposterior diameter in its upper portion than in its lower portion.

the viscoelastic properties of the articular cartilage and glenoid labrum.

There is a considerable degree of variability in joint geometry, based on the inclination and orientation of the glenoid (Baeyens, 1997; Galinat, 1988; Saha, 1973). The glenoid cavity is generally oriented slightly forwards. Its craniocaudal orientation is, however, strictly dependent on posture. The use of this parameter is consequently controversial (Baeyens, 1997).

The glenoid cavity generally shows slight posterior version of approximately 5–7° in relation to the mediolateral axis of the scapula. The scapula is principally oriented in an oblique frontal plane, with the lateral rim facing forwards. Limited posterior version of the glenoid cavity can be regarded as a functional adaptation, producing greater bone stability in the joint with the humeral head. If, however, ossification of the posterior portion of the glenoid cavity is deficient, posterior version may become more severe and may predispose to glenohumeral instability (Brewer, 1986) (Fig. 1.2).

The width and depth of the intertubercular groove of the humerus may vary substantially between humans, providing a groove that generally holds the biceps tendon (O'Brien, 1998). The small crest of the tubercle may be pronounced to a varying degree, particularly in its medial wall. In approximately 67% of shoulders, the groove is a prolongation of the crest of the humerus, and also has a supratubercular section (Hitchcock, 1948; Wood, 1998). Apparently, about half of all shoulders show an increase in tension at the arch of the crest, represented by the transverse humeral ligament, as demonstrated by the high frequency of traction on the medial rim of the crest (Michaud, 1990), in contrast with what happens in fewer than 5% of shoulders which do not show a supratubercular groove (Fig. 1.3).

Soft tissues of the glenohumeral joint

There are also many variants in the structure of the glenohumeral joint capsule and in its relationship to the structures that surround and strengthen it, such as for example, the glenoid labrum, the glenohumeral ligaments and the coracohumeral ligament, and the subcoracoid bursa (or bursae), and in its relationship to the glenohumeral joint space (Fig. 1.3).

The glenoid labrum and its relationship to the long head of the biceps tendon

The glenoid labrum is a fibrous tissue which surrounds and then expands the glenoid cavity. It does

observed in transverse section through its central part, but slightly eliptical if observed in oblique coronal section. The radius of curvature in the axial plane is a few millimetres smaller than the radius of curvature measured in the coronal plane. The radius of curvature of the glenoid cavity measured in the coronal plane is, on average, 2.3 mm + 0.2 mm longer than the radius of curvature of the humeral head. However, this is not in agreement with the results found by Hata (1992). In synovial joints, the radius of curvature of the concave joint surface is generally greater than that of the convex joint surface. The difference between the radii of curvature of the joint surfaces has an important role in joint congruity and may vary under load, according to

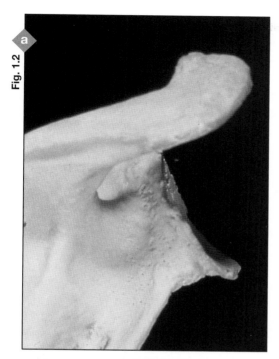

Fig. 1.2

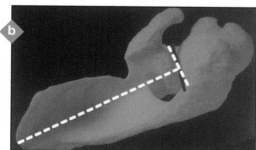

(a) Deficient ossification of the posterior part of the glenoid cavity may predispose to instability; **(b)** view of the scapula from above: the dashed lines represent the correct 'version' of the glenoid cavity, while the solid line indicates the posterior version which predisposes to instability.

consequently also presents considerable interindividual variation: from approximately 120–375% of the depth of the glenoid fossa alone. Based on these dimensions, the percentage cover of the cartilaginous surface of the humeral head by the glenoid fossa, if the labrum is also included, increases from 12–65% (Hata, 1992). Variations are also visible in the shape of the labrum, with triangular, obtuse and transverse, and crescent moon-shaped sections. Transverse images through the anterosuperior and middle labrum are mostly triangular, while transverse images through the anteroinferior labrum and the posterior labrum are often more rounded (Zlatkin, 1991). The lower halves of the labrum insert in the glenoid fossa, at the peripheral and central rims. Above the equator, the insertion may be the same or it may appear only along the peripheral rim, creating a type of meniscus. In the former case, this part of the labrum is firmly fixed, while in the latter case it is mobile and there is a small groove between the glenoid and the labrum: the superior sublabral recess (De Maeseneer, 2000).

At its upper apex, the glenoid labrum is closely associated with the tendon of the long head of the biceps brachii muscle. Next to its insertion in the supraglenoid tubercle, the tendon also inserts in the anterosuperior and posterosuperior parts of the glenoid labrum and in the base of the coracoid process (De Maeseneer, 1998). Extreme stresses on this insertion can cause detachment of the upper labrum, as happens in sports involving throwing which can lead to various types of superior labrum from anterior to posterior (SLAP) lesions. In some type II (peripheral) insertions, near to the insertion of the biceps tendon, there may be a relatively large sublabral recess. In 11% of shoulders, a section of the anterosuperior part of the labrum may not insert in the glenoid, thus creating a sublabral hole. This is not the same as a sublabral recess and should not be confused with a sublabral tear. The anterosuperior part of the labrum is absent in 1.5% of shoulders. In this case, the posterior labrum ends close to the cranial apex of the glenoid cavity, close to the biceps tendon, and, after a brief interruption, the point of origin of the anteroinferior labrum can be seen at 3 o'clock in the glenoid. The middle glenohumeral ligament (GHL) is cord-like and it takes origin at the end of the posterior labrum. This variant, known as Buford complex, and the presence of a sublabral hole must be distinguished from pathological pictures such as Bankart lesion (De Maeseneer, 2000; Wall, 1995).

Limited vascularization of the periphery of the glenoid labrum is provided by capsular and periosteal vessels, arising from the suprascapular, circumflex

not contain chondrocytes, except at the junction with the hyaline cartilage of the glenoid cavity. The inferior part of the labrum is larger than the cranial part, while the posterior part is normally larger than the anterior part. The width of the base of the labrum is significantly larger in the anterior and inferior parts of the joint (Hata, 1992). The height and width of the glenoid labrum vary from less than 2 to 14 mm. The depth of the fossa, which includes the labrum,

Anatomical variants of the shoulder

Fig. 1.3

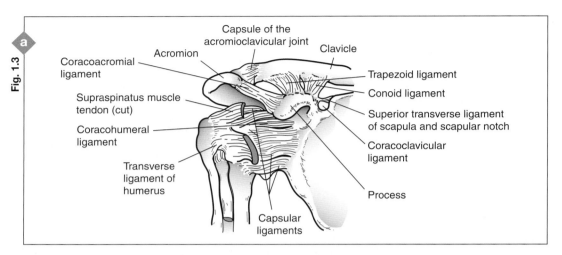

a

Coracoacromial ligament
Acromion
Capsule of the acromioclavicular joint
Clavicle
Trapezoid ligament
Conoid ligament
Superior transverse ligament of scapula and scapular notch
Supraspinatus muscle tendon (cut)
Coracohumeral ligament
Coracoclavicular ligament
Transverse ligament of humerus
Capsular ligaments
Process

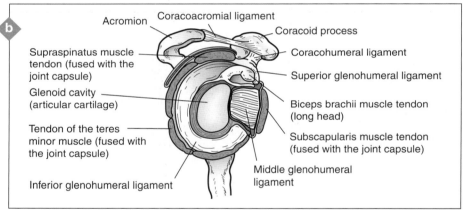

b

Acromion
Coracoacromial ligament
Coracoid process
Supraspinatus muscle tendon (fused with the joint capsule)
Coracohumeral ligament
Superior glenohumeral ligament
Glenoid cavity (articular cartilage)
Biceps brachii muscle tendon (long head)
Tendon of the teres minor muscle (fused with the joint capsule)
Subscapularis muscle tendon (fused with the joint capsule)
Inferior glenohumeral ligament
Middle glenohumeral ligament

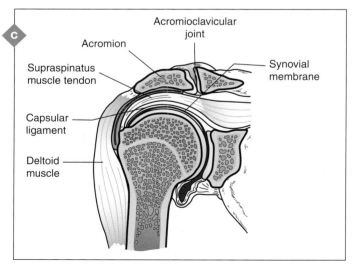

c

Acromioclavicular joint
Acromion
Synovial membrane
Supraspinatus muscle tendon
Capsular ligament
Deltoid muscle

Anatomical variants of the shoulder may affect structures and soft tissues. The figure illustrates from the top downwards the scapulohumeral complex in anterior view, the scapula in lateral view (humerus removed), and the scapulohumeral complex in frontal section. The arrows show the three types of ventral insertion of the joint capsule referred to in the text.

scapular and posterior circumflex humeral arteries (Cooper, 1992).

The joint capsule

The capsule of the glenohumeral joint takes origin, on the scapula, principally from the peripheral surface of the glenoid labrum and the part adjacent to the neck, except for the cranial part of the joint which takes origin from the base of the coracoid process, leaving the supraglenoid tubercle in the joint cavity. Zlatkin (1991) distinguishes three types of ventral insertion: the first immediately behind the glenoid labrum, the second in the neck of the scapula, and the

third at the transition point between the neck and body of the scapula (Fig. 1.4).

In the axillary region, the capsule is partly fused with the tendon of the long head of the triceps muscle, which inserts in the infraglenoid tubercle.

The capsule principally follows the anatomical neck of the humerus, with a small gap on the posterior side where there is an empty area between the rim of the cartilage and the insertion. Two types of insertion in the axillary part (V-shaped and C-shaped) occur with almost equal frequency. In the V-shaped insertion, the capsule descends 5–15 mm, and includes the medial part of the surgical neck in the cavity. The joint capsule in this section separates into two layers: a

Fig. 1.4

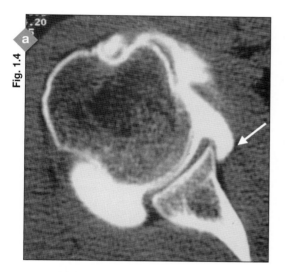

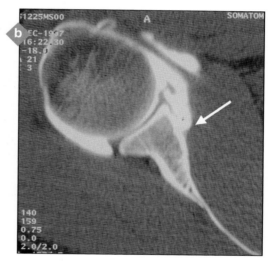

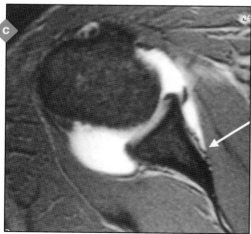

Variants of the anterior insertion of the glenohumeral capsule:
(a) insertion directly behind the glenoid labrum, **(b)** insertion in the neck of the scapula, **(c)** insertion in the body of the scapula.

longitudinal layer which inserts in the humerus, and a reflex layer which covers the periosteum and joins the rim of the cartilage. The joint capsule is thicker in this inferior part, though often mobile, and creates the axillary recess. This fibrous recess often contains bundles between the reflex layer and the synovial layer of the scapular side of the recess. These intracapsular bundles can limit the flexibility of the axillary recess, as well as the variable degree of fusion between the capsule and the triceps. It is unclear whether inflammatory processes influence the formation of bundles or the degree of adhesion to the triceps tendon; in the ring-shaped variant, the insertion is attached just below the rim of the joint surface (O'Brien, 1990).

The capsule of the glenohumeral joint has three expansions: subcoracoid, axillary and intertubercular. There are two to four openings in the capsule through which the joint is in continuity with the expansions. A fairly continuous recess surrounds the biceps tendon in the intertubercular groove, under the transverse humeral ligament. It may be very small, or absent altogether, if the tendon takes origin from the groove (Welcker, 1878). One or two often lobulated recesses, generally called subscapular bursae, are located between the scapula and the subscapularis muscle. These recesses communicate with the joint cavity through one or two openings in the GHL. When the middle GHL is absent, there is generally a single large opening. There is another opening, formerly called the sublabral hole, between the glenoid and the anterosuperior part of the labrum in 11% of shoulders. The other bursae will be dealt with below. Apart from the subcoracoid bursa, these do not communicate with the joint cavity (Tillmann, 1986).

The inferior part of the capsule forms the axillary recess, which has an important role in allowing ample elevation and abduction of the shoulder.

A slightly negative pressure in the capsule, compared to atmospheric pressure, contributes substantially to the functional stability of the joint, compensating for the lack of stability caused by the bone configuration (Kumar, 1985). The negative pressure results from the osmotic action of the synovia (Matsen, 1998).

The glenohumeral ligaments

The three GHL; the superior, middle and inferior; are generally described: they principally strengthen the anterior and inferior surfaces of the joint capsule. Their appearance may vary from well-structured ligaments to a tight bundle of collagen fibres, pointing in the same direction in the capsule. These ligaments run inside the capsule. At the point where the ligaments are covered by the subscapularis tendon and muscle, they can be observed better from inside the joint cavity, by athroscopy if appropriate. The GHLs may be absent, particularly the middle ligament, although there may be variations in the extension of the superior and inferior ligaments (Steinbeck, 1998). The medial origins of the GHLs differ between individuals. Consequently the origins are often identified using the time as shown on a clock around the glenoid cavity.

The superior GHL takes origin from the upper part of the glenoid cavity, in front of the origin of the biceps tendon. It may have a separate point of origin, at the anterosuperior apex of the glenoid cavity, or it may share a point of origin with the long head of the biceps or with the middle glenohumeral ligament. It runs over the lateral surface of the fovea capitis of the humerus, just above the lesser tuberosity (O'Brien, 1998). The ligament is fairly continuous (97%), however, it has a very variable consistency.

The middle GHL joins the superoanterior apex of the glenoid cavity, or neck of the scapula, to the humerus, and inserts medially to the lesser tuberosity. The middle GHL is the most variable, both in size and consistency. It may appear as a flat bundle or a cord. It is absent or veil-like, in 8–30% of shoulders (Craig, 1996; Ernlund, 2000; O'Brien, 1998; Speer, 1995). If well developed, the middle GHL makes a far greater mechanical contribution to the anterior stability of the shoulder than the superior ligament.

The anatomical variability of the superior and middle ligaments is also related to the presence of one or two openings communicating with the subscapular bursa, in the anterior part of the capsule (De Palma, 1949; Matsen, 1998; O'Brien, 1990, 1998). An opening above the middle and inferior GHL and one below have been found in 36–46% of shoulders. There is a single opening between the superior and middle GHL in 6–18% of cases. A single communication hole with the bursa between the middle and inferior GHL occurs less frequently. If the middle GHL is absent, there may be a large communication hole between the bursa and the capsule; the subcoracoid recess may, therefore, also be absent. This situation occurs more often when the anterior part of the capsule inserts very close to the anterior glenoid labrum (De Palma, 1949).

The inferior GHL has an anterior and a posterior bundle which contain a thickened intermediate part of the capsule of the axillary recess, the axillary bursa. The structure is known as the inferior GHL complex (O'Brien, 1998, 1990). The anterior bundle takes origin from the glenoid labrum, between 2 and 4 o'clock, while the posterior bundle takes origin between 7 and 9 o'clock. Running perpendicular to the transverse and oblique collagen fibres of the capsule, the medial portion of these bundles forms a structure that supports the humeral head during abduction of the arm. Both the bundles finally emerge, forming the C-shaped or V-shaped insertion, mentioned above, under the humeral head. The inferior GHL is, therefore, also likened to a hammock. This ligament has an important role in combined internal and external rotation movements during abduction of the shoulder, as often happens in throwing sports, tennis and swimming. This makes a substantial contribution to the capsular and ligamentous stability of the shoulder.

The anatomical relations between the joint capsule and the tendon of the long head of the biceps

Near to its point of origin, the tendon of the long head of the biceps is always inside the joint cavity, surrounded only by a synovial layer. The tendon may not be free in the joint capsule, in its more distal part, but situated between the synovial layer and the fibrous layer of the capsule, or it may insert in the capsule through a mesenteric-like fold (Wall, 1995). The point of origin is rarely solely on the supraglenoid tubercle, and is almost always also on the labrum, mainly the posterior part (Demondion, 2001; Vangsness, 1994). The intra-articular part of the tendon may be absent, if the point of origin is in the intertubercular groove, on one of the tuberosities, or if the long head of the biceps is absent. The tendon may be double (Adriao, 1933; Bergman, 1988; Le Double, 1897; Testut, 1884).

The rotator cuff 'cable'

A thickening, known to protect the rotator cuff from stresses, runs over the dorsal and upper surfaces of the capsule, perpendicular to the tendon of the long head of the biceps. It runs like a curved cord from the intertubercular groove of the humerus to the lower edge of the insertion of the infraspinatus muscle, in the greater tuberosity. This structure is not always visible in the shoulders of young people. It is more prominent in the shoulders of the elderly, probably because the critical preinsertion area of the cuff, between the cable and the insertion of the supraspinatus and infraspinatus muscles, becomes thinner with age (Burkhart, 1996).

The coracohumeral ligament

The coracohumeral ligament takes origin from the lateral surface of the base of the coracoid process. It covers obliquely the space between the cranial margins of the subscapularis and supraspinatus muscles and inserts in the tuberosity of the humerus, on both sides of the intertubercular groove, thus participating in the formation of its arch. The medial part of this ligament is free, while the lateral part adheres to the capsule. The length of the free part is rather variable and a bursa may be found underneath. Microscopic studies suggest that this ligament is often a folded capsular structure, rather than a true ligament with dense collagen fibres. The folded appearance may be explained by observing its inverted V-shaped point of origin in the base of the coracoid process (Cooper, 1993).

Coracoacromial arch

Bone structures of the coracoacromial arch

The shape of the acromion

The scapular spine and the acromion arise from many ossification centres: the most proximal is the basiacromion, followed by the mesoacromion, the metaacromion and the preacromion. The total, partial or failed development of the preacromial epiphysis leads to the acromion having different shapes (Nicholson, 1996). This accounts for the great interindividual variability that can be observed in 'normal' acromions and explains the presence of an abnormal morphology in cases with ossification defects. Absence of fusion between the various ossification centres may lead to a particular appearance of the acromial bone (Fig. 1.5).

Fig. 1.5

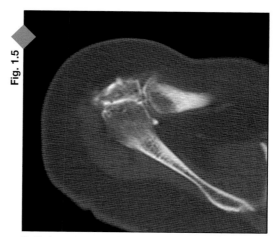

Particular appearance of the acromial bone due to failed fusion of the ossification centres.

Anatomical variants of the shoulder

Nicholson (1996) reports an incidence of 8%. Generally the mesoacromion centre and the meta-acromion do not fuse and the meta-acromion and the preacromion or the basiacromion and the mesoacromion do so far less frequently (Wood, 1998). This abnormal development should not be diagnosed as a fracture and it is often a cause of impingement.

The types of acromion

Variants of the acromion can be classified by the morphology and function of the coracoacromial arch, but also by the functional anatomy of the acromioclavicular joint. The classification of acromions (Bigliani, 1996) into three types – flat (type I), curved (type II) and hooked (type III) (Fig. I.6) – has been used extensively in studies of subacromial impingement (Neer, 1972). Although the reliability of Bigliani's classification has been criticized (Jacobson, 1995; Janssen, 1997; Zuckerman, 1997), studies have confirmed a link between a hooked acromion (type III) and rotator cuff pathology, although it has no predictive value (Farley, 1994; Saha, 1973). The unreliability of observations determining the type of acromion arises from the different interpretation of very slightly curved acromions and acromions with degenerative formations at the anterior surface. No longitudinal studies have been conducted into the effects of age on acromion morphology. A comparison of the incidence of the three types of acromion across different age classes revealed the possibility of changes in acromion type during one's life. Nicholson (1996) observed a statistically significant increase in the incidence of type II (curved) acromions and a significant reduction in type III (hooked) acromions in 420 scapulas of slim subjects in their sixth decade.

Fig. 1.6

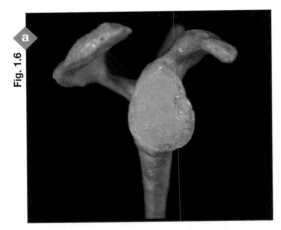

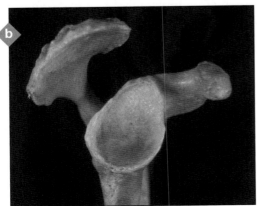

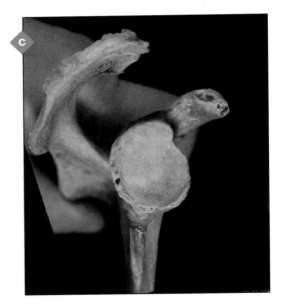

Bigliani's classification of the acromion: **(a)** type I – flat acromion, **(b)** type II – curved acromion, **(c)** type III – hooked acromion.

Wang and Shapiro (1997) also observed the influence of age on X-rays of the supraspinatus in 272 subjects with and without impingement. By comparing populations over and under 50-years-old, they found a significant reduction in the incidence of type I (flat) acromions, with a substantial increase in the incidence of type III (hooked) acromions in the population over 50.

A more cranial position of the humeral head in relation to the arch of the shoulder may lead to an area of impingement between the head itself and the acromion. The subacromial space is so small that the proximal end of the humerus, which moves near to the acromial arch, almost comes into contact with the inferior surface of the acromion. The eccentric position of the humeral tuberosities and the cranial translation of the humerus, caused by the contraction of the long head of the triceps muscle (and of the short head of the biceps muscle), or instability, give rise to areas of contact between the two bones and areas of traction on the insertions of the coracoacromial ligament. This situation occurs in the presence of spurs and in advanced age; the inferior surface of the acromion becomes cup-shape, until it forms a pseudarthrotic surface for the subacromial joint (Edelson, 1995; Nasca, 1984; Neer, 1972; Wuelker, 1995).

Figure 1.7 illustrates bone residues at the caudal surface of the acromion, and more specifically the degenerative alterations and subsequently the formation of facets.

A type IV acromion, characterized by an inferior convexity, has been observed on an oblique sagittal image obtained by MR in 14 out of 196 subjects (Farley, 1994). If this morphology represents a clear predisposing factor for impingement, it should be investigated in further studies.

The angle of the scapular spine and the angle of the coracoid process

Other aspects of the anatomical variability of the coracoacromial arch are determined by the angle of the scapular spine and the angle of the coracoid process, which give the scapula, viewed from the side, a characteristic Y-shape (Anetzberger, 1995). The spine creates an infraspinous fossa. It also creates a supraspinous fossa with the coracoid process. The presence should also be described of a subscapular fossa on the ventral surface of the scapula. Figure 1.8 shows various angles of the scapular spine and coracoid process.

Cranial and posterior coverage of the humeral head by the acromion

The inclination (not to be confused with the angle of the spine) and the length of the acromion determine

Fig. 1.7

a
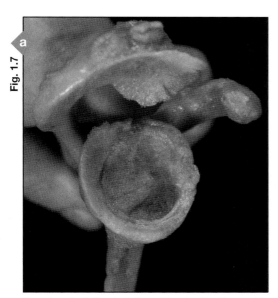

b
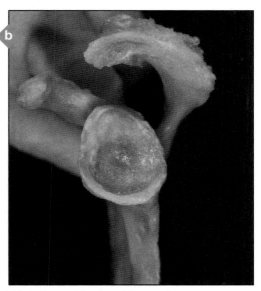

Examples of arthritic adaptations of the shoulder. Bone residues are visible on the caudal surface of the acromion. The degenerative alterations in the area of impingement form a pseudarthrotic surface for the subacromial joint.

Anatomical variants of the shoulder

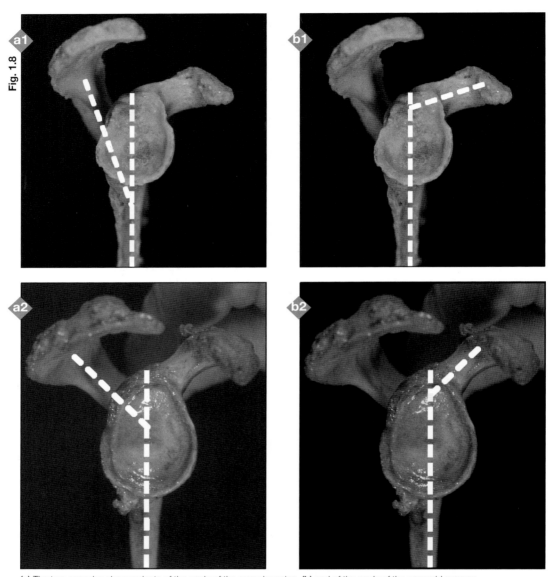

Fig. 1.8

(a) The two scapulas show variants of the angle of the scapular spine, **(b)** and of the angle of the coracoid process.

the posterior coverage of the humeral head (Edelson, 1993, 1992). Figure I.9 shows contrasting examples of the inclination of the acromion. Based on the length and inclination of the acromion, the rim of the acromion may or may not reach the upper apex of the glenoid cavity.

The cranial bone coverage of the humeral head is determined by the acromion-glenoid line and by the lateral acromial angle. The acromial line indicates the lateral extension of the acromion, in relation to the underlying glenoid cavity. The lateral acromial angle represents the degree of its lateral inclination (Banas, 1995).

The inclination of the coracoid process

The inclination of the coracoid process is a further morphological parameter which determines a spatial

Fig. 1.9

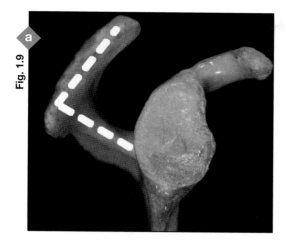

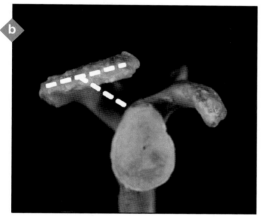

These two scapulas show variations in the inclination of the acromion, affecting cranial coverage **(a)** and posterior coverage **(b)** of the humeral head.

Fig. 1.10

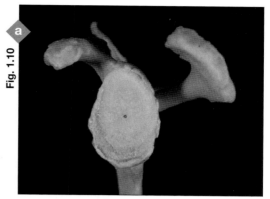

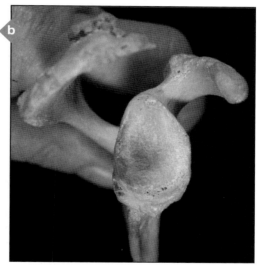

Different lengths of the acromion: **(a)** short acromion; the anterior edge remains posterior to the plane that runs perpendicularly through the superior apex of the glenoid cavity, **(b)** long acromion, extending over the superior apex of the glenoid cavity.

relation between the bone components of the lateral angle of the scapula and the coracoacromial arch (Anetzberger, 1995; Edelson, 1992). Figure 1.10 shows various inclinations of the coracoid process. Both the inclination and the length of the coracoid process determine the space available between the apex of the process itself and the anterior surface of the humeral head. A reduction in this space may lead to subcoracoid impingement.

The supraspinatus outlet

The supraspinatus outlet is an osteoligamentous ring formed by the scapular spine, the acromion, the

coracoacromial ligament and the coracoid process. It is an outlet for the passage of the supraspinous fossa into the subacromial space, through which the supraspinatus muscle runs from its point of origin to the greater tuberosity of the humerus (Neer, 1987). The proximal end of the humerus with its greater and lesser tuberosities, both of which are eccentric, moves with a considerable degree of freedom and amplitude in the subacromial space. The passage thus leads to the subcoracoid space, which is defined as a space between the coracoid process, the humeral head and the lesser tuberosity of the humerus (Dines, 1990; Gerber, 1987).

This opening may be in the form of an open or less open V, depending on the variations in orientation of the bases of the bone components. As a result of the differences in the length of the acromion and the coracoid process, the coracoacromial ligament, the only ligamentous component of the ring, may be shorter or longer, making the outlet more or less rigid.

Soft tissues associated with the coracoacromial arch

The soft tissues of the glenohumeral joint have been dealt with above. This section will focus on the rotator cuff, the extracapsular ligaments, the bursa and muscular variations in the subacromial and subcoracoid spaces.

The coracoacromial ligament

The coracoacromial ligament, which represents the soft tissues of the arch above the glenohumeral joint, joins the anterior edge of the acromion and the lateral part of the coracoid process. If the distance between the bone components of this arch increases, the coracoacromial ligament becomes very important in the architecture of the coracoacromial arch. As well as secondary thickening of the ligament and spurs resulting from an enthesopathic process at the upper apex of the coracoacromial ligament, other degenerative disorders may affect the acromion on both the lateral and medial surface (Edelson, 1992, 1993; Nicholson, 1996; Wang, 1997).

The rotator cuff

The rotator cuff is formed by the tendons of the muscles that insert in the greater and lesser tuberosities. The insertions of these tendons stretch progressively and interweave to form a single tendon around the upper end of the humerus and create the transverse humeral ligament, which covers the intertubercular groove. The tendons of the rotator cuff also insert in the joint capsule, close to the insertions in the humeral tuberosities (Welcker, 1878).

As confirmed by Macalister, the supraspinatus muscle is unusually invariable (Testut, 1884). Cases have been described, at most, of tendon or muscle bundles from the supraspinatus muscle or the omohyoid muscle and a separate small muscle belly, taking origin from the superior transverse scapular ligament (Frohse, 1908; Milianitch, 1926). The fibrous skeleton of the muscle and its tendons have been studied in recent years in detail, both anatomically and by magnetic resonance (MR). These studies have shown that the more cranial part of the tendon, which forms the posterior rim of the rotator cuff interval, has a denser and more rounded structure, twice as long as the remaining part of the tendon. It extends medially in the supraspinous fossa and takes origin from a separate bundle of the muscle in one-third of shoulders. A similar structure has been found in the subscapularis muscle: the more cranial part of its tendon extends medially and takes origin from usually single muscle bellies. This part of the tendon forms the anterior rim of the rotator cuff interval. These findings have been confirmed in vivo by MR (Duranthon, 2001; Volk, 2001).

The infraspinatus muscle has many more variants. Some muscles have bundles taking origin from the fascia infraspinata and join to the deltoid muscle, the teres major or the brachial fascia and are, therefore, remote from the shoulder (Gruber, 1879; Testut, 1884; Van Roy, 1993). The muscle has two layers in some cases: the surface layer (superficial infraspinatus muscle) is formed by the belly which takes origin from the medial edge of the scapula. A pseudofascicular appearance may be caused by a teres minor muscle which has a very extensive point of origin in the greater part of the fascia infraspinata. Milianitch and Spiridonovitch (1926) found that the muscle belly from which the spine of the scapula takes origin was completely independent in 5 out of 200 cases examined; this resulted in a smaller infraspinatus muscle, which represents an extreme form of strengthening of an edge of the tendon, similar to the strengthening visible in the supraspinatus and subscapularis muscles. Fusion, which is sometimes complete, between the infraspinatus and teres minor muscles is so common that some authors, including Luschka (1865), consider the second muscle to be the lower muscle belly of the infraspinatus muscle and consequently regard the presence of a teres minor muscle as an anatomical variant. The lack of differentiation between the two muscles has been confirmed several times during athroscopy (Wall, 1995). The 'costodeltoid' muscle may take origin from the inferior angle of the scapula, between the points of origin of the infraspinatus and teres minor muscles, and this muscle joins the posterior surface of the deltoid muscle. Calori was the first to describe the costodeltoid muscle in 1864 (Van Roy, 1993).

The teres minor muscle may be absent and divided into two muscle bellies, one of which inserts in the surgical neck or crest of the lesser tubercle, and is also known as the accessory teres minor. An additional muscle belly may take origin from the long head of the triceps and from the infraglenoid tubercle (Bergman, 1988; Frohse, 1908; Le Double, 1897; Milianitch, 1926; Testut, 1884). The teres minor and the additional belly are in close contact with the axillary pouch.

The subscapularis muscle can be divided into nine bellies, which can be grouped into two distinct strata. The lower muscle belly may be isolated and insert separately in the humerus, distal to the main part of the muscle (subscapularis minor muscle). Sometimes the muscle also has a muscle belly emerging through the coracoid process. In some cases, the axillary nerve runs through the subscapularis muscle, creating a potential entrapment site (Bergman, 1988; Frohse, 1908; Le Double, 1897; Testut, 1884). Other variants are complex fusions with the teres major or latissimus dorsi muscles.

Other muscle variants are abnormal insertions which reduce the subacromial space or the subcoracoid space. In approximately 20% of shoulders, the more cranial fibres of the pectoralis minor muscle continue beyond the coracoid process, and then insert in the coracohumeral ligament, the coracoacromial ligament or the joint capsule (Adriao, 1933; Wood, 1868). Sutton (Fick, 1904) regards the coracohumeral ligament as a phylogenic remnant of the initial insertion of this muscle in the greater tuberosity. The origin of the short head of the biceps may be widened by a lateral extension which leads beyond the coracoacromial ligament. The intra-articular part of the long head may be absent. Therefore it takes origin from the floor of the intertubercular groove, the lesser tuberosity or the ventral capsule. Up to three accessory heads may take origin from the lesser tuberosity or from the ventral capsule. The anterior circumflex artery of the humerus may run deeply to the accessory head of the biceps and may be compressed in this area (Vasquez, 2002; Warner, 1992). In some cases a small muscle belly of the pectoralis major muscle, generally the abdominal part or the more lateral bundles of the costal part, runs deeply to the muscle and then inserts in the ventral surface of the capsule, with the long tendon or with a type of lacertus (Harvey, 1907; Testut, 1884).

The periarticular bursa of the glenohumeral joint

Numerous bursae have been described in the region of the shoulder. Those which communicate with the joint cavity have been dealt with above. Some of the true bursae are located away from the joint. These are the subcutaneous bursa on the apex of the acromion, the bursae between the deltoid muscle and the scapular spine, the bursae nearest the inferior point of the scapula and the bursae between the scapula and the rib cage. Other bursae are located at the insertions of the latissimus dorsi, teres major and pectoralis major, and between the subscapularis muscle and the coracobrachial muscle or the short head of the biceps brachii. The subcoracoid bursa, the bursa deep to the coracohumeral ligament, the bursa between the coracoclavicular ligaments and finally the subdeltoid bursae are in close contact with the joint. The bursae mentioned above are frequently fused together and form a single large lobulated bursa, often called the subacromiodeltoid bursa (Fick, 1904; Testut, 1948). This is one of the few that can be identified in fetuses from the third month of pregnancy (Black, 1934).

The bursa has a typical synovial layer. In many places its fibrous layer cannot be distinguished microscopically from the surrounding layers, such as the peritendinous sheath of the rotator cuff or the deep fascia of the deltoid muscle, near to its insertion in the acromion. Many of these adhesions move quite a distance from one another. Particularly when there is a single lobulated bursa, these movements cause invaginations, traction and slipping of the internal layer and may lead to repeated microtraumas (Birnbaum, 1992). Histological degeneration can be found from the third decade of life, for example, stratification of the synovial layer and thickening of the connective tissue between tendons and bursa. Degenerative lesions are simultaneously present in adjacent tendons in more than 50% of cases. Almost continual movements occur for decades in the small subacromial space, with thickening at the same time, often in the absence of painful symptoms. These movements may lead to silent rupture of the rotator cuff, thus producing communication between the bursa and joint cavity. These points of communication are not anatomical variants, but friction lesions or 'Friktionsusur', as they were dubbed by Fick (1904; Uhthoff, 1984, 1991).

Organized fatty tissue is also present in the subacromial space, and extends medially along the supraspinatus muscle (Vahrensieck, 1996).

Acromioclavicular joint

Bone structures of the acromioclavicular joint

The AC joint shows many interindividual differences. While some joint facets are approximately parallel to

Anatomical variants of the shoulder

the lateral rim of the acromion, others have a more anterior or superior orientation (Fig. 1.11.a, b). The dimensions and curvature may also vary substantially (Fig. 1.11.c, d). The morphological variants may be partly explained by the different degrees of maturation of the distal epiphysis of the acromion (Bergman, 1988; Edelson, 1992, 1993). The hyaline cartilage initially present in the joint facets becomes fibrocartilage between the ages of 17 and 25 years (Rockwood, 1998).

A fibrous fold, or cartilaginous articular disc, may considerably alter the configuration of the joint. The articular disc is generally incomplete, crescent moon- or ring-shaped (Wood, 1868), and separates the upper part of the joint surfaces. Testut (1948) describes eight different joint configurations, based on the morphology of the articular disc. These configurations lead, along with the superior and inferior acromioclavicular ligaments, to a variety of joint types

ranging from a joint cavity with a meniscoid fold to a configuration with two separate joint cavities and one without cavities; the disc appears as an interosseous ligament in all cases. A complete disc from which two different cavities take origin is nevertheless rather exceptional (1%).

Changes in the articular disc very often occur in only the second decade. The articular disc may have a meniscoid configuration or may have a thinner fibrillar appearance (De Palma, 1963).

Keats and Pope (1988) describe four common configurations of the AC joint, based on the height of the acromion relative to the clavicle. The lower rim of the acromion and the clavicle were found to reach the same horizontal plane in approximately 81% of cases. The lower rim of the acromion was located more caudally in 7% of cases and more cranially in a further 7% of cases. In the remaining 5%, the clavicular facet overlapped the acromion. The authors note that

Fig. 1.11

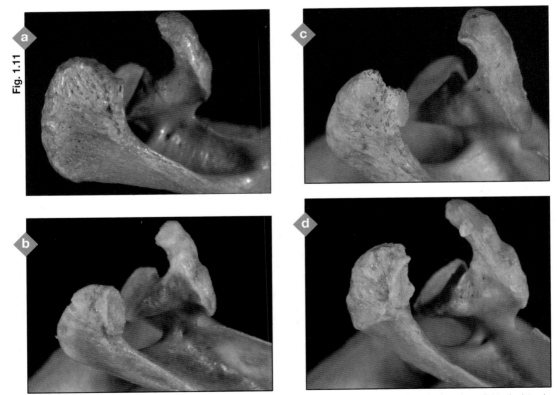

Variants of acromial joint facets: **(a)** joint surface of the acromion in vertical orientation, the joint facet is almost parallel to the lateral rim of the acromion; **(b)** joint surface of the acromion in oblique orientation, the large joint facet is in partial anterior and superior view; **(c)** relatively small joint facets of the acromion showing a small curvature; **(d)** large, concave joint facets of the acromion.

different heights of the corresponding joint surfaces may be misleading when evaluating post-traumatic acromioclavicular instability. The orientation of the joint space depends on the possible joint configurations and may be sagittal or oblique; an oblique orientation is undoubtedly present where the clavicle overlaps the acromion. Many aspects of anatomical variability may thus obstruct intra-articular injections into the AC joint. The use of fluoroscopy to monitor the joint cavity is, therefore, recommended.

The great interindividual variability of the intra-articular kinematics of the AC joint obviously goes hand in hand with the morphological variants of the joint (Baeyens, 1997) (also see Chapter 2).

Soft tissues of the acromioclavicular joint

Strong ligaments at a certain distance influence the mobility of the AC joint. The coracoclavicular ligament arises from the lateral trapezoid ligament and the medial and posterior conoid ligaments. These ligaments are generally independent to some degree, but they may be extensively fused, forming a single ligament with a strong medial rim. The ligaments may be partly or completely ossified, or may have cartilaginous nodules (Fick, 1904). These nodules should be regarded as an intermediate structure between the normal anatomy and a coracoclavicular joint. A coracoclavicular joint is very common in the Asiatic population, where the frequency is directly related to age. This means that it should be regarded as pseudarthrosis, comparable with that visible in kissing spine (Cho, 1998; Cockshott, 1979).

Additional ligaments may be found. The anterior coracoclavicular ligament, described first by Henle, is a strong rim of the fascia between the subclavius and pectoralis minor muscles. It may often be found simply by palpation. Caldani's ligament divides between the coracoid process on the one hand, and the clavicle and first rib on the other. It is probably a remnant of the retroclavicular muscles.

Muscle variants may reduce the space between the coracoid process and the clavicle, and may thus facilitate a further type of impingement, called kissing coracoid, between the coracoid process and the clavicle (Stenvers, 1981). The muscles which insert in the coracoid process are an accessory or inferior muscle belly, an anomaly of the omohyoid muscle, and an accessory head of the subclavius muscle. A series of retroclavicular and supraclavicular muscles, such as the sternoscapular, subclavius and tensor of the fascia of

the neck, take origin from the sternum, clavicle or superficial fascia of the neck, respectively (Bergman, 1988; Le Double, 1897; Testut, 1884).

Sternoclavicular joint

Bone structures of the sternoclavicular joint

Anatomically the sternoclavicular joint (SC joint) is often classified as a saddle joint, despite its characteristic three-dimensional (3D) movement. The joint allows elevation, lowering, extension and retraction movements, and rotation forwards and backwards. The fairly irregular morphology of the joint surfaces does not really correspond to a true saddle joint. An articular disc has an important role, not only reducing the obvious lack of congruity between the sternal and clavicular facets, but also dividing the joint into medial and lateral compartments, both involved in the mobility of the SC joint. A large part of the sternal end of the clavicle contains the insertion of the articular disc, also joined to the cartilage of the first rib. The sternoclavicular part of the joint is covered with fibrous cartilage, while the costoclavicular part has a hyaline cartilage lining. The joint surfaces may be characterized by the secondary internal growth of blood vessels in the fibrous cartilage (Barbaix, 2000).

Soft tissues of the sternoclavicular joint

The articular disc

The disc located in the SC joint is formed by two rather different sections: a roughly vertical fibrocartilage section between the clavicle and the manubrium of the sternum, and a thinner horizontal section between the clavicle and the cartilage of the first rib, which has a hyaline centre. An hourglass-shaped vascular area often divides the articular disc into two parts. Variations occur mainly in the horizontal part, although the vertical part was found to be entirely absent in one case (Fig. 1.12.). There is generally an avascularized biconcave hyaline area in the centre of this horizontal part, which deepens, suggesting that the inferior apex of the medial end of the clavicle, which often has conical thickening, rotates in this cup. This centre may be very thin or perforated (ring-shaped disc) and some parts may be missing, causing

Anatomical variants of the shoulder

Fig. 1.12

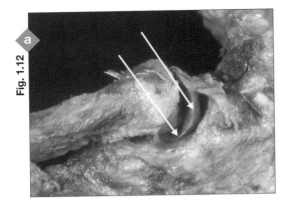

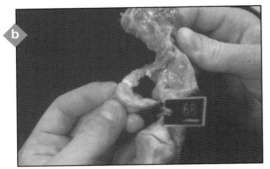

Articular discs of the sternoclavicular joint: **(a)** complete articular disc with thinner horizontal part, **(b)** incomplete articular disc; the horizontal part is absent.

it to resemble the shape of a meniscal disc. The description of the joint as a sternocostoclavicular joint by Testut (1948) gives a better anatomical background for explaining the details of the sternoclavicular and costoclavicular compartments of this joint and the possibility of movement in three dimensions. An additional well-vascularized synovial fold may delimit the disc (Barbaix, 2000). The articular disc seems to protect the SC joint from degenerative diseases for many decades, but perforation and degradation of the disc may occur from the seventh decade (De Palma, 1963).

The ligaments of the sternoclavicular joint

The joint capsule is strengthened by an anterior and posterior sternoclavicular ligament, which may in turn be covered by the sternoclavicular muscles; these muscles may extend laterally, and then insert in the coracoid process, for example, the sternoscapular

muscle (Debierre, 1890; Testut, 1884; Wood, 1868). A sternal muscle which extends in the direction of the clavicular insertion of the sternocleidomastoid muscle may also cover the anterior surface of the joint (Pichler, 1911). This muscle is found in approximately 3% of Europeans and can often be visualized in vivo (Pichler, 1917). The muscle is far commoner in the Asiatic population (11.5%) and among African Americans (8.4%) (Barlow, 1935).

The interclavicular ligament is fairly continuous, although its consistency is variable. The costoclavicular ligament may be formed by two components, separated by a bursa, or may be a single strong ligament. In exceptional cases a cartilaginous spiral, inserting between the clavicle and the first rib, replaces this ligament; a joint cavity may develop in this cartilage (Fick, 1904; Luschka, 1865).

The more lateral portion of the synovial membrane may protrude through the joint capsule, forming a recess which may be isolated (Fick, 1904).

Neurovascular bundle and adjacent structures

Anatomical variants may occur in or around the neurovascular bundle, which runs through the axillary region (Fig. 1.13). Anatomical dissections often find an abnormal configuration of the brachial plexus with a course along the blood vessels. In its upper projection, the bundle may be forced to run along or through variants of the scalene muscles or abnormal connective tissue configurations present in this area. In the more distal course, variants of the pectoralis minor muscle, or the presence of a muscular arch in the axilla, may form modified bridges over the neurovascular bundle.

Kerr (1919) has described 29 variants of the brachial plexus and nerves emerging from the latter. This may be responsible for many thoracic outlet syndromes. It may furthermore explain problems found during anaesthesia of the brachial plexus, as well as some disorders due to positioning of the patient during surgical procedures (Zeuke, 1985). The most extreme variants of the terminal rami are those concerning the median and musculocutaneous nerves. The respective roles of the lateral and medial fasciculi and the level of fusion between the two components, which take origin from the median nerve, are very variable. Fusion may frequently occur high up in the axilla or, by contrast, in the lower third of the arm. The musculocutaneous nerve not only creates frequent or multiple anastomoses with the median nerve, but may

Fig. 1.13

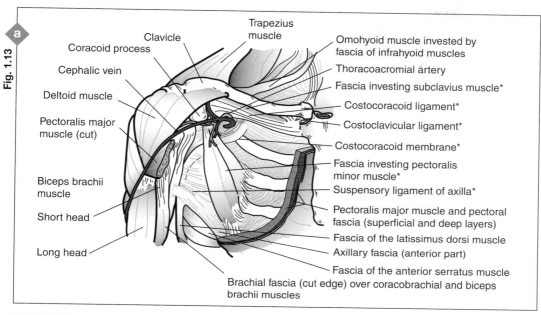

a

- Clavicle
- Coracoid process
- Trapezius muscle
- Cephalic vein
- Deltoid muscle
- Pectoralis major muscle (cut)
- Biceps brachii muscle
- Short head
- Long head
- Omohyoid muscle invested by fascia of infrahyoid muscles
- Thoracoacromial artery
- Fascia investing subclavius muscle*
- Costocoracoid ligament*
- Costoclavicular ligament*
- Costocoracoid membrane*
- Fascia investing pectoralis minor muscle*
- Suspensory ligament of axilla*
- Pectoralis major muscle and pectoral fascia (superficial and deep layers)
- Fascia of the latissimus dorsi muscle
- Axillary fascia (anterior part)
- Fascia of the anterior serratus muscle
- Brachial fascia (cut edge) over coracobrachial and biceps brachii muscles

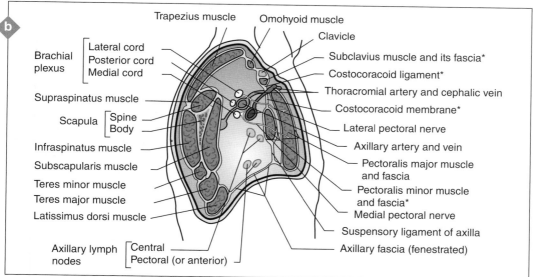

b

- Trapezius muscle
- Omohyoid muscle
- Clavicle
- Brachial plexus
  - Lateral cord
  - Posterior cord
  - Medial cord
- Supraspinatus muscle
- Scapula
  - Spine
  - Body
- Infraspinatus muscle
- Subscapularis muscle
- Teres minor muscle
- Teres major muscle
- Latissimus dorsi muscle
- Axillary lymph nodes
  - Central
  - Pectoral (or anterior)
- Subclavius muscle and its fascia*
- Costocoracoid ligament*
- Thoracromial artery and cephalic vein
- Costocoracoid membrane*
- Lateral pectoral nerve
- Axillary artery and vein
- Pectoralis major muscle and fascia
- Pectoralis minor muscle and fascia*
- Medial pectoral nerve
- Suspensory ligament of axilla
- Axillary fascia (fenestrated)

Normal anatomy of the shoulder with reference to relations between the neurovascular bundle and adjacent structures.
*Components of the clavipectoral fascia.

also be entirely absent, and in this case the flexor muscles of the elbow are innervated by median nerve rami (Buch, 1964; Choi, 2002).

Numerous variants have been observed of the adjacent structures. In some cases, they may reduce the space available for the plexus structures, cause changes in the course of the plexus, create entrapment sites or act as an anchoring point over which the plexus is stretched in certain positions of the shoulder and arm.

The supraclavicular part of the brachial plexus runs between the anterior and middle scalene muscles. The best-known variant in this segment is a cervical rib which may be osseous, ligamentous or mixed. This

Anatomical variants of the shoulder

Fig. 1.14

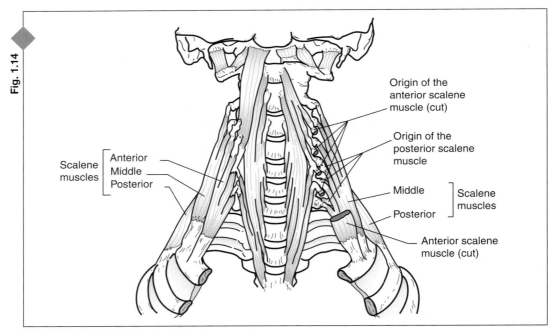

Origin of the
anterior scalene
muscle (cut)

Origin of the
posterior scalene
muscle

Middle

Posterior

Scalene
muscles

Anterior scalene
muscle (cut)

Scalene
muscles

Anterior
Middle
Posterior

Normal anatomy of the scalene muscles.

variant causes the course to be more cranial and the lower trunk and medial fasciculus are stretched as a result (Rayan, 1988).

Variations of the scalene muscles are far more common (Fig. 1.14). The subclavian artery, some structures of the brachial plexus and the thyrocervical trunk may run through the anterior scalene muscle (Bergman, 1988; Debierre, 1890; Delitzin, 1899; Luschka, 1862; Miller, 1939). Many supernumerary scalene muscles have been described. The pleural scalene muscle is a small muscle between C6, C7 and the pleural apex. The smallest scalene muscle (Table I.Ia, between p. 398 and p. 399) takes origin from C5, C6 and C7 and inserts on the first rib, between the subclavian artery and the brachial plexus. It is very common (according to some authors who report an incidence of more than 28%) and is regarded as the most usual cause of narrowing of the subclavian artery (Bergman, 1988; Sunderland, 1949; Testut, 1884). The name accessory scalene (Table I.Ib, between p. 398 and p. 399) has been used by various authors to indicate a duplication of the anterior scalene: a stronger supernumerary scalene between the anterior and middle scalene muscles, with a higher origin than the smallest scalene or the bundles that take origin from the middle scalene, which run through the plexus and then fuse with the anterior scalene muscle

(Bergman, 1988; Testut, 1884; Wood, 1868). All these muscles reduce the available space, particularly when they are hypertrophic, as happens in dancers and in respiratory diseases. A further supernumerary muscle is the costochondroscapular muscle, which takes origin from the upper rim of the scapula and from the transverse ligament of the scapula and runs over the pleural apex, passing through the anterior and middle scalene muscles and inserting on the first rib and its cartilage (Fedoroff, 1927).

The first potential compression site is between the clavicle and the first rib. The term intermediate scalene muscle is used to indicate duplication of the anterior scalene muscle, which inserts in the clavicle (Debierre, 1890). The lateral scalene muscle is supernumerary, takes origin from C6 and inserts on the lower surface of the lateral end of the clavicle (Meckel, 1816). Supernumerary bundles of the subclavius and omohyoid muscles, which run through the coracoid process and the posterior subclavius muscle, may reduce this space (Forcada, 2001; Wood, 1868). Bayon (1920) observed an ossified ligament between the clavicle, the first rib and the coracoid process, which may be regarded as a consequence of myositis ossificans of the subclavius muscle, which disappears. The levator claviculae sometimes has an additional insertion on the coracoid process (Barbaix, 1999).

The passage under the pectoralis minor muscle may be extended by bundles of the subclavius muscle which insert in the coracoid process through a clavian head of the pectoralis minor muscle or, at the distal end, by bundles from the latissimus dorsi which insert on the coracobrachial muscle and on the coracoid process (Adriao, 1933; Bergman, 1988; Testut, 1884; Wood, 1868). In 2003, we observed a supernumerary pectoral muscle, a lateral pectoral muscle, on the left side of a cadaver of a woman (Table I.IIa, between p. 398 and p. 399). The muscle took origin from the fifth and sixth ribs, ran laterally to the pectoralis minor, deeply to the pectoralis major, and inserted on the crest of the lesser tubercle and on the transverse ligament of the humerus cranially, at the insertion of the latissimus dorsi muscle. This, therefore, simulated the double structure of the deep pectoral, typical of the majority of mammals. The space under the pectoralis minor may be reduced by the presence of a pectoralis minimus muscle, which runs from the sternum and from one or two ribs to the coracoid process, or from a pectoralis quartus muscle, which takes origin from a bundle of the rectus abdominis muscle (Bonastre, 2002; Testut, 1884; Turgut, 2000).

A possible site of distal compression is between the tendons of the pectoralis major and the latissimus dorsi. In approximately 8% of people, a muscular bundle separates from the latissimus dorsi and then inserts with the pectoralis major muscle. This bundle may be muscle or tendon. It is the commonest form of Langer's muscle of the axilla, or axillopectoral muscle (Table I.IIb, between p. 398 and p. 399). In this case, the neurovascular bundle runs in a prismatic triangular space along with the biceps and the coracobrachial. This space is normally open on the medial side, thus allowing the bundle to migrate and to protrude from the space which narrows between the pectoral and latissimus dorsi muscles during abduction and external rotation of the arm. If this arch is present, the bundle is pushed into the corner between the latissimus dorsi muscle and the dorsopectoral muscle. The muscle can be compressed at this point, particularly if the arch is tendinous. The multiple variants of the arch include insertions on the fasciae of the coracobrachial muscle and on the coracoid process. The classic variants can be readily palpated and their effects on the brachial artery are clearly visible on ultrasound with Doppler recording of the blood flow in the artery (Clarijs, 1996).

The variants affecting the single nerves that emerge from the plexus are specific. The suprascapular nerve runs between the scapular notch, under the superior transverse ligament of the scapula. This ligament may undergo ossification or be congenitally osseous and thus make the notch into a generally smaller hole (Fischer, 1927; Wood, 1998). An accessory ligament was described by Delbet (Testut, 1948) and rediscovered by Avery (2002), and both named it the anterior coracoscapular. It is present in 50% of shoulders, situated just anterior and inferior to the transverse scapular ligament. It subdivides the scapular notch into two openings. The suprascapular nerve generally runs under this ligament, before crossing the notch. In this case, a sling forms which prevents the nerve sliding freely during sudden movements. The suprascapular artery, which normally runs over the superior transverse ligament of the scapula, occasionally passes across the notch.

As already mentioned, the axillary nerve may perforate the subscapularis muscle. The musculocutaneous nerve, however, cannot pass through the coracobrachial muscle, but may run behind it or between it and the short head of the biceps. The coracobrachial muscle may be divided into a normal and a short coracobrachial muscle, with the nerve interposed (El-Naggar, 2001). Wree (1983) has demonstrated a short coracobrachial muscle which inserts in the latissimus dorsi muscle and which compresses the radial nerve.

Conclusions

The anatomy of the shoulder girdle is largely subject to interindividual variations. Clinical treatments and investigations of the shoulder (for example, arthroscopy), as well as rehabilitation following shoulder girdle disorders and restriction, are viewed against a background of the anatomical variations of the main structures. The anatomical differences can already be recognized in the basic configuration of the glenohumeral joint, the coracoacromial arch, the AC joint and the SC joint, and can also be found in some of the surrounding soft tissues. Anatomical variability can probably explain differences in joint mobility, locking or freeing mechanisms and contact areas in the joints. These anatomical variants should, therefore, be taken into consideration, and biomechanical models of the shoulder refined. Some variants cause degenerative processes, while some may predispose towards the development of musculoskeletal diseases and degeneration.

Bibliography

Adriao M., Note sur quelques variations musculaires de l'épaule., *Comptes Rendus des Anatomistes* 28: 445–449, (1933)

Anatomical variants of the shoulder

Anetzberger H., 'Putz R. Die Morphometrie des subakromialen Raums und ihre klinische Relevanz.' *Unfallchirurg* 98: 407–414, (1995)

Avery B.W., Pilon F.M., Barclay J.K., 'Anterior coracoscapular ligament and suprascapular nerve entrapment.' *Clin. Anat.* 15: 383–386, (2002)

Baeyens J.P., 'Three dimensional arthrokinematic analysis of the late preparatory phase of handball throwing: a step by step clinical evaluation.' PhD thesis, Vrije Universiteit Brussel, (1997)

Banas M.P., Miller R.J., Totterman S., 'Relationship between the lateral acromion angle and rotator cuff disease.' *J. Shoulder Elbow Surg.* 4: 454–461, (1995)

Barbaix E., Van Roy P., Janssens V., Clarijs J.P., 'Observation de multiples variantes simultanées des muscles de la nuque et de la ceinture scapulaire, dont un M. levator claviculae.' *Morphologie* 83: 13–14, (1999)

Barbaix E., Lapierre M., Van Roy P., Clarijs J.P., 'The sternoclavicular joint: variants of the discus articularis.' *Clin. Biomech.* 15 suppl.: S3–S7, (2000)

Barlow R.N., 'The sternalis muscle in American whites and negroes.' *Anat. Rec.* 61: 413–426 (1935)

Bayon H., 'A case of ossified costocoracoid membrane fused with the clavicle.' *Anat. Rec.* 19: 239–240, (1920)

Bergman R.A., Thompson S.A., Afifi A.K., Saadeh F.A., *Compendium of human anatomic variation*, Urban and Schwarzenberg, Baltimore, (1988)

Bigliani L.U., Morrison D.S., April E.W., 'The morphology of the acromion and its relationship to rotator cuff tears.' *Orthop. Trans.* 10: 228, (1996)

Birnbaum K., Lierse W., 'Anatomy and function of the bursa subacromialis.' *Acta Anat.* 145: 354–363, (1992)

Black B.M., 'The prenatal incidence, structure and development of some human synovial bursae.' *Anat. Rec.* 60: 333–355, (1934)

Bonastre V., Rodriguez-Niederfüht M., Choi D., Sanudo J.R., 'Coexistence of a pectoralis quartus muscle and an unusual axillary arch: report and review.' *Clin. Anat.* 15: 366–370, (2002)

Brewer B.J., Wubben R.C., Carrera G.F. 'Excessive retroversion of the glenoid cavity.' *J. Bone Joint Surg.* 68-A: 724–731, (1986)

Buch C., 'Zur Variation der Innervationsweise des M. biceps brachii unter Beachtung der Astabgabe vom N. musculocutaneus und vom N. medianus.' *Anat. Anz.* 114: 131–140, (1964)

Burkhart S.S., 'Shoulder arthroscopy: new concepts.' *Clin. Sports Med.* 15: 635–654, (1996)

Cho B.P., Kang H.S., 'Articular facets of the coracoclavicular joints in Koreans.' *Acta Anatomica* 163: 56–62, (1998)

Choi D., Rodriguez-Niederführ M., Vasquez T., Parkin I., Sanudo J.R., 'Patterns of connections between the musculocutaneous and median nerves in the axilla and arm.' *Clin. Anat.* 15(1): 11–17, (2002)

Clarijs J.P., Barbaix E., Van Rompaey H., Caboor D., Van Roy P., 'The muscular arch of the axilla revisited: its possible role in thoracic outlet and shoulder instability syndromes.' *Man. Ther.* 1: 133–139, (1996)

Cockshott P., 'The coracoclavicular joint.' *Radiology* 131: 313–316, (1979)

Cooper D.E., Arnoczky S.P., O'Brien S.J., Warren R.F., 'Anatomy, histology and vascularity of the glenoid labrum.' *J. Bone Joint Surg.* 74-A: 46–52, (1992)

Cooper D.E., O'Brien S.J., Arnoczky S.P., Warren R.F., 'The structure and function of the coracohumeral ligament: an anatomic and microscopic study.' *J. Shoulder Elbow Surg.* 2: 70–77, (1993)

Craig E.V. 'Shoulder arthroscopy in the throwing athlete.' *Clin. Sports Med.* 15: 673–700, (1996)

Debierre C., 'Traité élémentaire d'anatomie de l'homme.' *Tome 1*, Ed. Alcan, Paris (1890)

Delitzin S., 'Ein Fall von Durchbohrung des M. scalenus anterior durch den Truncus thyreo-cervicalis.' *Arch. Anatomie und Entwicklungsgeschichte* 124–129, (1899)

De Maeseneer M., Van Roy F., Handelberg F., Shahabpour M., Osteaux M., 'Normal and pathologic labrum and bicipito-labral complex: a pictoral essay using plastic models.' *Radiology* 209: 615–616, (1998)

De Maeseneer M., Van Roy F., Lenchik L., Shahabpour M., Jacobson J., Ryu K.N., Handelberg F., Osteaux M., 'CT and MR arthrography of the normal and pathologic anterosuperior labrum and labral-bicipital complex.' *RadioGraphics* 20: S67–S81, (2000)

Demondion X., Maynou C., Van Cortenbosch B., Klein K., Leroy X., Mestdagh H., 'Etude des rapports entre le tendon du chef long du biceps brachial et le labrum glénoidal.' *Morphologie* 85: 5–8, (2001)

De Palma A.F., Callery G., Bennett G.A., 'Variational anatomy and degenerative lesions of the shoulder joint.' Am Academy Orthopaedic Surgeons Instructional Course Lectures 6: 255–281, (1949)

De Palma A.F., 'Surgical anatomy of acromioclavicular and sternoclavicular joints.' *Surg. Clin. N. Am.* 43: 1541–1550, (1963)

Dines D.M., Warren R.F., Inglis A.E., Pavlov H., 'The coracoid impingement syndrome.' *J. Bone Joint Surg.* 72-B: 314–316, (1990)

Duranthon L.D., Gagey O., Lassau J.P., Cabanis E.A., 'Le squelette fibreux de la coiffe des rotateurs. Apports de l'étude tridimensionnelle in vivo des tendons de la coiffe des rotateurs.' *Morphologie* 85: 9–12, (2001)

Edelson J.G., Taitz C., 'Anatomy of the coraco-acromial arch.' *J. Bone Joint Surg.* 74-B: 589–594, (1992)

Edelson J.G., Taitz C., 'Bony anatomy of coracoacromial arch: implications for arthoscopic portal placement in the shoulder.' *Arthroscopy* 9: 201–208, (1993)

Edelson J.G., 'The hooked acromion revisited.' *J Bone Joint Surg.* 77-B: 284–287, (1995)

El-Naggar M.M., Zahir F.I., 'Two bellies of the coracobrachialis muscle associated with a third head of the biceps brachii muscle.' *Clin. Anat.* 41(5): 379–382, (2001)

Ernlund L.S., Warner J.J.P., 'Gross anatomy of the shoulder: bony geometry, static and dynamic restraints, sensory and motor innervation.' In: Lephart S.M., Fu F.H. (Eds.), *Proprioception and neuromuscular control in joint stability*, Champaign, Human Kinetics, p. 89–97, (2000)

Farley T.E., Neumann C.H., Steinbach L.S., Petersen S., 'The coracoacromial arch: MR evaluation and correlation with rotator cuff pathology.' *Skeletal Radiol.* 23: 641–645, (1994)

Fedoroff D.N., 'Zur Morphologie der Muskelvarianten des Lateralgebietes des Halses.' *Anat. Anz.* 62: 338–346, (1927)

Fick R., 'Anatomie und mechanik der Gelenke', *1. Teil: Anatomie der Gelenke.* Fischer Verlag, Jena, (1904)

Fischer H., 'Quelques considérations sur la morphologie de l'omoplate. Echancrure coracoïdienne transformée en un canal par un pont osseux (Origine congénitale).' *Comptes Rendus de l'Association des Anatomistes* 5: 96–98, (1927)

Forcada P., Rodriguez-Niedenführ M., Llusa M., Carrera A., 'Subclavius posticus muscle: supernumerary muscle as a potential cause for thoracic outlet syndrome.' *Clin. Anat.* 14: 55–57, (2001)

Frohse F., Fränkel M., *Die Muskeln des menschlichen Armes*, Fischer Verlag, Jena (1908)

Galinat B.J., Howell S.M., Kraft T.A., 'The glenoid posterior acromion angle: an accurate method of evaluating glenoid version.' *Orthop. Trans.* 12: 727, (1988)

Gerber C., Terrier F., Zehnder R., Ganz R., 'The subcoracoid space. An anatomic study.' *Clin. Orthop.* 215: 132–138, (1987)

Gruber W., *Beobachtungen aus der menschlichen und vergleichenden Anatomie*, 2. Heft: Hirschwald Verlag, Berlin, pp. 39–48, (1879)

Harvey B.C.H., 'Insertion of the abdominal portion of the pectoralis major muscle in man into the capsule of the shoulder and the coracoid process.' *Anat. Rec.* 1: 66–67, (1907)

Hata Y., Nakatsuchi Y., Saitoh S., Hosaka M., Uchiyama S., 'Anatomic study of the glenoid labrum.' *J. Shoulder Elbow Surg.* 1: 207–214, (1992)

Henle J., *Handbuch der systematischen Anatomie des Menschen*, Ertser Band, Friedrich Vieweg und Sohn, Braunschweig

Hitchcock H.H., Bechtol C.O., 'Painful shoulder, observations on the role of the tendon of the long head of the biceps brachii on its causation.' *J. Bone Joint Surg.* 2A: 263–273, (1948)

Huber C.E., 'Zur form und grösse der cavitas glenoidalis.' *Anat. Anz.* Jena 172: 137–142, (1991)

Iannotti J.P. Gabriel J.P., Schneck S.L., Evans B.G., Misra S., 'The normal glenohumeral relationships.' *J. Bone Joint Surg.* 74-A, 491–500, (1992)

Jacobson S.R., Speer K.P., Moor J.T., Janda D.H., Saddemi S.R., MacDonald P.B., Mallon J., J., 'Reliability of radiographic assessment of acromial morphology.' *J. Shoulder Elbow Surg.* 4: 449–453, (1995)

Janssen E., Van Kessel W., 'Osteometry and observations of the scapula, especially the coracoacromial arch in relationship to the glenoid cavity.' MS thesis written in Dutch, Vrije Universiteit Brussel, p 86, (1997)

Keats T.E., Pope T.L., 'The acromioclavicular joint: normal variation and the diagnosis of dislocation.' *Skeletal Radiol.* 17: 159–162, (1988)

Kerr A.T., 'The brachial plexus of nerves in man, the variations in its formation and branches.' *Am. J. Anat.* 23: 285–395, (1919)

Kumar V.P., Balasubramaniam P., 'The role of atmospheric pressure in stabilizing the shoulder.' *J. Bone Joint Surg.* 67-B: 719–721, (1985)

Le Double A.F., 'Traité des variations du système musculaire de l'homme.' Tome 2, Schleicher Frères, Paris (1897)

Luschka, H. Von, 'Die anatomie des menschen in rücksicht auf die bedürfnisse der praktischen heilkunde. Erster band, erste abteilung: die anatomie des menschlichen halses', *Verlag der Laupp'schen Buchhandlung*, Tübingen, p. 440, (1862)

Luschka, H. Von, 'Die anatomie des menschen in rücksicht auf die bedürfnisse der praktischen heilkunde. Dritter band, erste abteilung: die anatomie der glieder des menschen', *Verlag der Laupp'schen Buchhandlung*, Tübingen, p. 495, (1865)

Matsen III F.A., Thomas S.C., Rockwood C.A., Wirth M.A., 'Glenohumeral instability.' In: Rockwood C.A., Matsen F.A. (eds.) *The shoulder*, vol. 2, Saunders, Philadelpha, pp. 611–754, (1998)

Meckel J.F., *Handbuch der menschlichen anatomie*, Zweiter Band, Buchhandlung des hallischen Waisenhauses, Halle und Berlin, (1816)

Michaud T., 'Biomechanics of unilateral overhead throwing motion: An overview.' *Chiropractic Sports Medicine* 3: 13–26, (1990)

Milianitch N., Spiridonovitch R., 'Variation de la morphologie et de l'innervation des muscles de l'Èpaule et du bassin chez les Serbes. Comptes rendus de l'Association des Anatomistes, IX Réunion', Liège, pp. 385–395, (1926)

Miller R.A., 'Observations upon the arrangement of the axillary artery and brachial plexus.' *Am. J. Anat.* 64: 143–163, (1939)

Nasca R.J., Salter E.G., Weil C.E., 'Contact areas of the "subacromial" joint', In: Bateman J.E., Welsch P. (eds.) *Surgery of the shoulder*, pp. 134–139, (1984)

Neer C.S., 'Anterior acromioplasty for the chronic impingement syndrome in the shoulder: a preliminary report.' *J. Bone Joint Surg.* 54-A: 41–50, (1972)

Neer C.S., Poppen N.K., 'Supraspinatus outlet.' *Orthop Transactions* 11: 234–237, (1987)

Nicholson G.P., Goodman D.A., Flatow E.L., Bigliani L.U., 'The acromion: morphologic condition and age-related changes. A study of 420 scapulas.', *J. Shoulder Elbow Surg.* 5: 1–11, (1996)

O'Brien S.J., Neves M.C., Arnoczky S.P., Rozbruck S.R., Dicarlo E.F., Warren R.F., Schwartz R., Wickiewicz T.L., 'The anatomy and histology of the inferior glenohumeral ligament complex of the shoulder', *Am. J. Sports Med.* 18: 449–456, (1990)

O'Brien S.J., Answorth A.A., Fealy S., Rodeo S.A., Arnoczky S.P., 'Developmental anatomy of the shoulder and anatomy of the glenohumeral joint.' In: Rockwood C.A., Matsen F.A. (eds.) *The shoulder*, Saunders, Philadelphia, pp. 1–33, (1998)

Pichler K., 'Ueber das vorkommen des M. sternalis. Nach untersuchungen am lebenden.' *Anatomischer Anzeiger* 39: 155–160, (1911)

Pichler K., '500 Fälle von sternalismuskel. Beobachtungen am Lebenden. Zweite Mitteilung', *Anatomischer Anzeiger* 50: 339–347, (1917)

Prescher A., Klümpen T., 'The glenoid notch and its relation to the shape of the glenoid cavity of the scapula.' *J. Anat.* 190: 457–460, (1997)

Rayan G.M., 'Lower trunk brachial plexus compression neuropathy due to cervical rib in young athletes', *Am. J. Sports Med.* 16: 77–79, (1988)

Renoux S., Monet J., Pupin P., Collin M., Apoil A., Jouffroy F.K., Doursounian L., 'Preliminary note on biometric data relating to the human coracoacromial arch', *Surg. Radiol. Anat.* 8: 189–185, (1986)

Rockwood C.A., Williams G.R., Young D.C., 'Disorders of the acromioclavicular joint', In: Rockwood C.A., Matsen F.A. (eds.) *The shoulder*, vol. 1, Saunders, Philadelphia, pp. 483–553, (1998)

Saha A.K., 'Dynamic stability of the glenohumeral joint,' *Acta Orthop. Scand.* 42: 491–505, (1971)

Saha A.K., 'Mechanics of evaluation of the glenohumeral joint', *Acta Orthop. Scand.* 44: 668–678, (1973)

Soslowski L.J., Flatow E.L., Bigliani L.U., Mow V.C., 'Articular geometry of the glenohumeral joint', *Clin. Orth. Relat. Res.* 285: 181–190, (1992)

Speer K.P., 'Anatomy and pathomechanics of shoulder instability,' *Clin. Sports Med.* 14: 751–760, (1995)

Steinbeck J., Liljenquist U., Jerosch J., 'The anatomy of the glenohumeral ligamentous complex and its contribution to anterior shoulder stability,' *J. Shoulder Elbow Surg.* 7: 122–126, (1998)

Stenvers J.D., Overbeek W.J., '*Het kissing coracoid (The kissing coracoid)*', De Tijdstroom, Lochem-Poperinge, (1981)

Sunderland S., Bedbrook G.M., 'Narrowing of the second part of the subclavian artery', *Anat. Rec.* 104: 299–307, (1949)

Testut L., *Les anomalies musculaires chez l'homme*, Masson, Paris (1884)

Testut L., Latarjet A., 'Traité d'anatomie humaine', *Tome I Ostéologie, Arthrologie, Myologie.* IX Ed., Doin & Cie, Paris (1948)

Tillmann B., 'Tichy P. Funktionelle anatomie der schulter', Unfallchirurg, 89: 389–397, (1986)

Turgut H.B., Anil A., Peker T., Barut C., 'Insertion abnormality of bilateral pectoralis minimus', *Surg. Radiol. Anat.* 22: 55–57, (2000)

Uhthoff H.K., Sarkar K., Hammond D.I., 'The subacromial bursa: a clinicopathological study,' In: Bateman J.E., Welsch P. (eds) *Surgery of the shoulder*, pp. 121–125, (1984)

Uhthoff H.K., Sarkar K., 'Surgical repair of rotator cuff ruptures. The importance of the subacromial bursa', *J. Bone Joint Surg*, 73-B: 399–401, (1991)

Vahrensieck M., Wiggert E., Wagner U., Schmidt H.M., Schild H., 'Subacromial fat pad', *Surg. Radiol. Anat.* 18: 33–36, (1996)

Van der Helm F.C.T., 'A finite element musculoskeletal model of the shoulder mechanism', *J. Biomech.* 27: 551–569, (1994)

Van Roy P. De, 'Anatomische Variabiliteit van de M. Deltoideus en van de Spieren van de Rotatorcuff, (Anatomical variation of the deltoid muscle and rotator cuff muscles),' *Geneeskunde en Sport* 26: 167–170, (1993)

Vangsness C.T. Jr., Jorgenson S.S., Watson T., Johnson D.L., 'The origin of the long head of the biceps from the scapula and glenoid labrum', *J. Bone Joint Surg.* 76-B: 951–954, (1994)

Vazquez T., Rodriguez-Niederführ M., Parkin I., Sanudo J.R., 'Accessory heads of the biceps brachii muscle,' *Clin. Anat.* 15 (1): 71–76, (2002)

Volk A.G., Vangsness C.T., 'An anatomic study of the supraspinatus muscle and tendon', *Clin. Orthop.* 384: 280–285, (2001)

Wall M.S., O'Brien S.J., 'Arthroscopic evaluation of the unstable shoulder', *Clin. Sports Med.* 14: 817–840, (1995)

Wang J.C., Shapiro M.S., 'Changes in acromial morphology with age', *J. Shoulder Elbow Surg.* 6: 55–59, (1997)

Warner J.J.P., Paletta G.A., Warren R.F., 'Accessory head of the biceps brachii. A case report demonstrating clinical relevance', *Clin. Orthop.* 280:179–181, (1992)

Welcker H., 'Die Einwanderung der Bicepssehne in das Schultergelenk. Arch. für Anatomie und Entwicklungsgeschichte', p. 21, (1878)

Wood J., Variations in human myology observed during the Winter session of 1867/68 at King's College, London. Proceedings of the Royal Society of London, 17: 483–525, (1868)

Wood V.E., Marchinski L., 'Congenital anomalies of the shoulder.' In: Rockwood C.A., Matsen F.A. (eds.) *The shoulder*, Saunders, Philadelphia, pp. 99–163, (1998)

Wree A., 'Kompression des nervus radialis durch einen musculus coracobrachialis minor. Eine anatomische studie,' *Anat. Anz.* 153: 459–464, (1983)

Wuelker N., Roetman B., Roessig S., 'Coracoacromial pressure recordings in a cadaveric model', *J. Shoulder Elbow Surg.* 4: 462–467, (1995)

Zeuke W., Linss W., 'Topographischen Untersuchungen zur Pathogenese postoperativer Paresen im Versorgungsgebiet des Plexus brachialis', *Anat. Anz.* 160: 243–250, (1985)

Zlatkin M.B., Iannotti J.P., Schnall M.D., *MRI of the shoulder*, Raven Press, New York, p. 170, (1991)

Zuckerman J.D., Kummer F.J., Cuomo F., Greller M., 'Interobserver reliability of acromial morphology classification: an anatomic study', *J. Shoulder Elbow Surg.* 6: 286–287, (1997)

BIOMECHANICS OF
THE SHOULDER

J.P. BAEYENS
P. VAN ROY

The glenohumeral joint is characterized by a low level of correspondence between the joint surfaces. In any position of the shoulder, only 25–50% of the humeral head is contained in the glenoid, and this is surrounded by a substantial capsuloligamentous structure which allows the glenohumeral joint a high degree of mobility. The glenohumeral joint thus remains stable throughout the wide range of movements involved in shoulder function, including intense repetitive movements such as throwing actions.

A decade ago the biomechanics of the shoulder were far less well understood than those of the knee. However, the creation of the International Shoulder Group (as part of the International Society of Biomechanics) and the *Journal of Shoulder and Elbow Surgery* resulted in a considerable increase in studies of the shoulder during the 1990s.

Stability of the glenohumeral joint

At the end of the wind-up or cocking phase of throwing, changes can occur due to anterior glenohumeral instability, ranging from subluxation to frank dislocation. The most important question here is: at which forces and moments is the glenohumeral joint sufficiently vulnerable to instability? Anterior subluxation/dislocation can be induced with the shoulder abducted at 90° and externally rotated, applying a direct force in the anterior direction and external rotation moment (Ovesen, 1986). Using inverse kinematics to study kinetic data on the shoulder obtained from healthy elite throwers, Fleisig (1995) identified a critical moment close to the final part of the wind-up phase

of throwing. Substantial loads are generated in the shoulder, including a twisting moment within the range $67 \pm 11\,\text{N}$ to $310 \pm 100\,\text{N}$ of anterior force.

Which, then, are the structures that limit these anterior destabilizing factors? The stabilizing structures of the shoulder can be divided into three subsystems: a passive subsystem, an active musculoskeletal subsystem and an afferent and efferent nerve subsystem, which consists of numerous transducers of force and movement and a nerve control centre.

The basic systems involved in passive glenohumeral stability are joint congruency, joint orientation, negative intra-articular pressure, and capsuloligamentous and labral stabilization. This section will examine the limits of these stabilizing factors.

Congruency of the joint heads

The articular surfaces of the humeral head and the glenoid which come into contact appear to roughly resemble cross sections of a sphere, with small deviations from a perfect spherical shape of less than 1% of the radius (Table 2.1; Soslowsky, 1992). The glenoid cartilage is thicker at the periphery (mean 3.8 mm) and thinner in the centre (mean 1.2 mm). The humeral cartilage, by contrast, is thicker in the centre (mean 2 mm) and thinner at the periphery (mean 0.6 mm). Consequently, measurements obtained from X-rays show that the radius is larger and the glenoid surface flatter.

The ratio of the radius of curvature of the cartilage surface of the humeral head to that of the articular surface of the glenoid is, on average, 0.99 ± 0.05

Table 2.1

Radius of glenohumeral curvature (from Soslowksy 1992)

	Radius of glenohumeral curvature (mm)			
	Cartilage surface		Bone surface	
	Male	Female	Male	Female
Humeral head	26.85 ± 1.40	23.27 ± 1.69	26.10 ± 1.41	23.15 ± 2.09
Glenoid	26.37 ± 2.42	23.62 ± 1.56	34.56 ± 1.74	30.28 ± 3.16

(range 0.89 to 1.09). Rozendaal (1996) correlates this situation with a two-link model. The first link causes the centre of the joint surface of the humeral head to move along a circle, the radius of which is the difference between the radii of curvature of the articular surfaces of the glenoid and the humerus. The second link is the arm itself, which can rotate freely around the centre of the articular surface of the humeral head.

The glenohumeral joint is well lubricated and has a friction coefficient of 0.002, which can be considered negligible (in contrast with the concavity-compression effect) (Collins, 1992). Consequently, in order to be stable, the joint can bear only reaction forces perpendicular to the articular surface. This limits the range of directions of the reaction forces that the glenohumeral joint can bear to a small conical section, 60° in the anteroposterior direction and 90° in the superoinferior direction. Lippitt (1993) and Lazarus (1996) have demonstrated that at 45° abduction and 35° external rotation the joint can withstand a compressive force of 100 N in the anterior, posterior, superior and inferior directions and tangential forces of approximately 30, 30, 50 and 50 N before dislocating. These data have been used to determine a range of directions of forces that can be sustained in the anteroposterior direction equal to 33° ($= \cotan^{30\,N}/_{100\,N} + \cotan^{30\,N}/_{100\,N}$) and in the superoinferior direction equal to 51° ($= \cotan^{50\,N}/_{100\,N} + {}^{50\,N}/_{100\,N}$). Dislocation may nevertheless occur even within these angles.

Pagnani (1996) has shown, in isolated cadaver shoulder models, that when a compressive force of 111 N is applied to a shoulder at 45°, the anterior and posterior translations induced by a translating force of 50 N are 30% of those caused by a compressive load of 22 N. The compressive load can be induced by muscles such as the rotator cuff muscles. The function of the rotator cuff is not, however, entirely understood. When a single oblique muscle antagonizes an abnormal external moment, the rotator cuff may shift the tangential force backwards, causing articular contact. Nevertheless, to obtain a shift inside the glenoid angles, the force of the rotator cuff must be considerably greater than the perpendicular component of the force of the joint reaction. More efficient compensation can be obtained by activating the oblique muscle so that the perpendicular component of the external force is just balanced. The equilibrium moment must, therefore, be provided by the rotator cuff muscles. There is, however, a small difference in the ability to generate the moment between the rotator cuff muscles and the other shoulder muscles, and it is based on a parameter defined by muscle volume divided by the area of the transverse section (Rozendaal, 1996). Co-contraction occurs during high levels of performance, for example, throwing, where the high level of muscle activation is maintained only briefly (Di Giovine, 1992).

Joint orientation

CT scans have failed to show significant differences in glenoid tilting in traumatic anterior, recurrent anterior, posterior and contralateral shoulder instability (Dowdy, 1994; Yanaga, 1995).

The dorsal tilt and retroversion of the humeral head have been explained as a teleological (i.e. goal-directed) characteristic of prehensile activity in humans. Analysis of CT scans has revealed no significant differences in dorsal tilt between healthy individuals and patients with traumatic or recurrent anterior instability (Yanaga, 1995). Kronberg and Broström (1990) found, using X-ray studies, significantly greater external rotation in the dominant and non-dominant shoulders of healthy volunteers than in the dominant and non-dominant shoulders of patients with recurrent anterior instability. A wide range of overlaps were, however, found.

Handball players show a significant increase in external humeral rotation in the arm used for throwing compared to the other arm (Pieper 1996). Pieper attributed these variations to a biopositive adaptation to the mechanical stimuli of constant strain on the extremities during growth. Torsional adaptations may reduce the specific strains of the sport on the capsuloligamentous complex, owing to an increase in the degree of external rotation.

In conclusion, no association between joint geometry (tilt and orientation of the glenoid, humeral torsion) and shoulder stability can be demonstrated. Furthermore, the mobility of the scapula in space orientates the glenoid independently of its tilt or orientation in relation to the scapula, even with valid and confirmed statistical differences between these joint geometries. Its significance is undoubtedly negligible, when compared with the kinematic potential of the scapula.

Negative intra-articular pressure

A layer of synovial fluid less than 1 mm thick is present in the normal glenohumeral joint. This joint fluid can, together with viscous and intermolecular forces, help to retain the articular surfaces. The normal intra-articular pressure is, moreover, slightly negative (-42 cm H_2O in a resting position). Gohlke (1994) found that the stabilizing effect of the negative intra-articular pressure decreased as abduction and rotation increased. Furthermore, although the effect of the articular pressure can be determined with certainty, the associated forces are small (in a resting position 20 N at 1.5 mm of inferior movement after increasing translation with one order of magnitude) (Gibb, 1991). The forces imparted during abduction of the glenohumeral joint without load produce tangential forces on the articular surface which massively exceed the resistance force caused by the intra-articular pressure.

Labrum

Avulsion of the anterior portion of the labrum has been found in 87% of cases of traumatic anterior instability (Hintermann, 1995). Although the aetiology of non-traumatic anterior instability is not yet entirely clear, various labrum anomalies have been observed in the majority of patients with non-traumatic instability (Altchek, 1990).

The labrum defect may be a classic Bankart lesion, an anterior labral periosteal sleeve avulsion (ALPSA) lesion, a bony Bankart lesion, a Perthe lesion, a glenolabral articular disruption (GLAD) lesion or a glenoid articular rim disruption (GARD) lesion. A GLAD lesion is a superficial anteroinferior tear of the labrum

(generally with an inferior flap) with undetectable anterior instability, while classic and bony Bankart lesion, Perthe lesion and ALPSA lesion are unstable lesions. In GLAD lesion, the deep fibres of the GHL are still strongly attached, but various degrees of damage to the articular cartilage in the anteroinferior quadrant are also present. If no anteroinferior lesion of the labrum is found during surgery, lateral avulsion of the GHL, also known as humeral avulsion of the glenohumeral ligament (HAGL) must be ruled out.

In 1923, Bankart defined detachment of the glenoid labrum and capsule from the anterior glenoid rim as the critical lesion in recurrent anterior instability; this type of lesion was subsequently dubbed 'Bankart lesion'. But can the clinical existence of GARD, GLAD and HAGL lesions cast doubt on the crucial impact of the labrum on anterior instability?

The labrum forms approximately 50% of the total depth of the glenoid cavity (Hata, 1992), consequently it was originally believed that the labrum served as a 'lock' controlling glenohumeral translation and extending the contact surface of the glenoid with the humeral head. Hata (1992) found in particular that the glenoid labrum is far thicker in the anteroposterior portion, and thus probably contributes to stability in the anteroinferior direction. One might wonder whether the labrum serves solely to increase the compressive effect of the cavity, since it is not formed of bone or cartilage like the remainder of the glenoid. A structure of medium rigidity is clearly more advantageous in preventing overload of the labral transition zone. Owing to its low elasticity, the labrum deforms very readily under load. Consequently the importance of widening the load zone as a stabilizing mechanism needs to be evaluated. This point of view is supported by the anatomical signs found by Nishida (1995) and Gohlke (1994), who suggest that the labrum is the site of insertion of the glenohumeral and capsule ligaments, rather than a fibrocartilaginous extension of the joint cavity, as maintained by Prodromos (1990). These authors concluded that the labrum is a superfluous fold of capsular (fibrous) tissue, with fibrocartilage present in only a thin transition zone, at the point where the labrum inserts in the glenoid rim.

Townley found as early as 1950 that removal of the anterior labrum did not cause anterior dislocation, unless the anterior portion of the capsule with the ligaments was cut or became detached from the glenoid rim. Anteroinferior detachment is generally associated with certain capsular lesions of the glenoid neck. This capsuloperiosteal separation creates laxity in a major stabilizing complex, the inferior glenohumeral ligament complex (IGHLC), which is closely connected

Biomechanics of the shoulder

to the labrum. Gohlke (1994) established that the very small change in anteroposterior translation, caused by an artificial Bankart lesion with a significant increase after a horizontal incision, indicated that avulsion of the labrum without a complex lesion of the capsuloligamentous structures produced only minor instability. In a simulation of Bankart lesion in a biomechanical study, Speer (1995) observed a multidirectional increase in the translation of the humeral head. These translations are small, however. The largest increase was 3.4 mm during inferior translation with abduction at 45°. Janevic (1992) evaluated surgical repairs of anterior glenohumeral instability in vitro, positioning the joints of cadavers at their maximum functional limits and measuring the resulting translation of the humeral head and the glenohumeral contact area, using a spatial connection. Janevic found that, in comparison with a normal joint, a Bankart lesion from 3 to 6 o'clock does not influence the translation of the humeral head or joint congruency at different limits of mobility (maximum abduction, flexion and extension, maximum internal and external rotation in a neutral position and anterior and posterior apprehension test).

Some clinical studies suggest that Bankart lesion is not the only cause of anterior dislocation. Further plastic deformation of the IGHLC, besides its medial disinsertion, is necessary to allow anterior dislocation or a predisposition to multidirectional instability.

This hypothesis is further supported by biomechanical studies aimed at evaluating the mechanical properties of the various areas of the IGHLC (Bigliani, 1992). The IGHLC was divided into three bone-ligament-bone (BLB) sections: the anterior bundle, the anterior axillary pouch and the posterior axillary pouch. The samples isolated were elongated until rupture with unidirectional traction with controlled stretching. Three rupture models were observed: at the glenoid insertion point, in the central section of the ligament and at the humeral insertion point. Rupture tests on the BLB samples showed that ligament lesions were predominant with rapid traction (10%/sec) and rupture at the insertion points were predominant with slower traction (0.1%/sec and 0.01%/sec). However, even when a lesion occurs at the glenoid insertion, this is secondary to significant elongation of the IGHLC. For the BLB samples tested at a stretch rate of 10%/sec, the mean rupture tension of the IGHL was 25.4 ± 6.0, which was significantly higher in the anterior axillary pouch (30.4 ± 4.3, $p < 0.05$). In glenohumeral subluxation-dislocation, the ligament may, therefore, stretch and become permanently elongated, regardless of whether rupture occurs at the insertion point.

Capsuloligamentous complex

The IGHLC consists of three functionally distinct parts: an anterior bundle and a posterior bundle with an axillary pouch in between (O'Brien, 1990). During abduction and external rotation, the anterior bundle fans open and the posterior bundle coils like a rope. During internal rotation, however, the posterior bundle fans open and the anterior bundle coils. Gohlke (1994) was able to identify the posterior bundle in only 62.8% of cases, since in the remainder it was fused with the surrounding tissues.

All types of concentric capsulorrhaphy shorten the circular structures of the capsuloligamentous complex, particularly the oblique bundle, and elevate the anterior portion of the IGHLC. Consequently the T-capsulorrhaphy used by Gohlke in experimental studies (1994), by adding translation and twisting forces, causes an equivalent reduction in internal and external rotation depending on the degree of abduction.

The role of the shoulder capsule and the glenohumeral ligaments in preventing instability is complex and varies according to the position of the shoulder and the direction of the translation force. Furthermore, the extreme rotation of the humerus seems to wind up the concentrically orientated fibres of the capsule, developing forces orientated towards the articular surfaces, thus increasing stability.

It is also useful to evaluate measurement of the glenohumeral angle in cadavers. If glenohumeral movement is considered along with the contribution of the scapulothoracic movement as far as complete abduction, this will show that glenohumeral abduction of 90° corresponds to abduction in vivo of 120–135°.

Biomechanical studies of the stabilizing effect of the capsuloligamentous complex have varied objectives, ranging from simulating the lesion mechanism, studying selective sectioning, studying stretching and changes in length, measuring forces and recording translations.

The in vitro results of the paired movements can be divided into three categories:
— if pure rotation of the glenohumeral joint is attempted in one plane, a rotation in two planes is obtained automatically (Terry, 1991);
— rotation of the glenohumeral joint in one plane requires an additional twisting force, to remain in two planes (Clark, 1990; Harryman, 1990); and
— anterior translation spontaneously produces internal rotation and posterior translation spontaneously produces external rotation, whereas external or internal rotation produces both posterior and anterior translation.

These induced movements are correlated with the quantity of forces applied, particularly at the limits of the movement (Gohlke, 1994). These studies show that, during the progression of glenohumeral rotation, something in the joint is tensed and causes the humeral head to translate and rotate in another direction. Therefore, although the relations between the humeral head and the glenoid cavity remain relatively constant throughout the arc of movement, the shoulder joint does not behave exactly like a sphere moving in a cavity. Rotation of the humeral head is associated with further translation in the glenoid. Howell and Kraft (1991) have, moreover, observed persistence of the normal antero-posterior glenohumeral translation in a group of patients who underwent selective nerve block of the supraspinatus and infraspinatus muscles. This suggests that the compressive forces of the rotator cuff are not responsible for these paired movements. The differences in capsuloligamentous tension nevertheless seem to influence paired translation.

The anterior portion of the IGHLC is the principal stabilizer, and limits the anterior translation and external rotation of the shoulder abducted at 90°. At lower angles of glenohumeral abduction, this limiting role is taken by the middle GHL.

At the maximum limit of the range of movement (ROM), the ligaments thicken and push the humeral head to translate and rotate. Magnetic resonance images with 3D reconstruction, obtained from asymptomatic volunteers who performed external and internal rotations with the arm abducted at 0° (Rhoad, 1998) and active and passive abductions (Graichen, 2000), were used to quantify the 3D translation of the humeral head in the glenoid in vivo. Howell (1988) chose axillary radiography as a means of measuring the antero-posterior excursion of the humeral head in the glenoid cavity, in both volunteers with healthy shoulders and patients with anterior instability. In the healthy volunteers, the movement of the arm in the horizontal plane causes slight translation (less than 1 mm), while the humeral head remains centred in the glenoid cavity, rotating little in the glenoid. Placing the arm in the cocking phase of throwing in abduction, horizontal abduction and external rotation of the humerus causes the posterior translation of the centre of the humeral head, in relation to the glenoid cavity, of approximately 4 mm. The humeral head is relatively recentred when the joint is placed in internal rotation.

With the arm in a flexed or internally rotated position, it has been observed that the humeral head undergoes anterior translation of 4 mm in relation to the centre of the glenoid cavity. In the event of anterior instability, placing the arm in the cocking

position of throwing, reduces posterior translation. Baeyens (2001) demonstrated, by means of computed tomography (CT) with 3D reconstruction, that by moving from 90° abduction and 90° external rotation to the final position (90° abduction with complete external rotation and horizontal extension) the humeral head in healthy shoulders does not rotate internally or externally in the glenoid. A substantial external rotation component has, nevertheless, been demonstrated in shoulders with minor instability. The geometric centre of the humeral head in healthy shoulders undergoes posterior translation in the glenoid, whereas in slight anterior instability, it undergoes central translation.

Active stabilization

The shoulder muscles stabilize the joint in four different ways:
— by passive resistance;
— by generating muscle tension which directs the reaction forces of the joint into the compressed glenoid angles;
— by moving the humerus in relation to the glenoid, thus increasing the static limits; and
— by limiting the arc of movement of the glenohumeral joint with antagonistic twisting moments.

Clinical cases of recurrent anterior dislocation of the shoulder have intraoperatively revealed laxity and rupture of the subscapularis muscle. In 9 of the 45 cases studied, Symeonides (1972) observed that the subscapularis slides superiorly over the humeral head, as the humerus dislocates from the glenoid. Symeonides also observed post-traumatic lesions of the subscapularis in 30 cases. A biopsy performed in 4 cases revealed the presence of healed post-traumatic lesions. It is clear from all these observations that the subscapularis is the principal anterior stabilizer of the glenohumeral. In this regard, it is useful to mention the 5-year follow-up published by Wirth (1994) of transposition of the pectoralis (major or minor) in the treatment of recurrent anterior glenohumeral instability with irreparable lesion of the subscapularis: according to the Neer classification, 82% of cases showed a satisfactory result.

The humeral head may, nevertheless, dislocate under the lower rim of the subscapularis tendon, following abduction with external rotation. The study by Turkel (1981) of the sequential sectioning of ligaments showed a mean increase of 18° in external rotation in the neutral position, after sectioning of the

Biomechanics of the shoulder

subscapularis. No significant increase was noted, however, in anterior translation at 45° and 90° abduction of the glenohumeral. At 90° of glenohumeral abduction in external rotation, it was noted that the lower rim of the subscapularis protruded beyond the lower rim of the humeral head, rendering this muscle incapable of counteracting the instability. Blasier (1992) simulated the forces generated in the rotator cuff muscles when the shoulder is abducted at 90° and static loads are applied to the tendon insertions along anatomical force lines.

A weight applied to any tendon of the cuff makes a significant, measurable contribution to anterior stability, measured on the basis of the force required to produce a standard movement of 10 mm. The contributions of the various tendons are not significantly different and do not depend on whether the humerus is in external rotation or a neutral position. The results of Blasier's studies do not, therefore, support the hypothesis that the subscapularis is the most important stabilizer of the cuff muscles, at least in abduction at 90°. Howell and Kraft (1991) have furthermore suggested that compressive forces, if applied symmetrically to the rotator cuff, are equivalent to the forces applied asymmetrically to a single portion of the cuff.

Capsuloligamentous and muscle limits in glenohumeral instability have been evaluated using a nonlinear approach. What is the force necessary to cause dislocation? To which directions of force is the glenohumeral joint particularly vulnerable? Which parameters limit the subluxation-dislocation of the glenohumeral joint? The glenohumeral joint may consequently appear to be constantly unbalanced between the rims of the glenoid cavity. These continual subluxation movements, constantly balanced by links induced by traction, can clearly not be tolerated. Which mechanisms balance the position of the humeral head in the glenoid so well? The idea of increasing proprioception and thus glenohumeral stability is very interesting in this context. A great deal of information has been acquired during the intermediate elevation of the shoulder, when the glenohumeral joint is principally stabilized by the action of the muscles. One might consequently wonder whether data concerning the late phase of cocking in throwing have been correctly extrapolated, when the capsuloligamentous complex (and in particular the IGHL) becomes the principal stabilizer of the glenohumeral joint.

Using surface electromyography (EMG), Wallace (1997) compared healthy and damaged shoulders in patients with recurrent post-traumatic monolateral anterior dislocation, to investigate differences in proprioception. The latency between the start of the movement and detection of the contraction of the infraspinatus and of the sternal portion of the pectoralis major was used as a sign of proprioception. No significant differences in latency were demonstrated between the healthy and the unstable shoulder, thus suggesting that there were no significant deficits in reflex activity. The capsule reflexes, though undamaged, were nevertheless too slow (3 m/sec) for muscle potentiation to be able to support the mechanical load to which the glenohumeral joint is subjected in the late cocking phase of throwing.

This partly explains why progressive specific muscle potentiation sessions, in studies by Burkhead and Rockwood (1992), have yielded few results in patients with post-traumatic instability. Only 16% of shoulders with traumatic subluxation obtained a good or excellent score on the Rowe scale.

Glousman (1988) examined the EMG activity of many shoulder muscles during the throwing movement in both asymptomatic throwers and throwers with chronic anterior glenohumeral instability. The eccentric activity of the pectoralis major, the subscapularis and the latissimus dorsi, associated with the internal rotation present in the terminal phase of cocking, was reduced in shoulders with anterior instability, whereas the external rotation and anterior translation of the shoulder remained the same or increased. This difference in neuromuscular control may have a key role in perpetuating chronic anterior instability in the shoulder in throwers. The increased activation of the infraspinatus seems to be an attempt at compensation. It is not possible, in any case, to establish whether these neuromuscular imbalances are primary or secondary to the instability.

Glousman (1988) correlated the reduced function of the anterior serratus with reduced protraction of the scapula, which starts during cocking. Since the humerus is abducted horizontally and simultaneously rotated externally, there may be additional tension on the anterior glenohumeral links. MacMahon (1996) compared the EMG activity of the scapular and rotator cuff muscles in patients with anterior instability and healthy volunteers while they were performing three movements common in daily activities (abduction, elevation and anterior flexion in the whole range of movement, divided into 30° intervals). The supraspinatus showed reduced EMG activity, in both elevation and abduction, between 30° and 60° in shoulders affected by anterior instability. In all three movements, the shoulders affected by anterior instability showed reduced EMG activity of the anterior serratus, in particular from 30° to 120° of abduction and from 0° to 120° of elevation and anterior flexion. None of the other muscles examined (infraspinatus, rhomboid and trapezius) showed alterations. Warner (1990) discovered, using Moire topography, that axioscapular muscle dysfunction is common in patients with anteroinferior instability. Static Moire evaluation revealed scapulothoracic asymmetry or an increased topography in 14% of asymptomatic individuals and in 32% of patients with instability. The dynamic Moire test demonstrated an abnormal pattern in 18% of asymptomatic subjects and in 64% of patients with instability. It remains to be determined whether these data represent a primary or secondary phenomenon.

Conclusions

Glenohumeral stability can be divided into three categories on the basis of shoulder position.

At rest and without active contraction of the muscle groups, the force of gravity pulls on the humeral head creating negative intra-articular pressure in the presence of an intact capsule. This vacuum acts as a stabilizing force.

During active intermediate elevation, the shoulder is stabilized dynamically by the action of both the muscles and the rotator cuff.

At the limits of the range of articular function, for example, at the end of the cocking phase of throwing in complete external rotation and horizontal abduction, the capsuloligamentous complex tightens and avoids excessive translation of the humeral head in the glenoid cavity.

Elevation of the arm

Osteokinematics

Glenohumeral rhythm

The movement of the humerus in relation to the movement of the scapula is generally known as scapulohumeral or glenohumeral rhythm. The main methodological problem of recording the movement of the shoulder is the movement of the scapula under the skin. Glenohumeral rhythm is consequently studied in two dimensions. De Groot (1999) showed that the range of scapulohumeral rhythm, expressed by the ratio of the angle of elevation of the arm (a) to the scapular angle (th), with a normal value of 2.1 to 3.6, can be obtained from the following tests:
— a/th ratio for the spine in frontal projection equal to 2.6, while for the medial crest it is 3.6;
— inaccuracy in identifying the spine means that the ratio varies from 2.1 to 3.3; and

— the ratio of 2.6 for the spine in the frontal plane becomes 3.6 in scapular projection.

It has, therefore, been concluded that two-dimensional (2D) analysis of a 3D movement is unreliable.

To solve this problem, Högfors (1991) studied glenohumeral rhythm in three dimensions by taking measurements on low-intensity X-ray stereograms in patients with radiopaque implants in contact with bone. The results show that, under normal conditions, the individual rhythm is very stable and largely insensitive to moderate loads (the study was confined to three patients). McQuade (1995) separately evaluated the effect of work by the upper and lower trapezius during 3D scapulothoracic movement at 135° of elevation in the scapular plane on scapulohumeral rhythm. A measurement device with 6° of freedom was used to mark the landmarks on the trunk and scapula, along with an inclinometer placed on the humerus. A 22% reduction in the mean frequency of the muscles examined, indicating muscle fatigue, was demonstrated, associated with an increase in the scapulohumeral ratio around the sagittal and coronal axes, ranging from 4.8/1 to 7.1/1 and from 5.3/1 to 8.3/1, respectively.

Glenohumeral osteokinematics

In an evaluation of the relation between the plane of elevation and of rotation, Nakagawa (1993) used a magnetic apparatus to measure the 3D angle of the humerus in relation to the trunk in 12 different elevation positions, at an interval of 15°. When the arm was elevated at 65°–70° anterior to the frontal plane, the rotation was small. The humerus rotates externally during the abduction and internal rotation associated with flexion. In the scapular plane (at approximately 30° anterior to the frontal plane), the most significant angle of rotation during maximum elevation was 49°. Using an electromagnetic apparatus, An (1991) conducted a cadaveric study of the 3D movements of the glenohumeral joint during elevation of the arm. An found that maximum elevation occurred anterior to the scapular plane (23°, range 10–37°). The results demonstrated the influence of axial rotation on elevation, i.e. the importance of external rotation anterior to the scapular plane and the need to rotate the arm internally to obtain maximum elevation posterior to the scapular plane. In the portion of movement just posterior to the scapular plane (29°, range 26–31.5°) there is an area that is subject to rotation. The axial rotation associated with elevation of the humerus has been linked to the mobility of the greater tuberosity. This is supported by the observation that there is a mean increase in elevation of 8° following surgical procedures such as acromioplasty and resection of the coracoacromial ligament.

To conclude, it is impossible to achieve maximum elevation either anterior or posterior to the scapular plane without adequate internal and external humeral rotation ranges. Any attempt to mobilize the glenohumeral joint, without paying attention to rotation, may be unsatisfactory. Moreover, any surgical procedure that limits rotation, reduces maximum elevation as a consequence.

Scapulothoracic osteokinematics

Scapular rotation around an axis approximately parallel to the spine of the scapula has been called flexion-extension, or anterior-posterior or forwards-backwards sliding. Movement around a vertical axis has been defined as anterior-posterior rotation, internal-external rotation or oscillation.

The contribution of the scapular muscles to the rotation movement has been studied using EMG on the throwing movement of baseball players (Di Giovine, 1992) and on a series of scapular exercises (Moseley, 1992).

Van der Helm (1994) and Meskers (2001) studied the shoulder girdle three-dimensionally during elevation, using a palpator device which recorded live the 3D positions of the bones by determining the locations of a number of clearly palpable bone landmarks. During forward flexion, the chest began to rotate in a posterior direction. This rotation continued through further movements. The chest was largely fixed up to 90° abduction, but then rotated in a posterior direction to a greater extent than during forward flexion. If, however, the elevation was bilateral, the lateral flexion of the trunk was negligible. The course of the lateral rotation of the scapula during abduction did not differ from that occurring during forward flexion of the humerus. Some differences were present at the start of elevation, because the scapula did not seem to rotate laterally during the first 40° of forward flexion. Furthermore, the scapula was orientated towards the same plane in which the humerus was elevated. Protraction of the scapula was visible during forward flexion, whereas the scapula was retracted during abduction of the humerus. The scapula tended to retract at the end of elevation. Rotation yielded largely the same results for the elevation of both humerus bones. Using a similar system, Ludewig (1996) demonstrated a general model for the scapula (which differed only in amplitude) for progressive rotation forwards, for a reduction in internal rotation and for

anteroposterior oscillation movements with static elevation in three positions (0°, 90° and 140°).

Osteokinematics of the clavicle

Inman and Saunders declared as early as 1944 that the clavicle also moves during abduction of the shoulder, since its lateral rim rotates in a superior direction at about 30° around the coronal plane. The authors measured the axial rotation of the clavicle by inserting pins in it. Inman and Saunders did not describe the insertion protocol, but Van der Helm (1994) maintained that, based on the photographs attached to the article, the pins had been inserted centrally close to the sternoclavicular joint (SC Joint). Inman and Saunders found that the lateral rim of the clavicle rotated in an anterior direction by 10° during only the first 40° of abduction of the shoulder, and then did not rotate any further until 130° of abduction, when it rotated a further 15° when the shoulder reached maximum abduction. When they had manually fixed the pin, which prevented rotation of the clavicle, elevation was limited to 110°. Inman and Saunders defined the axial rotation of the clavicle as the fundamental characteristic of elevation of the arm. By positioning two Kirschner wires in parallel 2.5 inches (approximately 6 cm) from the AC joint, in the superolateral rim of the clavicle and on the distal upper surface of the acromion, in young adults, Rockwood and Young (1990) demonstrated that the clavicle rotated axially 10° less than the scapula along the entire arc of elevation of the shoulder. This reduced axial rotation can be explained by the function of the conoid and trapezoid coracoclavicular ligaments, which force the clavicle to rotate around its major axis to follow the lateral rotation of the scapula, thus avoiding twisting in the AC joint capsule. By performing load and shift tests, Fukuda (1986) found that in small shifts, evidence that the acromioclavicular ligaments limit both posterior translation (89%) and superior translation (68%) was provided by the common pattern of the clinical lesions. In large shifts, the conoid ligament limited mainly superior translation (62%), while the acromioclavicular ligaments limited mainly posterior translation (90%).

Arthrokinematics

Glenohumeral arthrokinematics

In contrast with the studies mentioned on the translation behaviour of the humeral head on the glenoid, the following studies on the intra-articular behaviour of the glenohumeral joint stemmed from research into joint contact. Many published studies distinguished various patterns of contact in the glenohumeral joint, using the following techniques:

— black light lamp pointed at the humerus and impression of the contact on the glenoid;
— copper nails introduced in the humeral head and aluminium paper covering the glenoid in a polyethylene model of the shoulder;
— staining technique;
— pressure-sensitive film between the joint surfaces; and
— stereophotogrammetry.

Bowen (1992) used a pressure-sensitive film and compressive loads of 50 and 100 pounds (=22.5 and 45 kg) to demonstrate an increase in contact areas and a reduction in the corresponding contact pressures during elevation. In a resting position, glenohumeral contact did not conform to the humeral head, which touches the glenoid centrally in a histologically apparently thinner cartilaginous area called the loading area, in which there is an increase in subchondral trabecular bone density. Soslowsky (1992) used stereophotogrammetric measurements to evaluate contact patterns during elevation in the scapular plane. Elevation in the scapular plane was examined in 1° of external rotation, which allowed maximum elevation (40 ± 8°), and with the arm internally rotated by 20°, starting from an externally rotated position. The contact areas tended to be larger in middle elevation (from 60° to 120°) than at the limits of the range (0° or 180°). With the increase in elevation in the initial position of external rotation, the humeral head contact moved from an inferior to a superoposterocentral region, while the glenoid contact moved in a posterior direction. After positioning the humerus at 20° of internal rotation, starting from an externally rotated position, the humeral head contact moved from an inferoanterocentral to a superoposterocentral region, with a posterior shift in glenoid contact.

Physiotherapists should reconsider the traditional concave-convex rules used in therapy. With external rotation, posterior translation occurs outside the capsuloligamentous complex, particularly in the anterior portion of the IGHLC. Mobilization using anterior translation with external rotation accentuates an anomalous pattern of intra-articular movement. Increased interest has recently prompted studies investigating the relation between kinematic changes and clinical changes in the shoulder. Lukasiewicz (1999) found an 8–9° reduction in posterior inclination and an increase in the superior position of the scapula during elevation

in subacromial impingement. Ludewig and Cook (2002) observed a reduction in the forward rotation of the scapula, and an increase in the anterior inclination and medial rotation of the scapula in patients with subacromial impingement, associated with a reduction in anterior serratus activity and an increase in lower and upper trapezius activity.

Tyler (2000) demonstrated an increase in posterior capsule thickness and a reduction in internal and external rotation in cases of impingement of non-dominant limbs, whereas in impingement of dominant limbs, posterior capsule thickness was increased, associated only with a reduction in internal rotation. The thickness of the posterior capsule was inversely proportional to the internal impingement (r = −0.50; p = 0.006). Tyler calculated a posterior capsule thickness of 1 cm for each 4° of reduction in internal rotation. Using open magnetic resonance imaging (MRI), Graichen (2000) demonstrated that, in individuals with impingement, there was an increase in the superior and anterior position of the humeral head on the glenoid during abduction. Internal (subcoracoid) impingement has been hypothetically correlated in the literature with excessive external rotation with or without anteroinferior glenohumeral instability (Davidson, 1995). Baeyens (2001) demonstrated the impact of excessive glenohumeral external rotation, without anterior instability, on the development of internal impingement using a spiral CT scan with 3D reconstruction to evaluate the shoulder at 90° of abduction and 90° of external rotation.

Throwing movements

Kinematics of throwing

Throwing a heavy ball involves mechanical accommodation:

— reaching maximum external rotation early, which helps to achieve acceleration of internal rotation for a longer time;
— conduction with the elbow, i.e. an increase in the horizontal adduction of the shoulder and flexion of the elbow; and
— reduction in the contribution of the trunk and legs, which can be visualized as a shorter stride, a more upright position of the trunk and a smaller twisting angular velocity of the pelvis and trunk.

In the majority of throwing techniques (including three-quarter, side arm and underhand pitch), the angle of abduction of the shoulder remains fairly constant. The highest and lowest point through which the ball passes during the throw are reached more by tilting the trunk than by increasing and decreasing the angle of abduction of the shoulder in relation to the trunk. This suggests that an angle of abduction of 90° to 110° should be a very strong dynamic position for the arm and the shoulder. Deviations of more than 10° outside this range (less than 80° and more than 120°), during the ball release phase, should suggest that the arm position is abnormal.

Kinetics of throwing

Throwing involves a sequence of actions of the various bone segments, initiated by the actions of the legs and trunk and continued by the faster movements of the relatively smaller distal segments. The sequence of principal actions comprises rotation of the trunk, sternoclavicular protraction, extension of the elbow and flexion of the wrist and fingers; energy is thus transferred from the proximal to the distal portions. During the first phase of throwing, the proximal segments reach a maximum velocity less than that reached by the distal segments. The velocity of the segments decelerates significantly after reaching maximum values.

The instantaneous contributions of the rotation of the various segments to the linear velocity of the distal extremities, in a kinetic chain, have been studied by Feltner and Nelson (1996), who examined the penalty throw in water polo (where the distance from the goal is 4 m). The authors established that a continuum of techniques is required to transmit velocity to the ball at the moment of release.

The movements that contribute most to the velocity of the ball are extension of the forearm (26.6 ± 6.3%) and anticlockwise rotation of the trunk (24.2 ± 6.3%) (for a right-handed throw). Rotation of the arm makes a very variable contribution (13.2 ± 11.6%) and has a significant inverse relation to the horizontal adduction of the upper arm (8.9 ± 7.5%). As regards release of the ball, individuals with considerable internal rotation tend to bring their arm into smaller external rotation positions, increasing the velocity of the internal rotation. Individuals in whom the horizontal adduction of the arm makes a major contribution show greater velocity in this same movement and greater pronation positions of the forearm when the ball is released.

Using the opposite dynamic approach to the data for healthy adult pitchers, Fleisig (1995) identified two critical moments. The first occurred almost at the end of the cocking phase of the arm, when the first 64% of the time for which the foot is in contact with the ground has been completed, before releasing the ball and slightly before reaching maximum external rotation of the arm. During this period, the elbow is flexed by 95 ± 10° and the arm is externally rotated by 165 ± 11°, abducted by 94 ± 21° and adducted horizontally by 11 ± 11°. The shoulder is subject to a considerable load comprising 67 ± 11 N of twisting force due to internal rotation and 310 ± 100 N of anterior force. A shear strain of more than 250 ± 80 N, a compressive force of 480 ± 130 N and a twisting force due to horizontal adduction of 87 ± 23 N also occur.

The second critical moment for the shoulder occurs during the deceleration phase, shortly after release of the ball, when 108% of the time for which the foot is in contact with the ground has been completed, before release of the ball. During this period, the arm is hyperextended towards 'home base' (i.e. in the direction of throwing): the elbow is flexed by only 25 ± 10°, while one arm is externally rotated by 64 ± 35°, abducted by 93 ± 10° and adducted horizontally by 6 ± 8°. At this point, which is critical for the shoulder, a maximum compressive force of 1090 ± 110 N is generated. When this maximum compressive force is produced, a slight shear force is generated in the anterior direction (80 ± 180 N) and in the inferior direction (100 ± 130 N). During this period, the shoulder is subjected to a twisting force produced due to adduction of 26 ± 44 N, a twisting force due to horizontal abduction of 44 ± 51 N and a negligible twisting force due to internal rotation (7 ± 5 N).

Fleisig's study (1996), which compared the throwing movements of quarterbacks and baseball pitchers, found no significant differences as regards the forces in the anterior direction produced in the shoulder during the cocking phase of the arm. A possible explanation for the lower incidence of anterior labrum lesions in quarterbacks may be the greater glenohumeral stability, resulting from the greater horizontal adduction. The kinetic parameters of the trunk can be correlated with joint stresses. By limiting the movement of the legs, the rotation of the pelvis and the rotation of the upper part of the trunk, quarterbacks can regulate the energy that is transferred in a proximal-distal direction.

It is necessary, in order to understand the mechanisms of active stabilization, to examine the inverse kinematics along with the EMG data obtained from coordinated sequences of muscle events and their normalized amplitudes in relation to the upper limb during the throwing movement and to the positioning of the muscles and ligaments around the glenohumeral joint in different positions (for example, 90° of abduction, neutral horizontal adduction/abduction and 90° external rotation) (Turkel, 1981). During late cocking, the

Table 2.2

Kinetics and pathophysiology of throwing: the clinician should analyse the phases of throwing and the symptoms related to them

Phase	Symptoms	Likely causes
Between early and late cocking		Lesion of upper labrum or of the insertion of the biceps
End of late cocking	Smaller degree of instability or significant apprehension	Lesion of the anteroinferior labrum or IGHL
End of late cocking	Posterior pain and excessive external rotation	Lesion of the posterior labrum with internal impingement
	Pain during the deceleration phase	Anterior or anterosuperior lesion associated with fatiguing of the rotator cuff
	Pain during deceleration and subsequently	Lesion of the posterosuperior labrum and of the insertion of the biceps

humerus abducts horizontally by 18°–11° and rotates externally by 46°–170°, keeping its level of abduction constant. The stability of the scapula is guaranteed by the pairing of the forces generated by the adductors of the scapula (middle trapezius, rhomboids and levator muscle of the scapula) and by the anterior serratus (Table 2.2). When the humerus ends the abduction, during late cocking, the deltoid becomes less active. The supraspinatus is the least active of the muscles of the rotator cuff, but it is nevertheless fairly active. During late cocking, the supraspinatus is nevertheless in a posterior position and does not, therefore, contribute effectively to abduction. The subscapularis, pectoralis major and latissimus dorsi are in an anterior position in the late cocking phase.

The subscapularis and the pectoralis major (with the latissimus dorsi involved more in the acceleration phase) are activated during late cocking. The pectoralis major probably contributes to the twisting forces due to horizontal adduction generated during late cocking. Since the supraspinatus is in a posterior position, force may be partially generated in the cephalic direction by the subscapularis rotated upwards. The posterior muscles of the rotator cuff (infraspinatus and teres minor) are fairly active, working concentrically against a twisting force due to internal rotation.

During deceleration, the antagonist muscles of the shoulder are activated largely simultaneously. The trapezius, anterior serratus and rhomboids all demonstrate a high or very high level of activity. The middle and posterior heads of the deltoid are visibly very active. The teres minor demonstrates a very high level of activity, underlined clinically by a pain confined to the teres minor in the posterior portion of the rotator cuff, during deceleration. The latissimus dorsi is far more active than the pectoralis major. The subscapularis also has a surprisingly high level of activity. Di Giovine (1992) established that the role of the subscapularis, during deceleration, was to prevent subluxation of the humeral head during rapid internal rotation movement. The kinetic analysis by Fleisig (1995) shows only a small anterior translation force in the first half of the deceleration period, which is converted into a posterior translation force in the second half of the deceleration phase. The positioning of the subscapularis in late cocking may simply accentuate its shunt role.

Although the common mechanism of injury in a SLAP lesion is a fall on the abducted and flexed arm, SLAP lesions have also been found to occur during throwing (Snyder, 1990). It is not possible in the majority of these patients to recognize a traumatic episode, however, the lesion is the result of excessive repetition of the throwing action. A specific damaging mechanism has been attributed to the action of the long head of the biceps which, by contracting particularly during deceleration, tears the glenoid labrum in which it is inserted. Simulation of the contraction of the tendon of the long head of the biceps has shown that this action raises the glenoid labrum (Grauer, 1992). Arthroscopy has shown that, with the shoulder rotated internally, traction exerted on the tendon transmits stress to the posterior surface of the labrum, whereas with the shoulder rotated externally, the stress is transmitted to the anterior surface of the labrum.

EMG evaluation of the throwing action has revealed that the biceps brachii is active not only in the acceleration phase of the arm, but also in the deceleration phase (Di Giovine, 1992). The biceps produces great twisting forces, relative to flexion in the eccentric modality of contraction, during both the acceleration and deceleration phases of throwing, and these forces reach maximum values of $61 \pm 11\,\text{N}$ just before release of the ball (Fleisig, 1995). The biceps can produce a stabilizing compressive force that is far more pronounced at middle elevations (Pagnani, 1996). This is particularly effective when maximum compressive force is reached before release of the ball, since the reduction in external rotation allows the long head of the biceps to be aligned with the direction of compression (Fleisig, 1995). The level of EMG activity in the biceps is, moreover, greater in shoulders with chronic anterior instability, thus indicating the need, in the event of instability, for an increase in the compressive force of the shoulder (Glousman, 1988).

The validity of the long head of the biceps as a dynamic limitation in late cocking was demonstrated in numerous cadaveric studies by Rodosky (1994). The authors concluded that, in a position of abduction and external rotation, an increase in the force of the long head of the biceps increased the torsional rigidity $(\text{N}/°)$ of the joint. Biceps hypertrophy is commonly found after a rotator cuff lesion (Pagnani, 1996). An EMG comparison of professional and amateur pitchers found that the activity of the biceps was greater in the amateurs (Gowan, 1987). With an optimal deceleration mechanism, the maximum twisting forces due to flexion of the elbow are produced before the maximum compressive forces of the shoulder (Fleisig, 1995).

An inappropriate throwing rhythm may cause these two loads to be close together in time and to combine with the force created by the action of the biceps. This may lead to repeated overuse (see Chapter 16) during the throwing action which causes intrinsic destabilization of the shoulder with the consequent need for a stabilizing force requiring, in turn, greater involvement of the biceps, resulting in a vicious circle (see Premise to Section II, Chapters 3–4).

Bibliography

Altchek D.W., Warren R.F., Skyhar M.J., 'Shoulder arthroscopy', In: Rockwood C.A. Jr, Matsen F.A. III (eds.) *The shoulder*, WB Saunders, Philadelphia, pp. 258–277, (1990)

An K.N., Browne A.O., Korinek S., Tanaka S., Morrey B.F., 'Three dimensional kinematics of glenohumeral elevation', *J. Orthop. Res.* 9: 143–149, (1991)

Baeyens J.P., Van roy P., De Schepper A., Clarys J.P., 'Glenohumeral joint kinematics related to minor anterior instability of the shoulder at the end of the late preparatory phase of throwing'. *Clin. Biomech.*, 16: 752–757, (2001)

Bigliani L., Pollock R., Soslowsky L., Flatow E.L., Pawluk R.L., Mow V.C., 'Tensile properties of the inferior glenohumeral ligament'. *J. Orthop. Res.* 10: 187–197, (1992)

Blasier R.B., Guldburg R.E., Rothman E.D., 'Anterior shoulder stability: contributions of rotator cuff forces and the capsular ligaments in a cadaver model'. *J. Shoulder Elbow Surg.*, 1: 140–150, (1992)

Bowen M.K., Deng X.H., Hannafin J.A., O'Brien S.J., Altchek D.W., Warren R.F., 'An analysis of patterns of glenohumeral joint contact and their relationship to the glenoid "bare area"', *Trans. Orthop. Res. Soc.* 17: 496, (1992)

Burkhead W.Z., Rockwood C.A., 'Treatment of instability of the shoulder with an exercise program', J. *Bone Joint Surg.* 74(A): 890–896, (1992)

Cain P.R., Mutschler T.A., Fu F.H., Lee S.K., 'Anterior stability of the glenohumeral joint: a dynamic model', *Am. J. Sport Med.* 15: 144–148, (1987)

Clark J.M., Harryman D.T. II, Sidles J.A., Matsen F.A. III, 'Range of motion and obligate translation in the shoulder: the role of the coracohumeral ligament'. *Trans. Orthop. Res. Soc.* 15: 273, (1990)

Collins D., Tencer A., Sidles J., Matsen F. III, 'Edge displacement and deformation of glenoid components in response to eccentric loading', *J. Bone Joint Surg.* 74(A): 501–507, (1992)

Davidson P.A., Elattrache N.S., Jobe C.M., Jobe F.W., 'Rotator cuff and posterior-superior glenoid labrum injury associated with increased glenohumeral motion: a new site of impingement', *J. Shoulder Elbow Surg.* 4: 384–390, (1995)

De Groot J.H., 'The scapulo-humeral rhythm: effects of 2D roentgen projection', *Clin. Biomech.* 14: 63–68, (1999)

Di Giovine N.M., Jobe F.W., Pink M., Perry J, 'An electromyographic analysis of the upper extremity in pitching', *J. Shoulder Elbow Surg.* 1: 15–25, (1992)

Dowdy P.A., O'Driscoll S.W., 'Recurrent anterior shoulder instability', *Am. J. Sports Med.* 22: 489–492, (1994)

Feltner M.E., Nelson S.T., 'Three-dimensional kinematics of the throwing arm during the penalty throw in water polo', *J. Appl. Biomech.* 12: 359–382, (1996)

Fleisig G.S., Andrews J.R., Dillman C.J., Escamilla R.F., 'Kinetics of baseball pitching with implications about injury mechanisms', *Am. J. Sports Med.* 23: 233–239, (1995)

Fleisig G.S., Escamilla R.F., Andrews J.R., Matsuo T., Satterwhite Y., Barrentine S.W., 'Kinematic and kinetic comparison between baseball pitching and football passing', *J. Appl. Biomech.* 12: 207–224, (1996)

Fukuda K., CRAIG E.V., An K.N., Cofield R.H., Chao E.Y., 'Biomechanical study of the ligamentous system of the acromioclavicular joint', *J. Bone Joint Surg.* 68(A): 434–439, (1986)

Gibb T.D., Sidles J.A., Harryman D.T., Mcquade K.L., Matsen F.A. II, 'The effect of capsular venting on glenohumeral laxity', *Clin. Orthop. Rel. Res.* 268: 120–127, (1991)

Glousman R., Jobe F., Tibone J.E., Moynes D., Antonelli D., Perry J., 'Dynamic electromyographic analysis of the throwing shoulder with glenohumeral instability', *J. Bone Joint Surg.* 70(A): 220–226, (1988)

GohlkE F., Essigkrug B., Schmitz F., 'The pattern of the collagen fiber bundles of the capsule of the glenohumeral joint', *J. Shoulder Elbow Surg.* 3: 111–128, (1994)

Graichen H., Staumbeger T., Bonel H., Englmeier K.H., Reiser M., Eckstein F, 'Glenohumeral translation during active and passive elevation of the shoulder – a 3D open-MRI study', *J. Biomech.* 33: 605–613, (2000)

Grauer J.D., Paulos L.E., Schmutz W.P., 'Biceps tendon and superior labral injuries', *J. Arthroscopic Related Surg.* 8: 488–497, (1992)

Harryman D.T.I., Sidles J.A., Clark J.M., McQuade K.J., Gibb T.D., Translation of the humeral head on the glenoid with passive glenohumeral motion', *J. Bone Joint Surg.* 72(A): 1334–1343, (1990)

Hata Y., Nakatsuchi Y., Saitoh S., Hosaka M., Uchiyama S., 'Anatomic study of the glenoid labrum', *J. Shoulder Elbow Surg.* I: 207–214, (1992)

Hintermann B., Gächter A., 'Arthroscopic findings after shoulder dislocation', *Am. J. Sports Med.* 23: 545–551, (1995)

Högfors C., Peterson B., Sigholm G., Heberts P., 'Biomechanical model of the shoulder joint: II. The shoulder rhythm,' *J. Biomech.* 24: 699–709, (1991)

Howell S.M., Kraft T.A., 'The role of the supraspinatus and infraspinatus muscles in glenohumeral kinematics of anterior shoulder instability', *Clin. Orthop. Rel. Res.* 263: 128–134, (1991)

Inman V.T., Saunders J.B., Abbott L.C., 'Observations on the function of the shoulder joint,' *J. Bone Joint Surg.* 26: 1–30, (1944)

Janevic J.T., Engebretsen L., Lew W.E., 'Glenohumeral motion and contact force following anterior capsular repair', *Acta Orthop. Scand.* 63(Suppl): 248, (1992)

Kronberg M., Broström L.A., 'Humeral head retroversion in patients with unstable humeroscapular joints', *Clin. Orthop. Rel. Res.* 260: 207–211, (1990)

Lazarus M.D., Sidles J.A., Harryman D.T. II, Matsen F.A. III, 'Effect of a chondral-labral defect on glenoid concavity and glenohumeral stability', *J. Bone Joint Surg.* 78(A): 95–102, (1996)

Lippitt S., Matsen F., 'Mechanisms of glenohumeral joint stability', *Clin. Orthop. Rel. Res.* 291: 20–28, (1993)

Ludewig P.M., Cook T.M., Nawoczenski D.A., 'Three-dimensional scapular orientation and muscle activity at selected positions of humeral elevation', *J. Orthop. Sports Phys. Ther.* 24: 57–65, (1996)

Ludewig P.M., Cook P.M., 'Translations of the humerus in persons with shoulder impingement symptoms', *J. Orthop. Sports Phys. Ther.* 32: 248–59, (2002)

Lukasiewicz A.C., Macclure P., Michener L., Pratt N., Sennett B., 'Comparison of 3-dimensional scapular position and orientation between subjects with and without shoulder impingement', *J. Orthop. Sports Phys. Ther.* 29: 574–83, (1999)

Macmahon P.J., Jobe F.W., Pink M.M., 'Comparative electromyographic analysis of shoulder muscles during planar motions: anterior glenohumeral instability versus normal,' *J. Shoulder Elbow Surg.* 5: 118–123, (1996)

McQuade K.J., Wei S.H., Smidt G.L., 'Effects of local fatigue on three-dimensional scapulohumeral rhythm', *Clin. Biomech.* 10: 144–148, (1995)

Moseley J.B., Jobe F.W., Pink M., Perry J., Tibone J.E., 'EMG analysis of the scapular muscles during a shoulder rehabilitation program', *Am. J. Sports Med.* 20: 128–134, (1992)

Nakagawa T., 'Relation between elevation and rotation of the shoulder'. *J. Shoulder Elbow Surg.* 2(1), Part 2: S37/18 (Abstract), (1993)

Nishida K., Hashizume H., Toda K, 'Histologic and scanning electron microscopic study of the glenoid labrum', *J. Shoulder Elbow Surg.* 5: 132–138, (1995)

O'Brien S.J., Neves M.C., Arnoczky S.P., Rozbruck S.R., Dicarlo E.F., Warren R.F., Schwarts R., Wickiewics T.L., 'The anatomy and histology of the inferior glenohumeral ligament complex of the shoulder', *Am. J. Sports Med.* 18: 449–456, (1990)

Ovesen J., Sjobjerg J.O., 'Lesions in different types of anterior glenohumeral joint dislocation: an experimental study', *Arch. Orthop. Trauma Surg.* 105: 216–218, (1986)

Pagnani M.J., Deng X.H., Warren R.F., Torzilli P.A., O'Brien. 'Role of the long head of the biceps brachii in glenohumeral stability: a biomechanical study in cadavera', *J. Shoulder Elbow Surg.* 5: 255–262, (1996)

Pieper H.G., 'Torsional adaptation of the humeral shaft to unilateral strain in handball players', *J. Shoulder Elbow Surg.* 5(2), Part 2: S48/132 (Abstract), (1996)

Prodromos C.H., Ferry J.A., Schiller A.L., Zarins B., 'Histological studies of the glenoid labrum from fetal life to old age', *J. Bone Joint Surg.* 72(A): 1344–1348, (1990)

Rockwood C.A., Young D, 'Disorders of the acromioclavicular joint', In: Rockwood C.A., Matsen F.A. III (eds.) *The shoulder*, WB Saunders Company, Philadelphia, pp. 413–476, (1990)

Rozendaal L., 'Stability of the shoulder: intrinsic muscle properties and reflexive control,' Doctoral Thesis, Technische Universiteit Delft, (1996)

Snyder S.J., Karzel R.P., Del Pizzo, 'SLAP-lesions of the shoulder', *Arthroscopy* 6: 274–279, (1990)

Soslowsky L.J., Flatow E.L., Bigliani L.U., Pawluk R.J., Athesian G.A., Mow V.C., 'Quantitation of in situ contact areas at the glenohumeral joint: a biomechanical study', *J. Orthop. Res.* 10: 524–535, (1992)

Soslowsky L.J., Flatow E.L., Biliani L.U., Mow V.C., 'Articular geometry of the glenohumeral joint', *Clin. Orthop. Rel. Res.* 285: 181–190, (1992)

Speer K.P., Deng X., Torzilli P.A., 'Strategies for an anterior capsular shift of the shoulder: a biomechanical comparison', *Am. J. Sports Med.* 23: 264–269, (1995)

Symeonides P.O., 'The significance of the subscapularis muscle in the pathogenesis of recurrent anterior dislocation of the shoulder', *J. Bone Joint Surg.* 54(B): 476–83, (1972)

Terry G.C., Hammon D., France P., Norwood L.A., 'The stabilizing function of passive shoulder restraints', *Am. J. Sports Med.* 19: 26–34, (1991)

Townley C.O., 'The capsular mechanism in recurrent dislocation of the shoulder', *J. Bone Joint Surg.* 32(A): 370–380, (1950)

Turkel S.J., Panio M.W., Marshall J.L., Girgis F.G., 'Stabilizing mechanisms preventing anterior dislocation of the glenohumeral joint', *J. Bone Joint Surg.* 63(A): 1208–1217, (1981)

Biomechanics of the shoulder

Tyler T.F., Nicholas S.J., Roy T., Gleim G.W., 'Quantification of posterior capsule tightness and motion loss in patients with shoulder impingement', *Am. J. Sports Med.* 28: 668–73, (2000)

Van Der Helm F.C.T., 'Analysis of the kinematic and dynamic behaviour of the shoulder mechanism', *J. Biomech.* 27: 527–550, (1994)

Wallace D.A., Beard D.J., Gill R.H.S., Carr A.J., 'Reflex muscle contraction in anterior shoulder instability', *J. Shoulder Elbow Surg.* 6: 150–155, (1997)

Warner J.J., Micheli L.J., Arslanian L.E. et al., 'Patterns of flexibility, laxity, and strength in normal shoulder and shoulder with instability and impingement', *AJSM* 21:366–375, (1990)

Wirth M.A., Seltzer D.G., Rockwood C.A., 'Recurrent posterior glenohumeral dislocation associated with increased retroversion of the glenoid', *Clin. Orthop. Rel. Res.* 308: 98–101, (1994)

Yanaga K., Hirasawa H., 'Gleno-tilting angle and humeral retrotorsion angle in traumatic anterior instability of the shoulder', *J. Shoulder Elbow Surg.* 4(1), Part 2: S69/10 (Abstract), (1995)

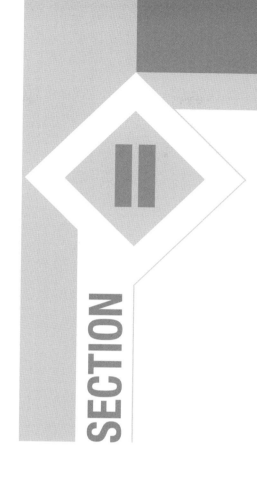

SECTION II

PATHOLOGY,
CLINICAL ASPECTS
AND DIAGNOSTIC
IMAGING

PREMISE

A. Fusco

Examination of the painful shoulder: interdisciplinarity and clinical rationale

The diagnostic and functional evaluation of painful shoulder in an athlete involves a rational process, requiring clinical experience and knowledge of concepts specific to various medical and technical professions within sport.

A correct diagnosis is essential for adopting effective treatment and this is closely related to identification of the cause of the disorder. A correct aetiological evaluation may help to identify programmes for the prevention of recurrent problems.

The diagnostic process must take into account that:
- the evidence available to date regarding diagnosis is not sufficient to determine a standard clinical examination;
- no single test or standardized examination protocol can provide certain or differential diagnoses;
- different shoulder disorders are inter-related (Jobe, 1991) (Fig. 3A.1) (Poppen, 1976);
- the shoulder, spine (Crawford, 1991; Culham, 2000; Solem-Bertoft, 1993), and lower limbs (Young, 1996) are functionally related;
- the epidemiology of shoulder disorders is related to the type of sport in which the individual takes part (Chapters 3, 5 and 16); and

Fig. 3A.1

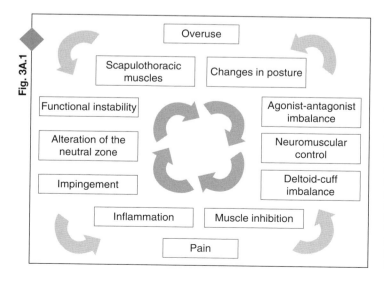

The pathogenetic cycle
The shoulder disorder may be part of a continuum leading from instability to impingement, via a cycle involving microtraumas, neuromuscular control deficit, occult subluxation or functional instability, weakness of the scapulothoracic muscles, muscle imbalance between the deltoid and rotator cuff, agonist-antagonist muscle imbalance caused by repetition of the adduction-internal rotation movement (an example of overuse), and alteration of the neutral zone.

Table 3A.1

The components of a correct diagnostic procedure for painful shoulder

The case history should include the following:
- an inventory of the patient's complaints
- how the disorder occurred
- its course over time
- factors influencing improvement and deterioration

The clinical examination starts with a basic functional examination (BFE) comprising the following:
- inspection
- general active and pain-provoking movements
- palpation
- active (movement) tests
- passive tests
- tests against resistance

Clinical decision based on the relationship between the case history and the basic functional history: one or more diagnostic hypotheses attributable to a structural or functional impairment; once a clinical decision has been made, the following may be carried out:
- an examination specific to the disorder (instability, impingement), aimed at confirming or ruling out the impairment by means of pathognomonic tests; this includes:
  — an indication for 'targeted' bioimaging
  — an interpretation of the correlation between bioimaging and clinical picture (differential diagnosis)
  — the identification of structural factors triggering or aggravating the impairment

Therapeutic clinical decisions resulting from the specific examination:
- an indication for surgery
- an indication for rehabilitative therapy; once a clinical decision has been made, the following may be carried out:
- a specific musculoskeletal examination (in manual therapy), aimed at confirming or ruling out the impairment, by means of specific manual tests. The aims of the specific musculoskeletal examination are the following:
  — identification of dysfunction at various sites: glenohumeral, acromioclavicular, scapulothoracic, sternoclavicular, cervicothoracic
  — identification of treatable aspects in the various areas according to the international classification of functioning (ICF)
- a functional sport-specific examination (Table 8.7). The aims of the functional sport-specific examination are the following:
  — identification of technical factors triggering or aggravating the impairment or disability (Chapters 3, 17)
  — a prognostic health profile (PHP) (Chapter 12)
  — identification of aspects that can be altered in the context of technique (Chapter 17)

- the forces applied to structures are related causally to the damage they cause (Wilk, 1997).

This book proposes developing a clinical rationale (Table 3A.1) starting from the case history (Wilk, 1997) and proceeding via a basic functional examination which may have content of common interest to both physiotherapists, general practitioners and specialists.

The relationship between the history and the basic functional examination may lead to a diagnostic hypothesis (Litaker, 2000), and this hypothesis may involve a structural lesion or a dysfunctional problem. The next part of the examination, therefore, involves confirming or disproving the diagnostic hypothesis by a combination of tests. If there is a suspected structural lesion, a clinical examination specific to the disorder (instability or impingement) can be carried out (Chapter 6), which may involve the use of 'targeted' bioimaging (Chapter 7). If the problem is dysfunctional,

<table>
<tr><td>

Table 3A.2

</td><td>

What is expected of the clinical examination: symptomatological difficulties in the clinical examination of an athlete with painful shoulder

- Not all the tests can be performed depending on the patient's condition
- Signs and symptoms attributable to several disorders may be found (e.g. pain)
- Objective signs not attributable to symptoms may be found (e.g. instability)
- Objective signs may not be found of symptoms reported (e.g. joint noise such as popping or grinding)
- There may be discrepancies between the imaging diagnosis and the clinical examination
- Clear symptoms of the lesions may not be found (e.g. partial lesions of the rotator cuff)

</td></tr>
</table>

a sport-specific functional examination may be carried out (Chapter 8) along with a specific musculoskeletal examination (Chapters 8 and 14).

Reaching a diagnosis should involve the identification of one or more causes of the disorder; examining the inter-relationships between disorders (Fig. 3A.1) shows that the term risk factors is preferable to aetiological factors (Chapter 4) and helps to decide whether treatment should be surgical (Section III) or rehabilitative (Section IV) (Fig. 15.2).

The risk factors can be identified by analysis of structural (predominantly anatomical) or functional aspects. Functional aspects involve biomechanics (osteokinematics, arthrokinematics), physiology (carriability of the athlete and ability to adapt to load), neuromotor aspects (proprioception, neuromuscular control), pathophysiology (tissue changes which cause stiffness or instability), and technique (athletic training, athletic actions).

To solve the problem of painful shoulder in an athlete, the clinical evaluation cannot, therefore, be separated from the rationale which determines its characteristics on an individual basis, nor can an interdisciplinary comparison be disregarded.

The major problems regarding the clinical and functional examination can be divided into observational difficulties (which are addressed in Chapters 6 and 8 and referred to in Chapter 17 as regards technique) and

symptomatological difficulties (which signs can be expected and what their significance is) (Table 3A.2).

These problems apply in addition to the current limits of validity of the tests used in the clinical examination and in the specific examination in manual therapy (Ellenbecker, 2002).

The lack of a language common to the various professionals in the worlds of medicine and sport technology is a final, but no less important, problem. The proposal made in this book, to reach points of convergence, is to use the biopsychosocial model (Chapter 12).

Promoting increased quality among medical professionals for greater efficacy of the clinical examination and interdisciplinary collaboration between the various professional figures seems to constitute a premise for the protection of the health of athletes.

Bibliography

Crawford H.J., Jull G.A., 'The influence of thoracic form and movement on range of shoulder flexion', *Physioth. Theory Practice* 9: 143–148, (1991)

Culham E., Laprade J., 'Biomechanics of the shoulder complex', In: Dvir Z. (eds.) *Clinical Biomechanics*, Churchill Livingstone, London, pp. 141–164 (2000)

Ellenbecker T.S., Bailie D.S., Mattalino A.J. et al., 'Intrarater and interrater reliability of a manual technique to assess anterior humeral head translation of the glenohumeral joint,' *J. Shoulder Elbow Surg.* 11(5): 470–475, (2002)

Jobe F.W., Pink M., 'Shoulder injuries in the athlete: the instability continuum and treatment', *J. Hand. Ther.* 4: 69–73, (1991)

Litaker D., Pioro M., El Bilbeisi H. et al., 'Returning to the bedside: using the history and physical examination to identify rotator cuff tears', *J. Am. Geriatr. Soc.* 48: 1633–1637, (2000)

Poppen N.K., Walker P.S., 'Normal and abnormal motion of the shoulder', *J Bone Joint Surg* 58A(2): 195–201, (1976)

Solem-Bertoft E., Thuomas K.A., Westerberg C.E, 'The influence of scapular retraction and protraction on the width of the subacromial space', An MRI study. *Clin Orthopaedics Related Res* 296: 99–103, (1993)

Whiting W.C., Zernicke, 'R.F. Biomechanics of musculoskeletal injury', *Human Kinetics*, pp. 177–189.

Wilk K.E., Andrews J.R., Arrigo C.A., 'The physical examination of the glenohumeral joint: emphasis on the stabilizing structures', *JOSPT* 25(6):380–389, (1997)

Young J.L., Herring S.A., Press J.M., Casazza B.A., 'The Influence of the Spine on the Shoulder in the Throwing Athlete,' *AJST* 7(1): 5–17, (1996)

SHOULDER INSTABILITY

A. Fusco
R. Zuccarino

The upper limb in human beings has undergone phylogenetic adaptations which have transformed its locomotion ability into a relational ability.

This transformation has required characteristics of stability and mobility to co-exist, and although these may appear to be opposites, they are both essential for correct shoulder joint function.

The throwing action is one of the relational activities mastered by humans during the course of their evolution, and has assisted in survival over several millennia in both defence and attack. In modern society, the throwing action predominantly occurs in play and sports.

The stability of the shoulder in such contexts seems to be a basic premise for correct shoulder function.

Since the ability of any joint to resist dislocation is in direct relation to its stability, what the shoulder gains in terms of mobility, it sacrifices in terms of stability. In contrast with many other joints of the human body, neuromuscular control, therefore, has a decisive role; the key considerations, as we have seen in Chapter 2, are the lesser importance of stabilization by the epiphyses and the relative weakness of the ligament system, particularly in the central sectors of joint movement.

The term instability, though current in the literature, appears to be difficult to define owing to the quantity of structures involved, the complexity of their interaction and the difficulty of controlling them centrally. Instability is nevertheless dealt with in the literature almost exclusively in relation to the glenohumeral joint.

The definition given by Matsen in this context is acceptable, i.e. a clinical condition in which unwanted translation of the humeral head in the glenoid compromises comfort and shoulder function (Matsen, 1991).

It is helpful from a clinical point of view to distinguish between structural and functional instability, where possible. In the first case there are objective signs that can be detected by clinical examination, which may or may not correspond to impairment or disability reported by the patient; in the second case there may or may not be signs and symptoms attributable to the impairment reported by the patient (different locations and types of pain, impaired joint mechanics, etc.).

Aetiopathogenesis

Shoulder stability depends on the efficiency of the joint, muscle and neurological stabilization mechanisms. Muscle function varies with joint position, the direction and amplitude of movement, and the extendibility of the periarticular structures (Comerford, 2001).

We have seen that the throwing action places great stress on stability. The stabilizing action by the muscles requires a capacity for precise control, and proprioception has an important role in this (Bender, 1996).

Shoulder disorders can be seen epidemiologically as a pathogenetic continuum or cycle, which can lead from instability to impingement (Jobe, 1991), involving the following: microtraumas, neuromuscular control deficit (Schenkman, 1994), occult subluxation or functional instability (Dugas, 1991; Garth Jr, 1987; Gross, 1993; Lombardo, 1977), weakness of the scapulothoracic muscles (particularly the anterior serratus) (Magarey, 2003), muscle imbalance between the deltoid and rotator cuff, agonist-antagonist muscle imbalance owing to repetition of the adduction-internal rotation

Shoulder instability

movement, and alteration of the 'neutral zone' (a concept introduced by Panjabi (1992) and revisited, in relation to the shoulder, by Hess (2000)).

The concept of a pathogenetic cycle deserves attention since it seems that it can begin from any phase (Fig. 3A.1). Some authors identify the mechanisms responsible for impingement, not only in overhead athletes but also in swimmers, as occult subluxation or functional instability (McMaster, 1986). This seems to correspond to the minor anterior glenohumeral instability syndrome which we saw in Chapter 2.

It is worth noting, for didactic purposes, some of the possible pathogenetic sequences:

— overuse may cause subacute inflammation, resulting in an increase in the volume of the periarticular tissues; this then causes a relative reduction in the subacromial space with subsequent impingement;

— overuse may cause adaptive 'shortening' of the scapulothoracic and glenohumeral motor muscles, which is compensated by overstrain of some structures or the occurrence of involuntary movements to guarantee function. Repeated movements under these conditions may cause inflammation of overstrained structures or arthrokinematic changes which may result in impingement;

— pain may cause a change in proprioception, due to the persistence of nociceptive impulses: this may result in an impaired motor response, with characteristics similar to instability;

— inadequate body and muscle training may cause early muscle fatigue, resulting in a reduction in the ability to control joint centring; this may cause functional instability and may involve microtraumas of the periarticular structures. The commonest consequences are a relative reduction in the subacromial space (or impingement, see first point) and pain, which leads to muscle inhibition (with potential instability) and compensation (with possible muscle imbalance or 'shortening');

— inappropriate athletic training, for example, repetitions of a technical action that primarily involves the agonist muscles, may lead to muscle imbalance; this may in turn involve alteration of the dynamic centring of the humeral head and defective neuromuscular control by the antagonistic muscles. The consequences may be impingement and chronic inflammation of the periarticular structures; and

— a change in posture, such as an increase in dorsal kyphosis, for example, which applies to many hypertrophic athletes, may present an obstacle to the physiological extension of the spine, impeding correct scapular sliding; the result of this is an increase in the flexion and external rotation requirement of the shoulder and subsequent stress on the anterior structures of the glenohumeral joint.

The factors influencing shoulder stability can be described and classified as structural or functional; structural factors determine the characteristics of passive mobility and simple movements, while functional factors govern dynamic mobility or complex movements. From a structural point of view, the system acts to allow the movement of the body, or of a part of the body; from the functional point of view, movement is the result of interaction between the structures that help to achieve it.

Structural factors and principles of classification

The anatomical structures responsible for shoulder stability are the joints, the periarticular connective tissue, and the muscles of the shoulder girdle joints.

All these structures are involved in and responsible for the stability of the shoulder complex and it is worth remembering that the only point of contact between the shoulder complex and the skeleton is the SC Joint.

We have seen in Chapter 1 that the conformation of the glenoid, particularly the depth of the glenoid cavity and the 'version' of the glenoid, is key to glenohumeral stability.

The most important interindividual variations in stability are the quality of the connective tissue and the biomechanical characteristics of the muscle, tendon and ligament tissue.

The concept of laxity, which is not itself a pathological condition, is associated fairly frequently but not invariably with the concept of instability; laxity corresponds to a factor of passive stabilization, i.e. the capsuloligamentous complex, whereas the concept of instability may often be secondary to functional deficits.

The concept of hypermobility should not be confused with instability for the same reason.

It seems useful, in this respect, to distinguish between end-range instability, in which capsuloligamentous stabilization has the major role, and mid-range instability, in which the slack of the capsuloligamentous complex and active (muscle) stabilization have a dominant role.

Reeves (1968) found a wide variability in the biological changes in the capsulolabral complex: the insertion of the labrum in the glenoid is slack in individuals under 25, and with advancing age it undergoes a progressive transformation with an increase in its tensile properties. The biomechanical behaviour of the capsuloligamentous structures is the opposite, becoming more prone to rupture with maturity (www. ortopedia.net). The concept of instability has only recently been associated with that of rigidity in the context of functional studies; a joint dysfunction appears, according to the author, because of an uncontrolled movement of a joint, which may occur in the presence of a more rigid, adjacent mobile segment (Sahrmann, 2002), i.e. one that is compatible with a movement restriction in one or more directions.

Minor changes in particular movements cause compensation actions around the joint. These actions allow movement in only one specific direction and may be sustained by other factors, such as changes in muscle length, force, extendibility, or activation patterns, which result from repeated movements and maintained postures (Comerford, 2001). This last aspect forms part of the functional factors of stability. Adequate elasticity of the muscle and tendon complex and appropriate extendibility of the capsuloligamentous and muscle tissues are important structural prerequisites for stability.

Athletic actions may be responsible for altering structural factors such as joint mobility and muscle extendibility. Such an alteration may occur as an adaptation of the tissues following prolonged repetitions, or as a consequence of particularly intense stresses.

Shoulder instability is, therefore, a complex issue, owing to the number of structures involved and the complexity of their interactions. It is nevertheless dealt with in the medical literature almost exclusively in relation to the glenohumeral joint.

Several structural factors have been identified as being responsible for the stability of the glenohumeral joint, i.e. the congruency of the contact surfaces of the joint, the orientation of the surfaces, negative intra-articular pressure, the containing action of the glenoid labrum, and the consistency of the capsuloligamentous sleeve. The role of these structures has been examined in Section I, Chapter 2.

There are few mentions in the literature of specific tests for the clinical examination of glenohumeral instability (Section II, Chapter 4), which is generally attributed to subluxation or dislocation.

Several authors, including Cofield and Irving (1987), while limiting their study to the glenohumeral component, nevertheless report a variety of forms ranging from a vague sense of discomfort to obvious fixed dislocation.

The difficulty in classifying shoulder instability is clear from the study referred to above, according to which 24 to 54 subdivisions are possible, representing a clinical continuum of traumatic and atraumatic forms of instability including traumatic unidirectional Bankart-lesion surgery (TUBS) and atraumatic

multidirectional bilateral rehabilitation inferior capsular shift (AMBRII) .

TUBS refers to a traumatic origin, leading to unidirectional anterior instability, resulting from a Bankart lesion; surgery is generally necessary to repair the lesion.

AMBRII is understood to denote an atraumatic origin of symptoms with multidirectional instability (MDI), maintained by bilateral glenohumeral laxity; rehabilitation has an important role in treatment.

A further term which seems of interest in this context is acquired instability by overuse syndrome (AIOS), which is typical of athletes.

The SLAP lesion concept, introduced by Snyder (1990), has a direct link with shoulder instability in athletes. The acronym stands for Superior Labrum from Anterior to Posterior, in other words lesions of the labrum and bicipital complex, which have been classified according to four levels of severity (Chapter 4). It is interesting to note, thanks to Laban (1995), that SLAP lesion is also present in 16% of rotator cuff lesions.

It is worth considering cases in which a rotator cuff lesion in its anterosuperior portion is associated with a SLAP lesion. This type of lesion has been called a superior labrum, anterior cuff lesion (SLAC) (Savoi, 2001); it occurs above all in patients involved in overhead sports and is manifested clinically with positive instability and cuff test results.

The number of acronyms related to shoulder disorders is continually increasing as epidemiological studies develop and ever more precise clinical classifications become necessary (Chapter 2): anterior labral periosteal sleeve avulsion (ALPSA) (Neviaser, 1952) refers to a Bankart lesion with associated avulsion of the periosteum; humeral avulsion of the glenohumeral ligament (HAGL) denotes a type of lesion, with avulsion, of the capsule in its anterior portion; the same situation affecting the posterior portion of the capsule is known as reverse humeral avulsion of the glenohumeral ligament (RHAGL) (Faletti, 2002).

Surgeons today seem to be leaning towards a pragmatic classification which takes a structural though simplified view of the instability in relation to the appropriateness of surgery and, where applicable, its rationale. Many modern shoulder surgery centres carry out preoperative triage, classifying the instability as unidirectional, multidirectional, painful and slack, minor due to overuse, or with laxity.

Functional factors and athletic actions

The functional factors responsible for shoulder stability are the interactions between the joint structures of the shoulder and the neuromuscular control of the muscle and joint structures which determine the spatial and temporal coordination of movement.

Athletic actions can be responsible for altering various functional factors. We shall try to identify some of these factors on an articular and neuromuscular level and then to examine the characteristics of individual athletic actions. A number of themes relating to athletic actions and their relation to athletic training will be developed in Section IV, Chapters 16 and 17.

On an articular level, the conditions should be optimal for distributing the load among the anatomical structures, thus reducing the stress on the joint; these conditions require the following:

— correct action of the spine, particularly of the cervical and thoracic section; and
— correct relative position of the various joints of the shoulder complex, for consistently correct dynamic centring of the glenohumeral joint.

Cervical and thoracic spine

The cervical and thoracic spine seems to have a key role in shoulder function. Cervical and thoracic posture does, in fact, have a considerable influence on the position and mobility of the scapula (Crawford, 1991; Culham, 2000; Solem-Bertoft, 1993). The morpho-functional characteristics of cervical and thoracic posture may cause variations in the distribution of load between the scapulothoracic joint and the glenohumeral joint (Magarey, 2003) and, according to other authors, alter the position and perception of the neutral zone of the shoulder (Panjabi, 1992).

The concept of a neutral zone refers to a mid-range position (intermediate in relation to the total amplitude of movement), in which the passive structures (capsuloligamentous complex and connective tissue) are virtually inactive. It is commonly believed to be the position closest to the ideal postural alignment.

A joint dysfunction is believed to occur owing to an uncontrolled movement of a joint, which may occur in the presence of a more rigid, adjacent mobile segment (Sahrmann, 2002). This aetiopathogenetic view refers to the concept of a neutral zone described above; in a pathological situation, impairment of this could be compatible with a movement restriction in one or more directions. It would appear acceptable to relate this phenomenon to impaired kinaesthetic perception.

Minor changes in particular movements cause compensation actions around the joint. These actions allow movement in one specific direction only and may result in repeated microtraumas and, in some cases,

macrotraumas. This condition is often present at the same time as a muscle imbalance. Impingement syndrome, which is the outcome of this situation, will be described in the following chapter.

As regards the role of the spine in throwing, various authors including Pappas (1985) suggest that it is impossible for the upper limb, at the level of the shoulder only, to generate the force necessary for the performances we have come to expect from athletes. The spine is a rotatory component in the kinetic chain, and it has the task of connecting the upper and lower limbs. It is a generator of force capable of accelerating the arm and a reducer of force capable of attenuating the forces that act on the glenohumeral joint during throwing; in addition, cervical and thoracic rotation and tilt facilitate the visual acquisition of the athlete's objective. Reduced extendibility of the hip muscles and weakness of the muscles that constitute the insertion of the thoracolumbar fascia have important effects on spinal function, and this increases the stress on the glenohumeral joint and on the rotator cuff.

A prevention programme for the shoulder should therefore include evaluation and an exercise routine for the lumbar, thoracic and cervical spine (Young, 1996).

Relative position of the joints and dynamic centring of the glenohumeral joint

Biomechanics suggest that the muscle stabilization of the glenohumeral joint and the scapulothoracic complex is obtained when the rotation moment is least; this means that control of stability can be obtained only with minimal muscle force, i.e. with a correct relative position of the various joints of the shoulder complex (sternoclavicular, acromioclavicular, cervical and thoracic spine, dorsal, and dorsolumbar).

At the neuromuscular level, the sensory afferences (particularly correct kinaesthetic, bathyaesthetic and baraesthetic perception) all contribute to the database used to construct an adequate motor response which, in turn, cannot exclude stabilization of the proximal structures of the body. The development of this mechanism, instant by instant, allows continual adjustment of control to achieve the high quality performance of an action in the most ergonomic manner; these conditions require the following:

— correct stabilization of the proximal structures;
— correct spatial recruitment of the muscle chains, which involves appropriate selection of agonistic muscles and relaxation of muscles not involved in

the action (distribution of tasks between muscles assigned to stabilizing and execution);
— correct temporal recruitment of the muscle chains (proximodistal or centrifugal sequence); and
— selection of agonistic muscles and correct balance between the agonistic and antagonistic muscles of the athletic action (fine and continual adjustment of movement variables).

Stabilization

Any impairment of the dynamic stabilization system seems to have major repercussions on the shoulder complex. The rotator cuff appears to have a deep stabilization role with regard to the glenohumeral joint, similar to the role of the transverse abdominal muscle with regard to the lumbar and pelvic complex, and the role of the oblique vastus medialis with regard to the knee.

The success of muscles in stabilizing the shoulder does not depend on the absolute force that muscles are capable of providing, but on whether the direction of the result of their action is congruent with the dynamic centring of the humeral head, known as effective force. The effective force of the rotator cuff is greater than that of the pectoralis major and the latissimus dorsi, which have a greater absolute force and are rotators in the late cocking position (Section I, Chapter 2).

It may be useful, from a didactic point of view, to report a recently proposed classification of the muscle subsystems, which seeks to go beyond the clinical limits of the divisions between local and global muscles and between stabilizer and motor muscles. The interaction between these two concepts produces an acceptable functional classification model (Comerford, 2001).

Local (primary or deep) stabilizers have the role of maintaining continual low intensity activity in all the positions in the ROM and in all directions of movement. It would seem that this activity increases segmental muscle stiffness, and is capable of resisting excessive physiological movements, particularly in the neutral zone. These stabilizers often act in advance of the load or the movement, to protect the joint.

The global (secondary or movement) stabilizers have the role of generating force and achieving eccentric control of the internal and external ROM (smaller or larger than the ROM according to the resting length of the muscles). To do this they must be capable of actively shortening within the entire arc of physiological movement. They should also be capable of eccentrically controlling or decelerating the rotator impulses occurring in the shoulder.

The global mobilizers (tertiary or load stabilizers) are the principal generators of movement force. They are biomechanically designed to produce rapid, wide-amplitude movements. These muscles are particularly efficient in the sagittal plane, but they are unable to contribute to rotator or segmental control. The stabilization role of these muscles is expressed in the presence of severe stresses or loads, when there is a biomechanical disadvantage, or when absorbing the countershocks of ballistic actions. These muscles must maintain adequate extendibility to allow the joint to move through the whole physiological and accessory (translation) range.

Spatial recruitment (stabilizer muscles and effector muscles)

Optimization of the muscle drive is more important than the amount of force that the muscles manage to recruit; the 'principle of the chronological coordination of impulses' (Hochmut, 1984 quoted in *Various Authors*, 1996) explains that it is only through the dynamic work of major muscle chains and the participation of all the joints (either working or fixed) that substantial quantities of impulse are obtained.

It is clear from the observation of technical actions by occasional athletes or beginners that the distal muscles are mainly used at the expense of the proximal muscles and the timing in the activation sequence of the muscle chains is incorrect.

There is evidence of a disturbance of stabilizer muscle function when pain is present. The anterior serratus and the lower trapezius are in fact believed to be inhibited in individuals with painful shoulder. This inhibition is manifested, first and foremost, as a non-specific response to any form of painful shoulder, involving disorganization of the normal activation or muscle recruitment pattern, and a reduced ability to produce force to stabilize the shoulder (Kibler, 1998). Kibler has described this phenomenon as 'scapular dyskinesia'.

Temporal (proximal-distal) recruitment

Professional throwers produce at least half the force from the lower part of the body, thus reducing the burden on the shoulder. The throwing action is a slingshot movement in which the acceleration generated in the proximal part of the body is transmitted in sequence to successive distal joints (Toyoshima, 1974).

The muscle actions that produce shoulder movements are based on a kinetic chain from the lower limbs and spine to the fingers (Kibler, 1991), with a

Shoulder instability

substantial contribution made by the lumbar and pelvic complex. Research into pelvic stability has demonstrated that shoulder movement is preceded by stabilizer muscle activity in the pelvic region (Hodges, 1996). The timing of the activation pattern may be altered, with the stabilizer muscles such as the cuff and the long head of the biceps acting later than the deltopectoral group, for example, (David, 2000).

Balancing the agonistic and antagonistic muscles in athletic actions

One of the aspects common to many sports is believed to be the high level of repetition of the adduction-internal rotation movement of the upper limb, regardless of the degree of abduction of the arm used (above or below 90°), the type of muscle contraction required by the technical action (concentric, eccentric, etc.), or the method of muscle contraction required (cyclic, explosive, etc.) (Berlusconi, 1990; Colonna, Magnani, 1992; Colonna, 1992; Warner, 1990). Some of the unique features peculiar to various athletic actions may have a variable influence on the occurrence of chronic shoulder disorders. The action of throwing is, however, believed to subject some of the periarticular structures to a specific risk of overuse.

The action of throwing is, in fact, particularly demanding as regards stability.

The use of different methods of muscle contraction, although the epidemiological influence of this has not yet been demonstrated, may have a role in muscle balance and, as we shall see, in the specific nature of training.

The agonistic muscles in throwing act mainly in a plyometric manner (pre-stretch followed by shortening); the antagonistic muscles act principally in an eccentric manner; this is the case particularly when the technical action is developed and correct.

The continual, fine adjustment of the variables of the movement is an important requirement for performing a correct technical action, completed, in turn, by the correct sharing of the workloads along all the structures involved in the kinetic chain. This results, otherwise, in exposure to microtrauma.

Repeated microtrauma is considered the principal mechanism responsible for overuse; we shall return to this concept in Chapter 16, along with the concept of overtraining.

The importance of analysing the technical action as part of the clinical examination thus becomes clear in order to identify any risk factors (or factors predisposing to injury) in this context.

A classification of sports disciplines and the types of equipment used is given in Chapter 16.

Athletic actions below 90° of abduction

Athletic actions which are performed mostly below 90° of abduction of the humerus have a low risk of injury from the point of view of joint biomechanics. The commonest disciplines of this type are golf, rowing, canoeing, sailing and Olympic windsurfing.

Factors which can potentially predispose towards overuse are:
— the large number of repeated actions typical of training in cyclic disciplines such as canoeing and rowing, which are believed to result in difficulty in neuromuscular control. The consequences could be instability, impingement, and muscle imbalance; and
— intrinsic factors such as age, which is higher on average in some sports such as golf, in which many former high-level athletes from other disciplines like to seek success; the incidence of impingement syndrome is higher, according to the literature (Chapter 5).

Athletic actions above 90° of abduction (overhead)

The epidemiological differences in overhead sports (Chapter 5) seem to suggest that functional and technical factors are important.

Functional factors

Functional factors include: the predominant method of muscle contraction and the muscle force required, the type of kinetic chain, and the antagonistic muscle action.

Predominant method of muscle contraction and muscle force required Overhead sports disciplines may involve technical actions characterized by concentric, eccentric or plyometric muscle contraction. Concentric contraction consists, in fact, of alternate concentric and eccentric contractions, as occurs in basketball, swimming or climbing.

The muscle force required (organic and muscular aspect) depends largely on the weight of the projectile which will influence the amount of acceleration the athlete can apply to it.

The predominant use of fast force, pure force and explosive force can be identified in the sports of basketball, shot put and volleyball, respectively.

Antagonistic muscle action is important in some technical actions, in other words a braking effect is necessary immediately following the throw, described as follow-through by US authors.

This action is generally performed with eccentric muscle contraction and is somewhat dependent on the characteristics of the projectile (technical aspects), which in turn influence the velocity or speed that the athlete can apply to it.

Plyometric contraction requires a pre-stretch cycle followed by shortening.

The technical actions of throwing or ballistic sports employ plyometric muscle contraction to obtain the desired effect and eccentric muscle contraction is used to regulate the action.

Type of kinetic chain

The kinetic chain may be open or closed; an open kinetic chain (OKC) involves the upper limb being free from limitations due to hanging or points of support. In the opposite case, such as in locomotion with four points of support or hanging from a hand-hold, this is a closed kinetic chain (CKC); in fact, the criteria apply strictly only when the limb is supported. One of the commonest sports disciplines with an OKC is swimming, while those with CKCs include competitive gymnastics and sports climbing.

Actions with CKCs are believed to favour glenohumeral joint stability and consequently have a lower incidence of injury compared to open chain actions. However, if the upper limb is used for locomotion-support, the substantial load in terms of weight on the glenohumeral joint must be taken into consideration, as must the caudocranial direction in which the load is applied; as shown in Chapter 4, this may result in subacromial impingement. An example of this occurs in gymnastics.

Technical factors

Characteristics of the projectile (weight, volume, shape)

The characteristics of the projectile (weight, volume, and shape) are variable depending on the sports in question.

The use of projectiles of moderate weight and small volume, such as a baseball, or of an aerodynamic shape, such as a javelin, requires the competitive 'thrower' to use predominantly fast or explosive force, which needs a significant antagonistic action.

As the weight of the projectile increases, the muscle force required by the athlete will be greater, and plyometric muscle contraction will be required, both of which have been addressed in the previous paragraph. The correct method of production of force, in turn, requires adequate joint mobility and appropriate temporospatial construction of the action, and this will be dealt with in Chapter 17.

Use of equipment (propulsion or impulsion)

The use in sports of propulsion equipment does not seem to be of particular interest as regards shoulder disorders; windsurfing perhaps requires further attention as regards overuse disorders, although recent developments in technique and equipment seem to be in line with ergonomic criteria.

The use of impulsion equipment (e.g. racquets), however, causes an increase in the inertial force moment, increasing the stresses on the stabilizing structures of the shoulder. Having said that, it is worth noting the importance of adequate joint mobility, muscle elasticity, coordinated agonistic action and effective antagonistic action.

Propulsion and impulsion equipment are defined in Section IV, Chapter 16.

Limitations imposed by the rules

The rules of some sports create conditions that can increase the risk of shoulder injury for athletes.

Such conditions may be related to the method of interaction between the athlete and others involved in the activity or between the athlete and the environment in which the sport is performed.

Conditions related to human interactions, which are important as regards epidemiological incidence, include pitting opponents against one another in team and combat sports. These conditions nevertheless seem to have a greater influence on the incidence of acute disorders than on the incidence of overuse or chronic disorders.

Conditions related to the environment include the characteristics and method of use of the support base; the support base both limits and supports the kinetic chain. These conditions may be important in increasing the risk of injury due to overuse.

In volleyball, for example, the presence of the net in front of the attacker, together with rule that the attacker may not touch the net during the action, requires a major antagonistic muscle action to prevent contact with the net. Although the attacking action occurs in the air, it helps achieve balance between the agonistic and antagonistic action; this could explain the lower epidemiological incidence observed in this overhead sport compared to other similar sports, such as handball or water polo, in which the incidence of injury is higher.

Ballistic sports and conditions prejudicial to stability

Some sports involve functional and technical conditions that make shoulder stability difficult. Such conditions are assumed to represent an increase in the pathogenetic risk factor.

We have seen that the disciplines mostly involved in disorders are ballistic sports (i.e. those involving a throwing action). It may be useful to clarify the correlation between factors influencing stability, the potential increase in the risk of injury and several sports, by way of illustration.

Functional factors

Predominant method of muscle contraction and muscle force required Plyometric muscle contraction seems to have greater pathogenetic influence owing to the greater stress on the shoulder and to the use of angular velocities which seem to be beyond neuromuscular control.

The muscle force required (organic and muscular aspect) depends to a large extent on the weight of the projectile. Sports which predominantly require an explosive force seem to involve a greater risk than those which predominantly use other types of contraction.

Technical actions with these characteristics include the attack in volleyball.

Antagonistic muscle action Correct balance and coordination between stabilizer muscles and motor or agonistic effectors, therefore, seem to be able to influence the incidence of injury and, as we shall see, the rehabilitation and prevention programme.

Muscle action is, in turn, influenced by the characteristics of the projectile (technological aspects), which thus determine the velocity or speed the athlete can apply to it.

Projectiles which are small in size or aerodynamic in shape allow greater acceleration and consequently require a more intense antagonistic action. This action is manifested as eccentric muscle contraction, and this represents a greater risk factor than concentric contraction.

These conditions occur during throwing a javelin or a baseball, for example.

Type of kinetic chain All overhead throwing activities use the OKC, which constitutes a greater risk to stability than the CKC.

Technical factors

Characteristics of the projectile (weight, volume, shape) Sports which use projectiles of moderate weight and small volume, such as a baseball, or with an aerodynamic shape, such as a javelin, involve the thrower reaching angular velocity values in the shoulder that are so high that they are theoretically incompatible with its stability. The mechanisms that are capable of limiting this incompatibility are the correct production of force and appropriate antagonistic muscle action.

Consequently, the more the arm can be accelerated due to the projectile's characteristics, the greater the corresponding risk factor seems to be.

Use of equipment It seems clear from the above that the use of impulsion equipment in overhead sports may increase the inertial force moment, causing an increase in the stresses imposed on the stabilizing structures of the shoulder. An example of an overhead action performed with impulsion equipment is the serve in tennis.

It should be noted that the technical characteristics of the equipment may, in turn, have a variable influence on the incidence of injury. The material of which the racquet is constructed, the material used for the strings and the tension of the strings are important variables worthy of multidisciplinary study.

Limitations imposed by the rules (environmental and human) The rules of the throwing disciplines in track and field athletics state that the athlete may not step outside the throwing area even after taking the throw; this requires a number of technical adaptations, such as 'rotary' techniques in the shot put and special 'pacing' in the javelin. The difficulties athletes encounter in the javelin to reconcile the maximum expression of explosive force with the stabilization of the whole body, and consequently the shoulder, are evident (Hodges, 1997).

In handball, the elevated throw, which is the conclusion in the majority of moves, takes place in the air, which makes it relatively difficult to stabilize the body and, as a result, the shoulder.

In water polo, the aquatic environment in which the sport is played causes difficulties that are apparently similar to those of the elevated throw in handball. The situation for the water polo player who is aiming at the goal is, in fact, made still more difficult by the need for the lower limbs, and the opposite arm to the shooting arm, to support the body and to stay afloat at the same time.

The problem lies in the search for the ideal position to cock the throw, depending on the playing action. Bearing in mind that the throw is hampered by the opponents, sometimes by placing their own upper limb in the throwing trajectory, sometimes with physical contact, the problem of stabilizing the shoulder becomes apparent: if the athlete wants to 'see' more space in the opponents' goal, the action will require height, i.e. leaving the water, losing stability and power.

Some sports require athletic performances which place the stability of the shoulder at particular risk owing to their intensity or duration, or to the presence of external variables. The rules and the performance context can sometimes help athletes to remain in correct articular balance, such as in the example described of the attack in volleyball. More often, however, they prove a further hindrance. Furthermore, in many sports training conditions and intensity may worsen a situation that is already critical (Section IV, Chapter 16).

The presence of one or more biomechanical aspects or techniques that may hinder shoulder stability may reasonably be considered a risk factor. Some sports involve just one of these factors, while others have several. Water polo is one of the sports which involves more than one risk factor; it combines instability of the support base with an overhead technique, performed with a relatively light projectile, with a possible disturbance of body stability caused by the action of the defender.

We have tried to illustrate the level of risk involved in some popular well-known sports: the risk is represented in the positive quadrant of the cartesian axes, increasing with one or more of the aspects mentioned (Fig. 3.1).

Conclusions

Shoulder instability, therefore, involves a complex, though not exhaustive, classification.

Overhead actions, repeated several times in the course of athletic activities, may be responsible for changes in structural factors, such as joint mobility and muscle extendibility, and in various functional factors.

Furthermore, the proposed approach for classifying shoulder problems in athletes requires an analysis of the characteristics of the individual as well as gross pathological observations.

It has been difficult to date to identify satisfactory therapeutic and prophylactic responses because studies on this subject have too often used too small a population.

Sometimes the approach is limited by the point of view which, as mentioned previously, relates almost exclusively to the glenohumeral joint; other studies fail to adequately consider structural and functional aspects, the most important of which is neuromuscular control. Studies may also focus either on evident mechanical pathological aspects, without sufficiently considering the cause of the problem, or on aspects of impairment, failing to take due account of the various psychosocial and participatory components, which are of paramount importance to athletes.

The various ways of addressing the problem can lead to classifications and pragmatic solutions which nevertheless require further interactive and integrational comparisons.
— The point of view of the surgeon currently seems directed at a comprehensive structural vision of the instability of the structure or structures susceptible to repair, i.e. unidirectional or multidirectional instability, painful slack instability, minor instability due to overuse, or instability with laxity.
— The point of view of other health workers, such as physiotherapists, is directed at a functional vision of shoulder disorders within a pathogenetic sequence or cycle leading from instability to impingement (or vice-versa) (Jobe, 1991), involving microtraumas, neuromuscular control deficit (Schenkman, 1994), occult subluxation or functional instability, weakness of the proximal muscles (Magarey, 2003), muscle imbalance between the deltoid and rotator cuff, agonist-antagonist muscle imbalance, and alteration of the 'neutral zone' (Panjabi, 1992; Hess, 2000).

What is of particular interest to our subject is that this dysfunctional cycle may start in any phase.

It is, therefore, logical to propose the following:
— there are close functional relations between the various components of the shoulder complex (sternoclavicular, scapulothoracic, acromioclavicular, glenohumeral, cervical and thoracic posture): these functional relations probably extend to most of the musculoskeletal system;
— there are links between various shoulder disorders in which instability forms part of an aetiopathogenetic continuum;

Shoulder instability

Fig. 3.1

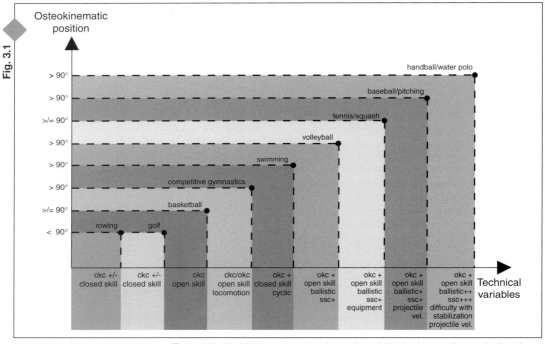

Level of risk of injury in athletic actions. The technical variables are plotted on the x-axis and the shoulder position predominantly used in each discipline on the y-axis.

The risk factor is minimal in actions with a CKC, with cyclic movements and with the arm abducted below 90°.

$<90°$ = the predominant athletic action occurs in an arm position with an angle of abduction of less than ninety degrees;

$>/= 90°$ = the predominant athletic action occurs in an arm position with an angle of abduction of ninety degrees or more;

$>90°$ = the predominant athletic action occurs in an arm position with an angle of abduction of more than ninety degrees (overhead);

CKC +/− = the predominant athletic action involves a CKC, but without support;

CKC = the predominant athletic action involves a CKC;

OKC+ = the predominant athletic action involves an OKC, even for the lower limbs;

closed skill = the athletic action occurs according to a repetitive rhythm;

open skill = the athletic action occurs according to a variable rhythm influenced by the context;

cyclic = the athletic action occurs according to a cyclic rhythm;

ballistic = the predominant athletic action is similar to throwing;

ballistic+ = the predominant athletic action is a type of throwing;

equipment = the predominant athletic action is similar to throwing and involves equipment which enhances the 'arm';

SSC = (stretch-shortening contraction) the athletic action requires plyometric muscle contraction;

SSC+ ++ +++ = the athletic action requires a plyometric muscle contraction substantially (+), predominantly (++), or almost exclusively (+++);

projectile vel. = the velocity of the projectile has a significant role in the athletic action, owing to its small size or weight;

difficulty with stabilization = the athletic action occurs in a context in which stabilizing the body is difficult.

— shoulder instability, in the form of impairment, seems to concern the glenohumeral joint more frequently, although evidence continues to emerge regarding the importance of the proximal stability of this joint (scapulothoracovertebral) as a requirement for distal (glenohumeral) stability;

— the throwing action (overhead sports) may be a triggering or worsening factor for shoulder disorders, consequently technical actions should be monitored and performed preferably in interdisciplinary sessions (technicians, sport injury doctors, and physiotherapists);

— neuromuscular control has a key role in the correct function of the shoulder complex; it can easily be disturbed, even in the absence of early symptoms;

— dealing with shoulder instability requires analysis of the athlete at various levels, in order to evaluate the influence of sociocultural and participatory aspects; the biopsychosocial model seems preferable to many health professionals; and

— using a correct clinical rationale and bearing in mind the factors predisposing to injury specific to overhead actions can help to identify the role of the various structural and functional components in shoulder disorders in athletes.

Acknowledgements

We are indebted to the following for their contributions to this chapter: Christine Grillet, independent professional, Toulouse (FRA), Tutor at Università degli Studi di Genova, Master of Rehabilitation of Musculoskeletal Disorders.

Francesca Coaro, independent professional, Vicenza, Università degli Studi di Genova, Master of Rehabilitation of Musculoskeletal Disorders.

Bibliography

Bender M., 'Case study,' *Manual Therapy* 2: 107–110, (1996)

Berlusconi M., 'La spalla dolorosa del nuotatore: inquadramento epidemiologico, clinico e strumentale,' *Proceedings XVI ANAN Convention*, Rapallo, pp. 29–37, (1990)

Cofield R.H., Irving J.F., 'Evaluation and classification of shoulder instability: With special reference to examination under anaesthesia,' *Clin Orthop Rel Res* 223: 32–43, (1987)

Colonna S., 'La valutazione isocinetica della spalla negli sport: pallavolo, pallanuoto, nuoto', In: Colonna S., Martelli G. (eds.), *Isocinetica* 91. Ghedini, Milan, pp. 93–98, (1992)

Colonna S., Magnani M., Guolo F. et al., 'Valutazione isocinetica della spalla in atleti affetti da sindrome da conflitto', In Colonna S., Martelli G. (eds.), *Isocinetica* 91. Ghedini, Milan, pp. 165–170, (1992)

Comerford M.J., Mottram S.L., 'Functional stability retraining: principles and strategies for managing mechanical dysfunction,' *Manual Ther* 6: 3–14, (2001)

Comerford M.J., Mottram S.L., 'Movement and stability dysfunction – Contemporary developments,' *Manual Ther* 6: 15–26, (2001)

Crawford H.J., Jull G.A., 'The influence of thoracic form and movement on range of shoulder flexion', *Physiotherapy, Theor. Practice* 9: 143–148, (1991)

Culham E., Laprade J., 'Biomechanics of the shoulder complex', In: DVIR Z. (ed.), *Clinical Biomechanics*, Churchill Livingstone, London, pp. 141–164, (2000)

David G., Margarey M., Jones M. et al., 'EMG and strength correlates of selected shoulder muscle during rotation of the glenohumeral joint', *J Clin Biomechanics* 2: 95–102, (2000)

Dugas RW , 'Anterior shoulder subluxation in the throwing athlete', *Orthopaedics* 14: 93–95, (1991)

Faletti C., Castagna A. Spalla, UTET, Milan, pp. 86–101 (reserved non-commercial edition), (2002)

Garth W.P. JR, Allman F.L., Armstrong W.S., 'Occult anterior subluxations of the shoulder in noncontact sports', *Am J Sports Med* 15: 579–585, (1987)

Gross M.L., Brenner S.L., Esformes I., Sonzogni, 'J.J. Anterior shoulder instability in weight lifters', *Am J Sports Med* 21: 599–603, (1993)

Hess S.A., 'Functional stability of the glenohumeral joint', *Manual Ther*, 5(2): 63–71, (2000)

Hodges P., Richardson C., 'Inefficient muscular stabilization of the lumbar spine associated with low back pain. A motor control evaluation of transversus abdominis', *Spine* 21(22): 2640–2650, (1996)

Hodges P.W., Richardson C.A., 'Feedforward contraction of transversus abdominis is not influenced by the direction of arm movement', *Exper Brain Res* 114: 362–370, (1997)

Jobe F.W., Pink M, 'Shoulder injuries in the athlete: the instability continuum and treatment', *J Hand Ther* 4: 69–73, (1991)

Kibler W.B., 'The role of the scapula in the overhead throwing motion', *Am Contemp Orthop* 22: 525–532, (1991)

Kibler W.B., 'The role of the scapula in athletic shoulder function', *Am J Sport Med* 26(2): 325–339, (1998)

Laban M.M., Gurin T.L., Maltese J.T., 'Slip of the lip tears of the superior glenoid labrum anterior to posterior (SLAP) syndrome: a report of four cases', *Am J Phys Med Rehabil* 74: 448–452, (1995)

Lombardo S.J., Jobe F.W., Kerlan R.K., Carter V.S., Shields C.L. JR., 'Posterior shoulder lesions in throwing athletes', *Am J Sports Med* 5: 106–110, (1977)

Magarey M.E., Jones M.A., 'Dynamic evaluation and early management of altered motor control around the shoulder complex', *Manual Ther* 8(4):195–206, (2003)

Matsen F.A. III, Harryman D.T., Sidles J.A., 'Mechanics of glenohumeral instability', *Clin Sports Med* 10: 783–788, (1991)

McMaster W.C., 'Anterior glenoid labrum damage: A painful lesion in swimmers', *Am J Sports Med* 14: 383–387, (1986)

Neviaser J.S., 'The pathologic anatomy of degenerative shoulder lesions', *Med Ann Dist Columbia* 21(4): 194–195, (1952)

Panjabi M., 'The stabilisation system of the spine. Part II. Neutral zone and instability hypothesis', *J Spinal disorders* 5(4): 390–397, (1992)

Pappas A.M., Zawacki R.M., McCarthy C.F., 'Rehabilitation of the pitching shoulder', *Am J Sports Med* 13: 223–235, (1985)

Reeves B., 'Experiments on tensile strength of the anterior capsular structures of the shoulder in man', *J Bone Joint Surg* 50(B): 858–865, (1968)

Sahrmann S.A., 'Diagnosis and treatment of movement impairment syndromes', Mosby, Philadelphia (2002)

Savoi F.H. III, Field L.D., Atchinson S., 'Anterior superior instability with rotator cuff tearing: SLAC-lesion', *Orthop Clin North Am* 32(3): 457–461, (2001)

Schenkman M., Rugo De Cartaya V., 'Kinesiology of the shoulder complex,' In: Andrews J.R., Wilk K.E. (eds.),

The Athlete's Shoulder, Churchill Livingstone, New York, Ch 2: pp 15–33, (1994)

Snyder S.J., Karzel R.P., Del Pizzo W. et al., 'SLAP-lesions of the shoulder', *Arthroscopy* 6: 274–279, (1990)

Solem-bertoft E., Thuomas K.A., Westerberg C.E., 'The influence of scapular retraction and protraction on the width of the subacromial space', An MRI study. *Clin Orthopaedics Related Res* 296: 99–103, (1993)

Toyoshima S., Hosikikawa T., Miyashita M. et al., 'Contribution of the body parts to throwing performance', In: Nelson R.C., Morehouse C.A. (eds.), *Biomechanics* IV. University Park Press, Baltimore, p. 169, (1974)

Various Authors, 'Corso per allenatori di pallanuoto di I livello', I, FIN Rome, pp. 148–149 (1996)

Warner J.J., Micheli L.J., Arslanian L.E. et al., 'Patterns of flexibility, laxity, and strength in normal shoulder and shoulder with instability and impingement', *AJSM* 21: 366–375, (1990)

Young J.L., Herring S.A., Press J.M., Casazza B.A., 'The Influence of the Spine on the Shoulder in the Throwing Athlete', *AJST* 7(1): 5–17, (1996)

www.ortopedia.net (ADRIANI E)

CHAPTER 4

IMPINGEMENT SYNDROMES: DEFINITION AND CLASSIFICATION

F. Odella
L. Pierannunzii
S. Odella

Most patients who complain of painful shoulder are currently diagnosed with impingement syndrome; this definition suggests a spectrum of anatomical and clinical alterations of the rotator cuff and subacromiodeltoid bursa, attributable to impingement between the humeral head and an equally rigid structure, consisting of the coracoacromial arch or, in specific cases, the posterosuperior rim of the glenoid. The tendon and bursa complex between the impinging bone components is progressively worn away, causing the characteristic pain and, in addition, in the event of tendon rupture, significant loss of function.

Although this aetiopathogenetic hypothesis currently has the most support, different pathophysiological interpretations have been suggested in the past. We owe to Duplay (1872) the definition of scapulohumeral periarthritis, still commonly though incorrectly used today, and used by this author to refer to post-traumatic pain. This original name had the merit of having identified the site of the pathological process, not in the scapulohumeral joint, but in the surrounding soft tissues. Duplay, however, specifically attributed the cause of the inflammation to alterations of the subacromiodeltoid bursa.

This hypothesis was initially confirmed by the first X-rays which showed calcifications, which Stieda (1908) regarded as intrabursal, in the gap between the humeral head and the acromiocoracoid arch; this gave rise to the concept of calcific bursitis. Scapulohumeral periarthritis and calcific bursitis soon became synonyms.

The first to focus attention on the supraspinatus tendon, separating it partly from the overlying bursa, was the US author Codman in the 1930s (1934). During the same period, Meyer (1931) had hypothesized that tendon ruptures in this area were attributable to friction of the rotator cuff against the overlying acromial process, thus anticipating the concept of impingement. Wrede (1912) had previously demonstrated the intratendon, rather than intrabursal, location of calcifications made visible by the advent of radiological diagnosis, thus signalling the decline of the concept of calcific bursitis.

We owe to Neer (1972) the modern definition of impingement syndrome, which contains the notion of microtraumatic mechanical pathogenesis.

The recognition by the same author of the existence of a continuum ranging from occasional painful shoulder in the young to massive rotator cuff ruptures in more elderly patients was subsequently illuminating.

Neer, therefore, proposed the following anatomical and clinical staging for impingement syndrome:
— *Stage I*: reversible oedematous and haemorrhagic alterations of the tendon and bursa complex, attributable to acute inflammation, produce pain after fatigue of the shoulder which disappears spontaneously with rest. Patients are under 25 years old on average;
— *Stage II*: chronic tendinitis, with possible intratendon and fibrous calcifications of the subacromiodeltoid bursa, causes pain when elevating the limb in patients usually aged between 25 and 40 years; and
— *Stage III*: partial or complete tendon rupture complicates the previous picture, causing fairly severe loss of function, typically in patients over the age of 40.

Impingement syndromes: definition and classification

The site of this type of rupture, when identified, is fairly constant and Codman had located it precisely in the supraspinatus tendon in 1934, approximately 1 cm from the insertion in the greater tuberosity, defining this site as the critical zone. This region is, in fact, the most affected by impingement between the acromion and the trochanter of the humerus, owing to its anatomical location.

Alternative hypotheses have been proposed to explain this preferential location, the most probable of which is clearly that of Lindblom in 1939, who suggested deficient vascular supply to the tendon close to its insertion. This hypothesis was, however, not confirmed by subsequent studies (Iannotti, 1989). After the theory of a microcirculatory defect on an anatomical basis was abandoned, there remained the possibility that functional occlusion of the vessels normally represented could contribute to the pathogenesis of the tendon lesion; either the tension of the tendon in adduction movements (Rathbun, 1970) or its compression against the coracoacromial arch in elevation movements (Sigholm, 1988) could 'squeeze' the intratendon vessels, thus producing potentially damaging recurrent ischaemia.

Aetiopathogenesis

It is difficult to attribute impingement syndrome to a clearly identified aetiological factor. More frequently it is merely possible to demonstrate a series of factors which, if considered individually, appear insufficient to account for the symptoms. For example, there are individuals who, although they have a 'hooked' acromion, i.e. one that protrudes towards the underlying supraspinatus outlet, have no symptoms at all. We can hypothesize, but this is a mere supposition, that if these individuals acquire further risk factors over the course of their lives, in addition to that already mentioned (such as working with arms raised, glenohumeral instability, etc.), they might develop shoulder pain more readily than individuals with a flat acromion with a more advantageous anatomical substrate.

Impingement is, in this respect, a multifactorial disorder in which only the synergic action of various risk factors can push the individual over the threshold of clinical symptoms.

It is consequently more correct to speak of risk factors than of aetiological factors.

The risk factors can, in turn, be divided into structural and functional factors. In the former the aetiopathogenetic trigger lies in dysmorphism of the anatomical structures involved; in the latter it lies, by contrast, in impaired function which is sometimes isolated and sometimes associated with an organic lesion (Table 4.I).

Table 4.1

Structural and functional factors in impingement syndromes.

Structural factors
- Acromion
- Coracoacromial ligament
- Coracoid
- AC joint
- Humerus
- Subacromiodeltoid bursa
- Rotator cuff

Functional factors
- Deficit of the depression mechanism of the humeral head
- Weight-bearing shoulder
- Scapular anomalies owing to position and mobility
- Posterior capsule rigidity
- Instability

Structural factors

Anatomical alterations can affect all the components of the coracoacromial arch (acromion, AC joint, coracoacromial ligament, and coracoid), the proximal epiphysis of the humerus or the contents of the space between them (bursa and rotator cuff). Alterations of the humerus and arch act by reducing the gap available for the soft tissues, known as the supraspinatus outlet. The resulting impingement will, therefore, be defined as outlet impingement. Alterations of the soft tissues here will, however, result in thickening and then in an increase in the pressure inside this space, which is unable to expand because it is delimited by bone surfaces. This second type of impingement is, therefore, termed non-outlet impingement.

Acromion

The acromion was suspected by Hamilton as early as 1875 of causing painful shoulder conditions. Neer (1972) subsequently demonstrated the possible role of alterations of the shape and slope of the acromial process, in particular its anteroinferior portion, thus accounting for the efficacy of anterior acromioplasty which this author proposed and which is still performed successfully today.

Hyperostosis, which is frequent around the insertion of the coracoacromial ligament in the direction of the underlying bursa, contributes to impingement, but is almost certainly not the primary cause. It can probably be interpreted as a reactive phenomenon caused by mechanical irritation of the acromion, related in particular to the traction exerted by the coracoacromial ligament, in which context these bone spicules often develop. It is not easy to understand why a similar enthesopathy does not also affect the coracoid insertion of the ligament, but the justification offered by Edelson and Taitz (1992) is, in our opinion, feasible; these authors maintain that the triangular shape of the ligament, with a broad area of attachment to the coracoid and a minimal area of attachment to the acromion, disperses the tension on the coracoid side and concentrates it on the acromial side.

Acromial morphology is, however, a congenital factor, except for rare dysmorphisms due to poor post-traumatic consolidation. From studies on the anatomy table of 139 shoulders, Bigliani (1986) identified three clearly-defined acromial morphotypes: flat or type I, curved or type II, and 'hooked' or type III (Fig. 4.1).

In the population examined by Bigliani, 17% were type I, 43% type II, and 40% type III.

Although a type III acromion is not sufficient to cause an impingement syndrome, it is understandable why this may constitute a predisposing factor. This morphotype is, in fact, significantly associated with complete rotator cuff ruptures in the study mentioned above.

A subsequent study (Morrison, 1987) found, based on radiographic projections for the study of the supraspinatus outlet, that 80% of shoulders with tendon rupture had a type III acromion, a percentage well above that in the general population.

Besides the profile of the acromial process, it is important to note its slope, defined as the angle, open anteriorly and lying in a vertical plane perpendicular to the scapular plane, between the acromion and the horizontal axis (Fig. 4.2). A correct lateral projection of the scapula allows this angle to be measured sufficiently precisely. It has, in fact, been observed that the more horizontal the acromion, the more likely impingement is. A post-mortem study has shown that acromions with a slope of more than 41° do not have degenerative alterations suggesting impingement, while 75% of acromial processes with these alterations have a slope of 35° or less (Edelson, 1992).

The thickness of the acromion has also been analysed, in addition to the profile and slope. Wuh and Snyder (1992/3) proposed measuring this thickness at the border between the middle third and the anterior third of the process, and thus identified three categories: type A, with a thickness of less than 8 mm; type B, with a thickness of between 8 and 12 mm; and type C, with a thickness of more than 12 mm. The value of this classification is, in our opinion, limited to preoperative planning, providing an indication of the thickness that can be removed during acromioplasty without causing iatrogenic fractures.

The length of the acromion is not entirely irrelevant from the point of view of the pathogenesis of impingement (Fig. 4.2). A long apophysis provides the underlying humeral head with greater bone cover than a short apophysis, in which the less rigid coracoacromial ligament has a more important role.

Fig. 4.1

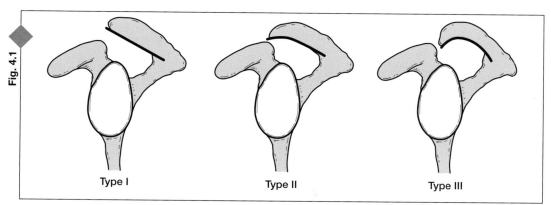

Type I   Type II   Type III

The three acromial morphotypes according to Bigliani.

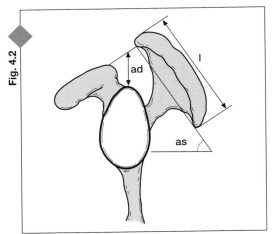

Fig. 4.2

Acromial biometry.
ad: arch distance (distance between the coracoacromial arch and the supraglenoid tubercle); l: length of the acromion; as: acromial slope.

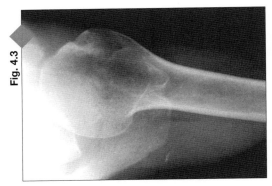

Fig. 4.3

Acromial bone.

It is, therefore, clear that a long acromion, particularly if it tends to be horizontal, is a risk factor for impingement. This has been confirmed by Edelson and Taitz, who also recognized three acromial morphotypes detectable on the anatomy table or approximately from an axillary projection: cobra-shaped and long (6.2 cm on average), with the joint facet with the clavicle 5–10 mm behind the anterior rim of the process, and frequently associated with impingement; square-tipped and short (5.2 mm on average), with the joint facet located at the anterior end of the apophysis, and rarely associated with impingement; and an intermediate form, characterized by a weaker correlation with impingement than the former but a stronger correlation than the latter (Edelson, 1992).

Acromial bone is a congenital anomaly represented by a lack of fusion between two of the three ossification nuclei (preacromion, mesoacromion, and metacromion) of this apophysis; this results in a bipartite acromion, the mobile portion of which is termed the acromial bone, while the transition zone constitutes congenital pseudarthrosis. Although the acromial morphology can be better visualized in outlet view, it is easier to diagnose from an axillary projection (Fig. 4.3).

Acromial bone is a very significant risk factor for impingement syndrome, either because it is depressed by the action of the deltoid, or because the pseudarthrosis focus may be hypertrophic and thus invade the subacromial space (Norris, 1983). The same considerations obviously apply to post-traumatic pseudarthrosis of the acromial process.

Coracoacromial ligament

The role of the coracoacromial ligament in the pathogenesis of impingement is not entirely clear. When the arm is flexed at 90° and completely internally rotated, the supraspinatus tendon and the long head of the biceps are in contact with this ligament. It has been hypothesized that thickening of the ligament, caused in turn by continual microtraumas, leads to impingement (Soslowsy, 1994).

Subsequent histological studies (Sarkar, 1990) have not confirmed this hypothesis, finding regressive but not hypertrophic alterations of the ligament.

It is in any case possible that the increased consistency of the ligament, although with no increase in its volume, may contribute to the impingement. This is the justification given by those who usually combine resection of this fibrous band with acromioplasty. The tendency has recently been to preserve and reinsert it, and this has not compromised the efficacy of subacromial decompression procedures.

It is worth noting, in our opinion, that a short coracocacromial arch, measured along the craniocaudal axis between the supraglenoid tubercle and the coracoacromial ligament, is a risk factor for impingement (Fig. 4.2); a cadaveric study has shown that degenerative alterations suggesting impingement are never found if this distance exceeds 15 mm, while 75% of shoulders with these lesions have a distance of 12 mm or less (Edelson, 1992).

Coracoid

The coracoid apophysis may be responsible for impingement, although less frequently than the acromial process (Gerber, 1985).

There are several distinctive clinical features: pain elicited by flexion-internal rotation is typically antero-medial and notably spreads along the limb.

The causes of this impingement include congenital dysmorphisms and the more frequent acquired dysmorphisms of the apophysis. Besides post-traumatic consolidation defects, acquired dysmorphisms include the sequelae of coracoid transposition procedures performed to treat anterior instability, and also the sequelae of the less frequent osteotomy procedures of the scapular neck to treat posterior instability.

Acromioclavicular joint

When the AC joint is affected by degenerative processes, it may present exuberant osteophyte formation, capable of interfering with the underlying rotator cuff (Fig. 4.4). This hypothesis, proposed by Neer in 1972, was subsequently taken up by Watson who identified the underestimation of acromioclavicular arthropathy as a cause of failure of conventional acromioplasty (Watson, 1978).

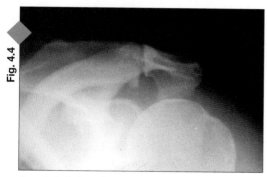

Fig. 4.4

Acromioclavicular arthropathy.

Although it is neither useful nor advisable to carry out routine resection of the end of the clavicle in the surgical treatment of common impingement syndromes, the indication should be evaluated clinically and radiologically in each individual patient; the presence of lower osteophytes, the reduced efficacy of the subacromial infiltration of lidocaine and the good efficacy of lidocaine if infiltrated in the AC joint, all suggest the need to combine the removal of the lateral 15 mm of the clavicle with acromioplasty.

Humerus

The proximal apophysis of the humerus may have an abnormally prominent trochanter which runs into the coracoacromial arch during common flexion-internal rotation movements of the arm. This dysmorphism may be congenital or acquired, and if acquired it may be the result of a poorly consolidated fracture, or a prosthesis implanted too deeply in the metaphysis, resulting in protrusion of the greater tuberosity beyond the head.

Rotator cuff

The rotator cuff is an aponeurotic structure, arising from the confluence of four tendons (supraspinatus, infraspinatus, teres minor and subscapularis) which surround the humeral head, providing it with not only a motor function but also a basic stabilization function. From the anatomical point of view, the cuff consists of fibrous connective tissue with a high content of type I collagen, highly resistant to traction. It is more highly vascularized on the bursa side than on the capsule side and has a laminar structure with overlapping layers.

For the supraspinatus in particular, we can recognize from the surface inwards the coracohumeral ligament, the layer of parallel tendon fibres, the layer of arched tendon fibres, and finally a layer of slack connective tissue which allows it to glide over the underlying joint capsule.

In impingement syndrome, the rotator cuff is subjected to microtraumas which are reflected in a gross pathological picture of tendinitis and fibrosis, often accompanied by calcifications (Neer's stage II).

These alterations, together with those of the bursa which always occur in addition, are sufficient to increase the thickness of the tissues that occupy the space between the humeral head and the acromial profile, further worsening the impingement. In this way an impingement that is initially of the outlet type and, therefore, extrinsic (i.e. originating outside the tendon), secondarily also becomes intrinsic. Primary tendinopathy (e.g. calcific tendinitis such as that illustrated in Fig. 4.5) can obviously, though less commonly, also cause impingement to occur.

When impingement results in partial tendon rupture (stage III), the muscle retraction and irregularity around the lesion contribute to the localized thickening of the cuff. It is, however, worth remembering that rupture of the cuff contributes to impingement syndrome mainly because of the severe functional repercussions (see the section on Deficit of the mechanism of depression of the humeral head) and only slightly through the structural alterations mentioned.

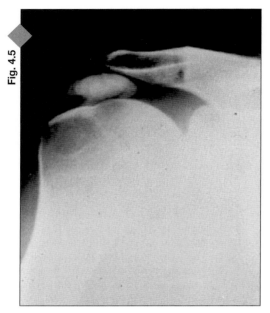

Fig. 4.5

Calcific tendonitis.

Subacromiodeltoid bursa

The sclerotic changes that occur in the chronically inflamed bursa of a painful shoulder contribute to the thickening of the soft tissues and thus to the self-perpetuation of the impingement mechanism. It is also theoretically possible, though rare, for primary bursitis (rheumatoid, due to infection, etc.) to trigger impingement.

The formation of scar tissue deserves particular mention in shoulders that have undergone surgery to remove the subacromiodeltoid bursa. Excessive new connective tissue may form, perhaps following a very traumatic surgical technique or as a reaction to the suture materials used, and may in turn become a cause of impingement and, therefore, of recurrence.

Functional factors

Functional factors do not always lack an anatomical substrate; if one is present, it does not participate directly in the pathogenesis of the impingement, but only via the impaired function it causes.

Deficit of the mechanism of depression of the humeral head

This mechanism depends essentially on the synergic action of all the muscles forming the rotator cuff, in particular the teres minor and the infraspinatus owing to the unique direction of their force vectors.

All the conditions involving reduced efficacy of these muscle motors are associated with ascent of the humeral head, resulting in subacromial overpressure and the possibility of symptoms of impingement (Fig. 4.6).

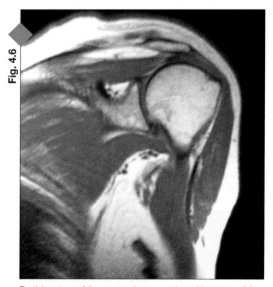

Fig. 4.6

Partial rupture of the supraspinatus tendon with ascent of the humeral head. The MRI shows a hypointense, thin tendon (black arrow), suggesting partial rupture, and discontinuity of the arch formed by the lower profile of the scapular neck and the lower profile of the anatomical neck of the humerus (white arrow), indicating moderate ascent of the humeral epiphysis.

In this respect, tendon lesions depending on chronic impingement can, in turn, accentuate the impingement, with a mechanism that is self-perpetuating on a functional basis, as well as on a structural basis (see the section on Rotator cuff) (Ogata, 1990). Lesions of the long head of the biceps also partly compromise the mechanism of depression, with similar adverse consequences.

Cuff lesions are often, for the reasons given above, a complication of impingement syndrome capable of worsening the syndrome further. We can nevertheless acknowledge that these lesions sometimes exist prior to the disorder and may induce it; tendon ageing, with the depauperization of vascularity, the degeneration of cell components and collagen fibres, reduced resistance to tension and microruptures are a likely mechanism of damage in the elderly, just as traction overuse is a plausible mechanism in athletes under

40 years old. Finally we should not overlook traumatic ruptures and ruptures resulting from calcific, rheumatic and metabolic tendinopathy, though these are rare.

The principal disorders that affect muscles are paralysis of the suprascapular nerve and C5-C6 radiculopathy.

In sports and activities that require the frequent or prolonged elevation of the upper limbs, the weak external rotators may be fatigued more than the deltoid and the greater pectoralis, resulting in relatively greater hyposthenia of the depressors than of the elevators of the humeral head (Bigliani, 1997). This situation may easily result in impingement due to the ascent of the humeral head.

In throwing disciplines, this overuse syndrome has two aetiopathogenetic triggers: the first is in the late cocking phase, when the subscapularis muscle contracts to stop the external rotation; the second is in the deceleration phase (after the throw), when the vigorous eccentric contraction of the supraspinatus prevents excessive internal rotation-adduction of the limb and antagonizes the diastasis of the joint heads. Besides muscle fatigue of the rotators, these movements are also believed to cause tendon damage due to traction overuse, which is responsible for partial rotator cuff lesions sometimes observed in athletes. Lesions of this type typically affect the capsule side of the tendon, probably because it is less vascularized.

Hence the importance of adequate strengthening of the rotators in order to prevent painful disorders in participants of high-risk sports (baseball, swimming, volleyball, tennis, etc.). The same principle also forms the basis of physiotherapy programmes used in the conservative treatment of impingement syndromes.

Weight-bearing by the shoulder

Impingement syndrome is fairly common in paraplegic individuals or those who depend almost exclusively on their upper limbs for weight-bearing. The reason for this is believed to be the upward forces acting on the humeral head when walking with the aid of elbow crutches, and when using a self-propelling wheelchair and getting up from it.

These forces cause subacromial overpressure, which is responsible for the symptoms (Bayley, 1987).

Scapular anomalies owing to position and mobility

Anomalies of the scapula are observed, when not congenital, in extreme thoracic kyphosis and in the sequelae of complete acromioclavicular separation. Anomalies of mobility are, however, observed in paralysis of the relevant muscles, fascioscapulohumeral muscular dystrophy, and adhesions of the scapulothoracic pseudoarticulation.

The ultimate outcome of all these conditions is disturbance of the scapulohumeral rhythm, limiting scapulothoracic excursion, and overuse of the glenohumeral joint, with development of subacromial and sometimes internal impingement (see the section on Internal impingement and anterior instability).

Posterior capsule rigidity

Posterior capsule rigidity is believed to be responsible for impingement syndromes via a rather complex mechanism, according to which the constricted posterior capsule wall acts during flexion like the cord of a yo-yo, to use a fitting example suggested by Matsen and Arntz (1990). If the tissue is slack and extendible, the torsion induced by the flexion movement of the arm does not involve any decentring of the humeral head; if, however, the tissue is fibrotic and not very extendible, torsion causes the humeral head to ascend towards the coracoacromial arch, like a yo-yo rotating upwards along its cord.

There are many causes of this, and they are often attributable to a previous painful condition limiting mobility. In these cases, the onset of rigidity worsens the impingement further, creating a vicious circle which progressively aggravates the clinical picture. Impingement is for the same reasons common in the context of retractile capsulitis (Fig. 4.7); this is more likely, the more the disorder has affected the posterior sector of the capsule, and this situation becomes apparent on objective examination in the form of a marked limitation in internal rotation and cross-body adduction.

Thrower's shoulder represents a separate case since, besides risking overuse syndrome (see the section on Deficit of the mechanism of depression of the humeral head), a degree of anterior laxity and posterior constriction frequently develops in response to the stress in abduction-external rotation produced in the late cocking phase.

This change in capsule tension is manifested on objective examination by a limitation of internal rotatory excursion and an increase in external rotatory excursion (with the arm abducted at 90°). This condition is considered acceptable as long as the sum of the two angles, and, therefore, the entire range of rotation of the humerus, is at least equal to 180° (180° rule). At the point where the internal rotation deficit

Impingement syndromes: definition and classification

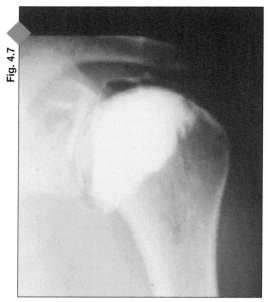

Fig. 4.7

Retractile capsulitis. Arthrography shows a marked reduction in capsule volume in cases which have not yet been clinically diagnosed.

becomes so much greater than the gain in external rotation as to reduce the total excursion to below this threshold, there would be a specific risk of developing pain (Morgan, 1998).

Based on similar pathophysiological considerations, we consider posterior capsule stretching to be an essential component of both a physiotherapy programme for the treatment of impingement, and athletic training for throwers, in order to prevent possible morbid sequelae.

Instability

A study by Tibone (1985) revealed that the benefits of anterior acromioplasty were exceptionally scarce in 35 shoulders of young athletes suffering from impingement syndrome: a good or excellent result was obtained in only 42% of cases. Because the study was retrospective, some of the preoperative clinical data (e.g. the apprehension test) were not available and might have helped to interpret these results. It is, nevertheless, extremely likely that the explanation for this is the high frequency of glenohumeral instability that often goes unrecognized in this category of patients.

Subacromial decompression is not believed to provide real benefits in this case and could be advantageously substituted by a capsuloplasty procedure. It is obvious that hypermobility of the humeral head may facilitate the occurrence of impingement phenomena (Glousman, 1993), but it is not yet entirely clear whether such impingement is predominantly against the coracoacromial arch or rather against the posterosuperior rim of the glenoid.

There is no doubt that a lesion of the inferior glenohumeral ligament (IGHL) delays the activation of the scapulothoracic pseudoarticulation in elevation movements of the limb; when this ligament complex is intact and therefore mechanically effective, it is in tension in abduction movements and thus draws in the scapula, initiating physiological scapular excursion. Lesion of the IGHL will, therefore, delay scapular rotation, advancing impingement between the trochanter and acromion as a result.

If, therefore, the occurrence of subacromial impingement as a result of instability is generally accepted, it is no less likely that an unstable shoulder will also develop other forms of impingement, particularly internal impingement.

Internal impingement and anterior instability

Internal impingement is a relatively recent concept which emerged in the early 1990s from the work of Walch (Walch, 1992) and Jobe (1993). Jobe, in particular, demonstrated that when the arm is abducted at 90° and completely externally rotated, the internal surface of the supraspinatus tendon close to its insertion is pressed against the posterosuperior rim of the glenoid and the labrum adhering to it (Fig. 4.8).

The continual repetition of a similar microtrauma in the late cocking phase of throwing is believed to account for many cases of painful shoulder in throwers, in whom arthroscopy reveals fibrillation of the posterosuperior segment of the labrum with, in some cases, partial rupture of the supraspinatus tendon.

These patients are frequently found to have laxity of the anterior portion of the glenohumeral ligament or anteroinferior disinsertion of the glenoid labrum; this additional lesion is believed to depend on the separation of the anteroinferior capsuloligamentous complex, caused by overuse in abduction-external rotation (Fig. 4.8).

The lesion mechanism proposed by Jobe is based on insufficiency of the subscapularis, i.e. the muscle responsible for stopping humeral 'hyperangulation' in the late cocking phase. Alternative causes are believed to be reduced retroversion of the humeral head and reduced movement of the scapular bascule owing to impaired scapular mobility (see the section on Scapular anomalies owing to position and mobility).

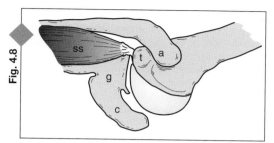

Fig. 4.8

Internal impingement. View from above of the left scapulohumeral joint in abduction-external rotation. Note the location of the supraspinatus tendon (ss), squashed between the trochanter (t) and the posterosuperior rim of the glenoid (g). Neither the acromion (a), nor the coracoid (c) are involved in the impingement mechanism.

The clinical picture contains a number of peculiarities which, together with a positive history of throwing sports, can provide clues to this condition. First of all, the apprehension test, i.e. forced abduction at 90° with external rotation of the arm, does not produce real apprehension in these patients, although it does cause pain, probably as a result of impingement. Secondly, the relocation test yields results that are the mirror image of those expected in anterior instability, i.e. anteroposterior pressure on the humeral head accentuates the pain because it intensifies impingement, whereas posteroanterior pressure provides relief because it reduces impingement.

The treatment proposed by the author (Jobe, 1996) is essentially conservative, with 2–4 weeks' rest from the sport and adequate strengthening of the subscapularis and rotators of the scapula. Only refractory cases will require surgical treatment comprising anterior capsuloplasty, after confirmation of anteroinferior instability has been obtained by physical examination under anaesthesia and diagnostic arthroscopy.

SLAP lesion and superior instability A radically different pathophysiological hypothesis to account for painful shoulder in throwers has emerged from studies by Morgan (1998) and Burkhart (1998). These authors concentrated on the frequent observation in these patients of a type II SLAP lesion. A SLAP lesion is understood to mean a lesion of the superior segment of the labrum located at the site of insertion of the tendon of the long head of the biceps (Snyder, 1990).

Arthroscopic examination of these lesions has been used to classify them into four types: type I is a substantially degenerative alteration of the bicipital anchor; type II – which will be described in greater

detail below – involves its complete detachment; type III is a bucket handle rupture of the superior labrum which does not involve disinsertion of the long head of the biceps; and type IV is an extension of the above tear through the proximal portion of the tendon.

Type II SLAP lesions are clearly the most frequent, consisting in detachment of the labrum-tendon complex from the glenoid margin and the supraglenoid tubercle (Table 4.I, between pages 398 and 399). This disorder is characteristic of throwers in whom, according to the classic theory of Andrews (1985), the mechanism of injury is acknowledged to be the sudden overload of tension to which the bicipital anchor is subjected following the eccentric contraction of the biceps in the deceleration phase. This contraction firstly prevents the diastasis of the glenohumeral joint heads, by acting in synergy with the contraction of the supraspinatus, and secondly stops the elbow extending.

The repetition of this microtrauma with every throw is believed to cause the gradual tearing away of the labrum-tendon complex.

Burkhart and Morgan (1998) recently proposed a further mechanism of injury which, although it may possibly cause SLAP, is more probably implicated in propagating it; this is the peel-back mechanism. This occurs when the arm is in extreme abduction-external rotation in the cocking phase. It causes torsion of the tendon of the long head of the biceps close to its base and tends to detach the adjacent labrum, subsequently propagating the lesion.

This pathogenetic hypothesis would explain the more frequent posterosuperior location of type II SLAP in throwers than in the general population, in whom this lesion is very rare and generally anterosuperior.

The pathogenesis in the general population appears to be mostly macrotraumatic, i.e. related to a single traumatic event (elongation strain on a contracted biceps brachii), rather than microtraumatic, as in athletes.

It is interesting to note, returning to the subdivision of type II SLAP lesions in anterior (or anterosuperior), posterior (or posterosuperior) and combined positions (or with both components), that lesions in throwers are purely posterior in 47% of cases and combined in 34%, while lesions found outside this category are anterior in 57% of cases and combined in 29% (Morgan, 1998).

From a symptomatological point of view, it is very important to note that the classic signs of SLAP (Speed's test and O'Brien's test) are generally clearly positive in anterior lesions, whereas they tend to be negative in posterior lesions; Jobe's relocation test has, however, proved sensitive and specific in posterior lesions, understood as specifically defined in the previous section (Morgan, 1998).

The same study also demonstrated that posterior type II SLAP lesions present an objective picture suggesting anteroinferior instability, but no corresponding anatomical findings on arthroscopy.

The study by Huber and Putz (1997) has demonstrated histologically that the labrum, the glenohumeral ligaments, and the biceps and triceps tendons are connected to a single system of periarticular collagen fibres which act synergically to contain the humeral head.

It is, therefore, likely that a posterosuperior lesion will involve pseudolaxity in the opposite, i.e. anteroinferior, location, by interrupting a circular system.

The frequent gross pathological finding of a rotator cuff lesion in a posterior location starting from the deep surface of the tendinous lamina could be ascribed to primary posterosuperior instability, which is difficult to diagnose on the basis of symptoms, via the acromial stop which prevents superior dislocation of the head, but which could progressively wear the cuff from the inside until it causes true rupture.

The excellent results reported by Morgan and Burkhart (Morgan, 1998) using arthroscopic reinsertion of the posterosuperior segment of the labrum and the bicipital anchor and tenorrhaphy of the cuff, if damaged, suggest that this aetiopathogenetic interpretation of shoulder pain in throwers is reliable. It is proposed as a counterargument to the theory of posterosuperior glenoid impingement suggested by Jobe (see the section on Internal impingement and anterior instability) and we can currently merely note the similarity of the two hypotheses. Since the therapeutic strategies suggested for internal impingement according to Jobe and for type II SLAP are, however, radically different while having a similar objective, and assuming that both hypotheses are true (an assumption contested by the respective authors) and consequently correspond to different disorders, the problem arises of making an accurate differential diagnosis. Only arthroscopy currently seems to meet this requirement adequately.

Principles of classification

Impingement syndromes may be classified in different ways and the fact that numerous taxonomic systems are found in the literature, none of which is completely exhaustive, confirms the impression that this definition hides a complex spectrum of heterogeneous disorders among which it is difficult to separate the unifying features from the distinguishing features.

In the light of the multifactorial nature of the aetiology, the distinction between functional and structural impingement appears impracticable, though theoretically interesting, except in a small group of cases; it is, in fact, common to find many risk factors, some of which are structural and others functional, in the same patient. Furthermore, the same factor may act simultaneously via a structural alteration and a functional aberration. This is the case, repeatedly, with rotator cuff lesions in which localized thickening is accompanied by a deficit of the mechanism of depression of the humeral head.

The distinction already mentioned between outlet and non-outlet impingement constitutes a fundamental step in the diagnosis. Outlet impingement includes all cases in which the supraspinatus outlet is anatomically constricted owing to structural alterations of the coracoacromial arch or the humeral epiphysis, the respective roof and floor of the osteoligamentous channel through which the supraspinatus tendon runs. It is clearly this category of patients who can benefit most from a subacromial decompression procedure.

An outlet impingement can only be confirmed from a good radiographic projection (outlet view), obtained with the X-ray beam at a tangent to the scapular plane and tilted in the caudal direction at approximately 10° in relation to the horizontal axis. By using this angle, the acromial profile can be evaluated along with its contribution to the restriction of the outlet (Fig. 4.9).

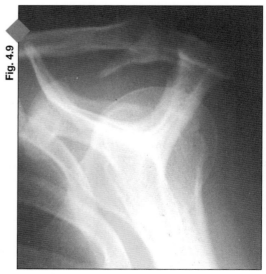

Fig. 4.9

Outlet view. The 'hooked' (type III) acromial morphology is clear.

It is therefore an essential requirement for the preoperative planning of an acromioplasty procedure.

The group of non-outlet impingements includes all cases in which the supraspinatus outlet is normal in shape and dimensions, and in which the impingement may consequently depend on a volumetric increase in the contents of this space (tendon and bursa alterations) or on functional causes.

A further classification distinguishes intrinsic from extrinsic impingement syndromes. In intrinsic impingement, the principal aetiopathogenetic trigger is a cuff disorder (degenerative tendinopathy in the elderly, rupture due to traction overuse in athletes, calcific tendinitis, traumatic rupture, rheumatic and metabolic tendinopathies, etc.), while in extrinsic impingement, non-tendon alterations (e.g. outlet impingement) may subsequently cause rotator cuff disorder.

This classification is, in our opinion, rather speculative, since it is impossible to state with certainty, when dealing with an elderly patient with chronic impingement syndrome, rotator cuff lesion and constricted supraspinatus outlet, whether the tendon rupture resulted from the outlet impingement (extrinsic form) because it is fairly likely that a picture of degenerative tendinopathy will have cast doubt upon the mechanism of depression of the head, subsequently producing impingement with the resulting acromial hyperostosis (intrinsic form).

The pathogenetic mechanism is circular, and it is accordingly more difficult to recognize the starting point, the longer the period since the onset of the disease (Fig. 4.10).

Finally, the separation of primary forms from secondary forms cannot be disregarded in a description of impingement syndrome.

Impingement is defined as secondary when a pre-existing disorder can be identified as capable of causing it; in the vast majority of cases this is instability or cuff rupture.

The diagnosis of secondary impingement is extremely important when determining the correct therapeutic indication. The priority in these cases is to treat the underlying disorder, resolution of which is generally accompanied by remission of the symptoms of impingement.

We have already mentioned the study by Tibone (1985) who reports the poor results obtained with acromioplasty in the treatment of impingement syndrome in athletes: the most reliable interpretation of these data is that in the study population, impingement is frequently secondary to unrecognized glenohumeral instability. Subacromial decompression is not believed to provide real benefits and could, however, be advantageously substituted by capsuloplasty.

Furthermore, primary forms are predominant in the adult and elderly population, in whom it is either impossible to find any reason for the development of the impingement (idiopathic forms), or the reasons identified do not constitute a disorder as such.

This is the case with the type III 'hooked' acromion. It does not constitute a dysmorphism in the strict sense, but is merely a morphological variant within the normal range. It is not a cause of impingement syndrome, but simply a risk factor. As mentioned above, it is possible to have a type III acromion without ever experiencing shoulder pain.

Conclusions

It appears clear from the above that the diagnosis of painful shoulder is not concluded by finding an impingement syndrome, since this is not a disease, but merely a set of symptoms. It is, therefore, essential to try to identify the functional or structural factors that have combined to cause it by means of the history, an objective examination and instrumental tests, so that the treatment offered is aimed as far as possible at

Fig. 4.10

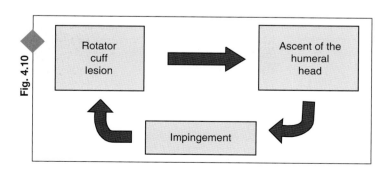

Circular pathogenetic mechanism.

stopping the mechanism of injury, and not merely at suppressing the symptoms.

From this point of view, the classification of impingement syndrome, understood as the specification of all the factors presumed to have a role in its pathogenesis and the identification of the causal links between these and the syndrome itself, is not a sterile diagnostic exercise, but a key requirement of targeted therapy.

An analysis of the principal aetiopathogenetic triggers has demonstrated the basic role of the mechanism of depression of the humeral head in preventing impingement phenomena. The same can be said of correct articular function. This is of primary importance when designing a therapeutic programme; the majority of impingement disorders resolve with adequate physiotherapy, aimed at strengthening the rotators and maintaining/recovering correct articular excursion, obviously combined with excluding the actions responsible for the impingement from work or athletic activity.

According to a recent study by Morrison (1997), conservative therapy is effective in 67% of cases.

A surgical solution should, therefore, be considered only if conservative therapy has failed. In any case, even if a valid rehabilitation programme has not led to the complete remission of the symptoms, it is the ideal preparation for surgery.

As regards surgical methods, all that has been said about the role of the anteroinferior rim of the acromion justifies anterior acromioplasty, as proposed by Neer in 1972. The more destructive acromionectomy and lateral acromioplasty should no longer be employed.

The four-in-one arthroplasty, described in 1982 by Neviaser, extends the above procedure by combining it with resection of the coracoacromial ligament, removal of the lateral end of the clavicle and tenodesis of the long head of the biceps. Neviaser reports excellent results in terms of regression of pain and recovery of articular function, but no other major clinical parameters were taken into consideration, such as resuming work or leisure and sport activities, patient satisfaction and muscle force. We agree with Bigliani and Levine (1997) that this procedure is too invasive to be used routinely in any patient with impingement. Although the debate regarding the value of resection of the coracoacromial ligament is still open, the same does not apply to the other two surgical procedures. Excision of the lateral end of the clavicle does not seem justified, unless acromioclavicular arthropathy is present and can be confirmed clinically and radiologically, while tenosynovitis of the long head of the biceps, a frequent complication of impingement

syndromes owing to the anatomical location of the tendon, is, in our experience, reversible with adequate subacromial decompression. It is only in cases of subluxation, rupture or evident degeneration of the tendon that its intra-articular segment should be removed and tenodesis performed at the bicipital groove.

Arthroscopic acromioplasty, introduced by Ellman towards the end of the 1980s, is a development of Neer's procedure with a view to reducing the surgical trauma (Ellman, 1987). Since the principle is the same, there is no reason to regard this technique as less satisfactory than the previous one, provided that the surgeon has acquired sufficient experience in performing shoulder arthroscopy. A comparative anatomical study in cadavers has demonstrated that the two techniques are entirely comparable (Gartsman, 1988). The considerable acceleration of the postoperative recovery permitted by the arthroscopic approach has made this method the gold standard in the treatment of impingement syndromes.

In conclusion, owing to the variable nature of impingement syndromes, it is necessary to implement full diagnostic testing, aimed at identifying the structural and functional factors involved in each patient in the pathogenesis of the disorder before moving on to the therapeutic phase. It is only by proceeding in this manner that the most suitable treatment can be chosen on a rational basis from among the many available, and this treatment can be termed aetiological rather than simply symptomatic.

Unresolved problems for research

The increasing use of arthroscopy to evaluate indistinct pictures of painful shoulder in athletes, where clinical examination and imaging have not proved conclusive, has led to the discovery of new pathological conditions. Internal impingement, hitherto unanimously accepted in the posterosuperior location, has recently been extended to the anterosuperior segment of the joint in forms of SLAC lesion (Savoi, 2001) and anterosuperior impingement of the subscapularis (Gerber, 2000). The list of intra-articular disorders connected with microinstability is likely to grow longer over the coming years.

Further reading

Bigliani L.U., Levine W.N., 'Current concept review. Subacromial impingement syndrome', *J. Bone Joint Surg.* 74A(12): 1854–1868, (1997)

Jobe C.M., 'Superior glenoid impingement', *Clin. Orthop.* 330: 98–107, (1996)

Morgan C.D., Burkhart S.S., Palmeri M., Gillespie M., 'Type II SLAP-lesions: three subtypes and their relationship to superior instability and rotator cuff tears', *Arthroscopy* 14(6): 553–565, (1998)

Morrison D.S., Frogameni A.D., Woodworth P., 'Non-operative treatment of subacromial impingement syndrome', *J. Bone Joint Surg.* 79A: 732–737, (1997)

Bibliography

Andrews J.R., Carson W., McLeod W., 'Glenoid labrum tears related to the long head of the biceps', *Am. J. Sports Med.* 13: 337–341, (1985)

Bayley J.C., Cochran T.P., Sledge C.B., 'The weight-bearing shoulder. The impingement syndrome in paraplegics', *J. Bone Joint Surg.* 69A(5): 676–678, (1987)

Bigliani L.U., Levine W.N., 'Current Concept Review. Subacromial Impingement Syndrome', *J. Bone Joint Surg.* 74A(12): 1854–1868, (1997)

Bigliani L.U., Morrison D.S., Apri E.W., 'The morphology of the acromion and its relationship to rotator cuff tears', *Orthop. Trans.* 10: 228, (1986)

Burkhart S.S., Morgan C.D., 'The peel-back mechanism: its role in producing and extending posterior type II SLAP-lesions and its effect on SLAP repair rehabilitation', *Arthroscopy* 14(6): 637–640, (1998)

Codman E.A., 'Rupture of the supraspinatus tendon and other lesions in or about the subacromial bursa', *The shoulder*, Thomas Todd, Boston (1934)

Duplay S., 'De la périarthrite scapulo-humérale et des raideurs de l'épaule qu'en sont la conséquence', *Arch. Gen. Méd.* 20: 513–525, (1872)

Edelson J.G., Taitz C., 'Anatomy of the coraco-acromial arch. Relation to degeneration of the acromion', *J. Bone Joint Surg.* 74B: 589–594, (1992)

Ellman H., Arthroscopic subacromial decompression: analysis of one- to three-year results', *Arthroscopy* 3: 173–181, (1987)

Gartsman G.M., Blair M.E. JR, Noble P.C., Bennet J.B., Tullos H.S., 'Arthroscopic subacromial decompression. An anatomical study', *Am. J. Sports Med.* 16: 48–50, (1988)

Gerber C., Sebesta A., 'Impingement of the deep surface of the subscapularis tendon and the reflection pulley on the anterosuperior glenoid rim: a preliminary report', *J. Shoulder Elbow Surg.* 9(6): 483–490, (2000)

Gerber C., Terrier F., Ganz R., 'The role of the coracoid process in the chronic impingement syndrome', *J. Bone Joint Surg.* 67B(5): 703–708, (1985)

Glousman R.E., 'Instability versus impingement syndrome in the throwing athlete', *Orthop. Clin. North America* 24: 89–99, (1993)

Hamilton F.H., 'Fractures of the scapula', In: *A Practical Treatise on Fracture and Dislocations.* 5th eds. Henry C. Lea, Philadelphia, pp. 209–221, (1875)

Huber W.P., Putz R.V., 'The periarticular fiber system (PAFS) of the shoulder joint', *Arthroscopy* 13: 680–691, (1997)

Iannotti J.P., Swiontkowski M.F., Esterhafi J., Boulas H.J., 'Intraoperative assessment of rotator cuff vascularity using laser Doppler flowmetry', *Abstract AAOS* 1989 Meeting, Las Vegas (1989)

Jobe C.M., 'Superior glenoid impingement', *Clin. Orthop.* 330: 98–107, (1996)

Jobe C.M., SIDLES J., 'Evidence for a superior glenoid impingement upon the rotator cuff', *Abstract. J. Shoulder Elbow Surg.* 2 (Suppl): S19, (1993)

Lindblom K., 'On pathogenesis of ruptures of the tendon aponeurosis of the shoulder joint', *Acta Radiol.* 18: 91–93, (1939)

Matsen III F.A., Arntz C.T. In Matsen III F.A., Rockwood C.A. JR (eds). *The shoulder*, WB Saunders Co., New York, Vol. 2, p. 627, (1990)

Meyer A.W., 'The minuter anatomy of attrition lesions', *J. Bone Joint Surg.* 13: 341–360, (1931)

Morgan C.D., Burkhart S.S., Palmeri M., Gillespie M., 'Type II SLAP-lesions: three subtypes and their relationship to superior instability and rotator cuff tears', *Arthroscopy* 14(6): 553–565, (1998)

Morrison D.S., Bigliani L.U., 'The clinical significance of variations in acromial morphology', *Orthop. Trans.* 11: 234, (1987)

Morrison D.S., Frogameni A.D., Woodworth P., 'Non-operative treatment of subacromial impingement syndrome', *J. Bone Joint Surg.* 79A: 732–737, (1997)

Neer C.S. II., 'Anterior acromioplasty for the chronic impingement syndrome in the shoulder. A preliminary report', *J. Bone Joint Surg.* 54A: 41–50, (1972)

Neviaser T.J., Neviaser R.J., Neviaser J.S., 'The four-in-one arthroplasty for the painful arc syndrome', *Clin. Orthop.* 163: 107–112, (1982)

Norris T.R., Fisher J., Bigliani L.U., 'The unfused acromial epiphysis and its relationship to impingement syndromes', *Orthop. Trans.* 7(3): 505, (1983)

Ogata S., Uhthoff H.K., 'Acromial enthesopathy and rotator cuff tear. A radiologic and histologic postmortem investigation of the coracoacromial arch', *Clin. Orthop.* 254: 39–48, (1990)

Rathbun J.B., Macnab I., 'The microvascular pattern of tre rotator cuff', *J. Bone Joint Surg.* 52B: 540, (1970)

Sarkar K., Taine W., Uhthoff H.K., 'The ultrastructure of the coracoacromial ligament in patients with chronic impingement syndrome', *Clin. Orthop.* 254: 49–54, (1990)

Savoi F.H. III, Field L.D., Atchinson S., 'Anterior superior instability with rotator cuff tearing: SLAC-lesion,' *Orthop. Clin. North Am.* 32(3): 457–461, (2001)

Sigholm G., Styf J., Corner L., Herberts P., 'Pressure recording in the subacromial bursa', *J. Orthop. Res.* 6(1): 123–128, (1988)

Snyder S.J., Karzel R.P., Del Pizzo W., Ferkel R.D., Friedman M.J., 'SLAP-lesions of the shoulder', *Arthroscopy* 6: 274–279, (1990)

Soslowsy L.J., An C.H., Johnston S.P., Carpenter J.E., 'Geometric and mechanical properties of the coracoacromial ligament and their relationship to rotator cuff disease', *Clin. Orthop.* 304: 10–17, (1994)

Stieda A., 'Zur Pathologie der Schulter gelenkschlembeutel', In: Langenbeck B. (eds). *Archiv fur Klinische Chirurgie*, August Hirschwald, Berlin, p. 910, (1908)

Tibone J.E., Jobe F.W., Kerlan R.K., Carter V.S., Shields C.L., Lombardo S.J., Yocum L.A., 'Shoulder impingement in athletes treated by an anterior acromioplasty', *Clin. Orthop.* 198: 134–140, (1985)

Walch G., Boileau P., Noel E., Donell S.T., 'Impingement of the deep surface of the suprapinatus tendon on the posterosuperior glenoid rim: an arthroscopic study', *J. Shoulder Elbow Surg.*, 1: 238–245, (1992)

Watson M., 'The refractory painful arc syndrome', *J. Bone Joint Surg.* 60B(4): 544–546, (1978)

Wickiewicz T.L., 'Glenohumeral kinematics in a muscle fatigue model: a radiographic study. *Orthop. Trans.* 18: 178–179, (1994)

Wrede L., 'Ueber Kalkarblagerungen in der Umgebung des Schultergelenks und ihre Beziehungen zur Periarthritis', In: *Archiv fur Klinische Chirurgie*, August Hirschwald, Berlin, p. 259, (1912)

Wuh H.C.K., Snyder S.J., 'A modified classification of suprapinatus outlet view based on the configuration and the anatomic thickness of the acromion', *Orthop. Trans.* 16: 767, (1992)

CHAPTER 5

EPIDEMIOLOGY OF SHOULDER LESIONS IN SPORT

E. REGGIANI

Many sports are characterized by specific athletic actions involving repeated movements of the upper limb above the head: these are generally termed overhead sports.

These sports all have the biomechanical model of throwing in common, for example, as performed by baseball and softball pitchers, volleyball and water polo players and javelin throwers, but also by tennis players, swimmers and, in some exercises, by gymnasts.

There is a particularly high incidence of shoulder injuries in overhead athletes, the shoulder being particularly susceptible to injury owing to its intrinsic lack of static stability and the complexity of its dynamic stability, which depend on its unusual anatomy and its very extensive range of possible movement. Technical overhead actions require a delicate balance between muscle activity and capsular and ligament containment when, as often happens, they are performed at the extreme limits of glenohumeral mobility, and at very high angular velocity and torque. The shoulder structures, when subjected to repeated stresses of this nature, will consequently easily be damaged by wear due to these multiple microtraumas.

The aetiopathogenetic importance of chronic functional overuse is also confirmed by the increase in the incidence of shoulder disorders in overhead athletes with advancing age and competitive level.

These epidemiological findings, which are generically unexceptionable, are not reflected precisely in the various types of lesion reported by a very extensive medical literature. The cases reported are non-specific, owing mainly to the various pathological classifications of lesions which make it impossible to compare data reliably. Furthermore, the diagnostic precision made possible by the advent of MR and arthroscopy has cast doubt on previous attempts at statistical analysis, while not as yet offering the scope for a new analysis.

Consequently any current attempt at classification can merely aim to make retrospective data uniform, as far as possible, with a view to a more precise epidemiological classification in the future. In this respect, the statistical data can be related both to the type of lesion and the type of sport.

Types of lesion

Shoulder lesions can be divided into macrotraumatic (rotator cuff ruptures, dislocations, some lesions of the glenoid labrum and fractures) and microtraumatic, which are more frequent and insidious, and which form the subject of this chapter.

Microtraumatic lesions include glenohumeral instability and subluxations (posterior, anterior and multidirectional), internal and subacromial impingement, bursitis, tendinitis and lesions of the glenoid labrum. They also include less common disorders such as vascular compression, neurological syndromes, exostosis, spontaneous fractures and others.

Glenohumeral instability

Shoulder instability is regarded as the underlying cause of the majority of disorders complained of by overhead athletes (Silliman, 1991), and there is, therefore, insufficient information on its actual incidence. This is attributable to numerous factors, such as the difficulty of discriminating between a physiological

Epidemiology of shoulder lesions in sport

increase in glenohumeral translation as an expression of functional adaptation and asymptomatic patho-logical laxity (Bigliani, 1997), the relative novelty of the concept of occult instability related to painful shoulder (Jobe, 1989), and objective diagnostic and interpretational problems (Pappas, 1995).

There are, furthermore, no quantitative data on glenohumeral translation to help determine, in the vari-ous forms of instability, how much is due to insuffi-ciency of the active or passive stabilizer muscles, both labral and ligamentous, although some observations suggest alterations of the latter in atraumatic forms (Von Eisenhart-Rothe, 2002).

Radiological studies in athletes with persistent shoulder disorders due to transient subluxation have shown that in 89.6% of cases there are various degrees of injury of the glenoid labrum, including anterior fractures (69.2%), posterior fractures (7.6%) and local degenerative alterations (23.2%) (Rossi, 1991).

Lesions of the glenoid labrum

Pain and pseudo-obstruction in the cocking phase of throwing with the limb abducted at 90° and externally rotated are due, in the vast majority of cases, to a type II SLAP lesion of the glenoid labrum (Jobe, 1995).

This affects overhead athletes in more than half of observations and consists of posterior labrum lesions in 47% of cases and combined anteroposterior lesions in 37% (Morgan, 1998).

Impingement

The cocking position with the limb abducted at 90° and in maximum external rotation may also cause internal impingement of the rotator cuff against the posterosuperior glenoid (Walch, 1993), which is responsible for the appearance of posterior shoulder pain. Internal impingement has been documented in water polo players (Giombini, 1997), baseball players and quarterbacks (Paley, 2000). Arthroscopy has demonstrated a partial rupture of the deep portion of the rotator cuff in 90% of cases, associated almost invariably with lesions of the glenoid labrum. The rup-ture affected the supraspinatus (53%), the supraspina-tus and the infraspinatus (32%) or the infraspinatus alone (4%). The labrum had a meniscal appearance (45%) or a non-meniscal appearance (55%) or appeared to be normal (18%), fringed (38%) or fis-sured (52%). In 88% of cases the lesions affected the posterosuperior portion of the labrum and in 36% the anterior portion (Paley, 2000; Riand, 2002).

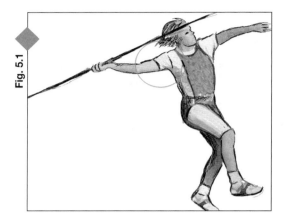

Fig. 5.1

External impingement of the rotator cuff between the humeral head and the coracoacromial arch causes worsening inflammation of the tendon and bursa struc-tures (Neer, 1983), correlated with recurrent micro-traumas associated with the repetitive nature of the athletic action. External impingement syndrome there-fore frequently affects older athletes. Studies show a relative prevalence of 58–64% in baseball players, 9–14% in tennis players, 4–12% in swimmers and a lower prevalence in javelin throwers (Fig. 5.1), volleyball players and players of American football (Roye, 1995; Tibone, 1986).

Exostosis

Posteroinferior glenoid exostosis, often associated with rotator cuff and labrum lesions and known as 'Bennett lesion' (Bennett, 1941), has been found in 33–100% of cases of posterior shoulder pain in top level baseball players (Barnes, 1978; Lombardo, 1977; Meister, 1999).

Vascular pathology

Chronic vascular lesions with occlusion, thrombosis or aneurysmatic dilation due to compression of the axil-lary artery by the pectoralis minor muscle or of the sub-clavian artery by the anterior scalene in hyperabduction of the upper limb have been described in a small num-ber of cases concerning baseball pitchers and volley-ball and water polo players (McCarthy, 1989; Nuber, 1990; Sereni, 1982; Tullos, 1972).

Reports of combined compression of the humeral circumflex artery and the axillary nerve in 'quadrilateral space syndrome', as it is called, are equally rare (Cahill, 1983).

Nerve pathology

Entrapment of the suprascapular nerve in the scapular notch with isolated atrophy of the infraspinatus muscle causes a disorder that is usually pain-free, and observed frequently in volleyballers (Ferretti, 1998). A smaller number of reports relates, however, to baseball players (Cummins, 1999).

Fractures

The stress caused by sudden, violent torque may cause spontaneous fractures of the humerus in throwers, particularly if they are over the age of 30 and relatively unfit (Branch, 1992). The case of an acute stress fracture of the proximal humeral epiphysis has, however, been reported in an elite junior badminton player, suffering from chronic shoulder pain following particularly intense training (Boyd, 1997).

Types of sports

The complex dynamics of throwing may be critical to the integrity of the glenohumeral structures, particularly during the acceleration and deceleration phases which come before and after the release of the equipment.

Volleyball

Shoulder injuries account for 8–20% of lesions affecting volleyball players (Goodwin-Gerberich, 1987; Schafle, 1990) and usually consist of tendinitis of the rotator cuff or biceps (Schafle, 1990). The great susceptibility of the shoulder is due to the repeated movements of abduction and external rotation, followed by extension and internal rotation of the upper limb, the compressive effect of which on the intra-articular structures is accentuated in the smash by the impact with the ball at the point of maximum abduction of the arm (Fig. 5.2).

An unusual condition in the general context of disorders due to wear, but one which affects more than 32% of elite volleyballers, is compression of the suprascapular nerve by the infraspinatus muscle at the spinoglenoid notch (Ferretti, 1998; Holzgraefe, 1994). This condition occurs particularly in the 'floating' serve, where the player stops the arm movement immediately

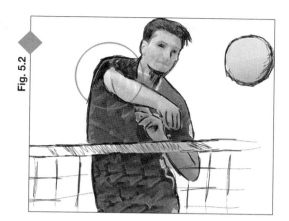

Fig. 5.2

after hitting the ball, to give it the desired effect, thus causing a forced eccentric contraction of the infraspinatus muscle. In many cases, this condition goes unrecognized or is marked at most by weakness in external rotation and slight hypotrophy of the infraspinatus muscle. In other cases, concomitant tendinitis causes severe pain, which may require surgical decompression (Ferretti, 1987; Takagishi, 1994).

Tennis

Racquet sports, such as tennis, have biomechanical characteristics similar to throwing and it should consequently not be surprising that the shoulder has proved to be the primary site of over use lesions. The incidence of such lesions ranges from 22–24% of cases in junior athletes (Kibler, 1988; Lehman, 1988) to 50% in middle-aged players (Lehman, 1988), and 56% in top level players (Priest, 1976), related to the number of serves and smashes that occur in the course of training sessions and competitions (Fig. 5.3).

The clinical examination of competitive tennis players with painful shoulder has demonstrated, in the majority of cases, subacromial impingement, which is almost invariably isolated and involves the biceps tendons and rotator cuff muscles (Lehman, 1988; Priest, 1976; Richardson, 1983). Some players, however, exhibit frank shoulder instability (Hawkins, 1983; Richardson, 1983), and glenoid labrum lesions (Lehman, 1988).

Posterior labrum tears may additionally occur during the cocking phase of the service, while anterior ruptures are possible during the acceleration and deceleration

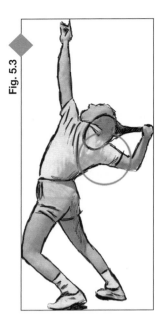

Fig. 5.3

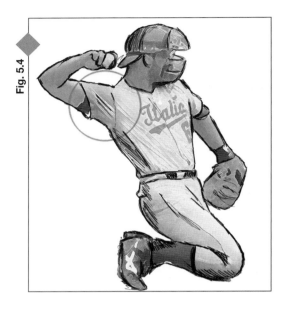

Fig. 5.4

phases of the service itself and the smash (Gregg, 1998).

These same actions may also cause a stress lesion of the long thoracic nerve in particularly susceptible individuals (Gregg, 1979).

The repeated tensions exerted by the supraspinatus on the greater tuberosity and by the subscapularis on the lesser tuberosity of the humerus may give rise to 'Osgood-Schlatter disease' of the shoulder involving pain, swelling, signs of impingement and radiographic alterations of the ossification of the proximal apophysis of the humerus. The problem occurs particularly during early adolescence, when ossification happens more rapidly (Gregg, 1998).

The induction of excessive muscle development may similarly cause osteochondrosis of the end of the acromion, where the deltoid tendon inserts, and of the end of the coracoid process, owing to traction of the short head of the biceps and the coracobrachial (Gregg, 1998).

Baseball and softball

In baseball and softball, which can be seen as typical examples of overhead sports, there is a significant association between the number of pitches performed

in a game and in a season and the incidence of shoulder pain (Lyman, 2002) (Fig. 5.4). The risk of injury consequently increases with age and competitive level (Oberlander, 2000).

The incidence of shoulder lesions among the young varies from 15–22% of cases seen in medical consultation. Furthermore, approximately 20% of lesions sustained by junior players affect the shoulder, with a peak of 21.6% among pitchers (16.3% of softball pitchers) (Powell, 1999). The percentage rises to 24–34% among senior players (Loosli, 1992; McFarland, 1998) and more than 56% among professional pitchers (Barnes, 1978).

Curve balls increase the risk of shoulder pain by 52% (Lyman, 2002). In any case, the complex kinematics of the pitch and in particular the torque and compression forces on the glenohumeral joint structures developed at the ends of the movement arc (Fleisig, 1995) create the potential for shoulder injuries, particularly in the presence of an imbalance between joint stability and flexibility (Gowan, 1987; Otis, 1990; Pappas, 1985).

Excessive translation of the humeral head, encouraged by capsule laxity, muscle weakness or fatigue, may thus cause entrapment and anterior or posterior labrum tears (McLeod, 1986); the deceleration forces of the abducted and internally rotated upper limb may cause impingement of the rotator cuff or the biceps against the coracoacromial arch owing to the superior translation of the humeral head (Andrews, 1988), or

SLAP type labrum ruptures owing to the violent contraction of the long head of the biceps (Jobe, 1984; Moynes, 1986; Sisto, 1987).

Water polo

The few data available on shoulder injuries in water polo players mention an incidence of 33% in members of the US team, attributing the disorders in the vast majority of cases to tendinitis of the rotator cuff and, in the remaining cases, to degeneration of the AC joint (Rollins, 1985). It has been demonstrated more recently that the principal cause of painful shoulder in water polo players is posterosuperior glenoid impingement, which occurs during the phase of maximum abduction and external rotation of the upper limb when shooting (Giombini, 1997) (Fig. 5.5).

Rare injuries include the case of a player affected by isolated paralysis of the anterior serratus muscle of odontogenic focal origin, which subsequently developed into a picture of compression of the cervicobrachial nervovascular bundle, owing to compensatory hypertrophy of the pectoralis minor muscle (Sereni, 1982).

Pain referred to the shoulder could finally be due to radiculitis owing to cervical osteoarthritis, caused by continual hyperlordosis stresses, related to the characteristic swimming style with the head out, and sudden rotations and flexions of the head occurring at various times during play. This type of cervicobrachialgia affects 15% of water polo players (Rettagliata, 1968).

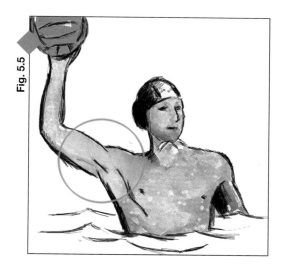

Fig. 5.5

Swimming

Although they are not throwers, swimmers share a number of biomechanical techniques with throwers and consequently suffer many of the same shoulder injuries.

According to US studies, the prevalence of painful shoulder (males vs. females) ranges from 10–13% in junior swimmers to 21–25% in seniors, and to 18–35% in national team athletes. However, according to a survey, the incidence of episodes of painful shoulder increases overall to 47%, 66% and 73%, respectively (McMaster, 1993).

Specialization in one style, with the possible exception of butterfly, and racing distance does not seem to influence the incidence of episodes of painful shoulder (Greipp, 1985), which seem to be related more to competitive level and years of activity (McMaster, 1993). An elite swimmer undergoing typical daily training may move his shoulder to the limits of the movement arc in approximately 2 million strokes in the course of one year, accounting for 75–90% in freestyle (Ciullo, 1989; Kammer, 1999). Furthermore, competitive swimmers usually start at around 7 years old.

This results in chronic functional overload with repeated microtraumas, which frequently leads to shoulder lesions (McMaster, 1996), often aggravated by excessive or inappropriate 'dry' training based on stretching and strength exercises with weights, and, in water, by the use of paddles and kickboards (Greipp, 1985; McMaster, 1996; McMaster, 1986; Stocker, 1995), too medialized entry of the hand, breathing on one side only, insufficient kick, and loss of roll and buoyancy, typical of tired swimmers (Kenal, 1996; McMaster, 1986).

Most lesions are related to shoulder instability (Bak, 1997; McMaster, 1998), particularly in the anterior and inferior direction, which could represent a congenital characteristic of elite swimmers (Zemek, 1996), but which can also result from two specific requirements to improve swimming performance, i.e. increasing the amplitude of the movement arc, and strength in adduction and internal rotation of the upper limb (Weldon, 2001). To stabilize the humeral head in the glenoid cavity, swimmers with abnormal shoulder laxity increase the tension of the rotator cuff muscles, and this irritates the supraspinatus tendon in particular, which may be subject to acute inflammation; local oedema reduces the subacromial space further, causing secondary compression and in some cases subacromial bursitis. The degenerative effects of impingement of the supraspinatus are aggravated by the repeated 'squeezing' of its blood supply during adduction, which occurs at the end of the traction phase and at the end of the stroke (Kenal, 1996).

Among swimmers, 70% with painful shoulder show signs associated with impingement and glenohumeral instability, whereas cases of laxity without impingement are fairly uncommon (11%) (Bak, 1997).

Gymnastics

Although gymnastics is included as an overhead sport, there have been few reports of shoulder injuries among gymnasts. A study of 13 elite gymnasts has shown that 6 (43%) complained of shoulder pain, manifested acutely during the ring exercise (Fig. 5.6) and in one case on the parallel bars. Electromyography has shown that there is a 'critical phase' of fairly slight muscle activity around the shoulder while the gymnast is hanging from the rings, which may increase joint stress related to exercise. This could explain the occurrence of glenoid labrum lesions, including labrum detachment, observed arthroscopically (Caraffa, 1996).

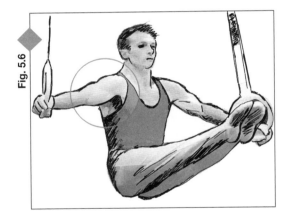

Fig. 5.6

Golf

Although golf is not included as an overhead sport, it is also characterized by a technical action (swing) that is potentially pathogenic for the shoulder structures, particularly during the back swing, at the apex of which the non-dominant upper limb is in a forced position in internal rotation, flexion and maximum adduction (Fig. 5.7).

A competitive golfer adopts this position more than 2000 times a week, and this predisposes the athlete to wear lesions; complete adduction overloads the AC

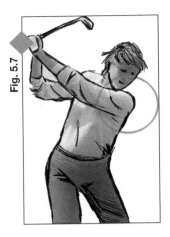

Fig. 5.7

joint and causes subacromial impingement, while internal rotation and flexion force the greater tuberosity of the humerus against the anterior acromion. A total of 10–15% of golfers suffer from acromioclavicular osteoarthritis or rotator cuff lesions. Finally, the entire back swing creates the conditions for posterior instability of the non-dominant shoulder, which increases the risk of joint lesions (Hovis, 2002).

Bibliography

Andrews J.R., Angelo R.L., 'Shoulder arthroscopy for the throwing athlete', *Tech. Orthop.* 3: 75–81, (1988)

Bak K., Faunl P., 'Clinical findings in competitive swimmers with shoulder pain', *Am. J. Sports Med.* 25: 254–260, (1997)

Bak K., Magnusson S.P., 'Shoulder strength and range of motion in symptomatic and pain-free elite swimmers', *Am. J. Sports Med.* 25: 454–459, (1997)

Barnes D.A., Tullos H.S., 'Analysis of 100 symptomatic baseball players', *Am. J. Sports Med.* 6: 62–67, (1978)

Bennett G.E., 'Shoulder and elbow lesions of the professional baseball pitchers', *JAMA* 117: 510–514, (1941)

Bigliani L.U., Codd T.P., Connor P.M. et al., 'Shoulder motion and laxity in the professional baseball players', *Am. J. Sports Med.* 25: 609–613, (1997)

Boyd K.T., Batt M.E., 'Stress fracture of the proximal humeral epiphysis in an elite junior badminton player', *Br. J. Sports Med.* 31: 252–253, (1997)

Branch T., Partin C., Chamberland P. et al., 'Spontaneous fractures of the humerus during pitching: a series of 12 cases', *Am. J. Sports Med.* 20: 468–470, (1992)

Cahill B.R., Palmer R.E., 'Quadrilateral space syndrome', *J. Hand Surg.* 8: 65–69, (1983)

Caraffa A., Cerulli G., Rizzo A., Buompadre V., Appoggetti S., Fortuna M., 'An arthroscopic and electromyographic study of painful shoulders in elite gymnasts', *Knee Surg. Sports Traumatol. Arthros.* 4: 39–42, (1996)

Ciullo J.V., Stevens G.G., 'Prevention and treatment of injuries to the shoulder in swimming', *Sports Med.* 7: 182–204, (1989)

Cummins C.A., Bowen M., Anderson K. et al., 'Suprascapular nerve entrapment in the spinoglenoid notch in a professional baseball pitcher', *Am. J. Sports Med.* 27: 810–812, (1999)

Ferretti A., Cerullo G., Russo G., 'Suprascapular neuropathy in volleyball players', *J. Bone Joint Surg.* (Am) 69: 260–263, (1987)

Ferretti A., De carli A., Fontana M., 'Injury of the suprascapular nerve at the spinoglenoid notch. The natural history of infraspinatus atrophy in volleyball players', *Am. J. Sports Med.* 26: 759–763, (1998)

Fleisig G.S., Andrews J.R., Dillman C.J., Escamilla R.F., 'Kinetics of baseball pitching with implications for injury mechanisms', *Am. J. Sports Med.* 23: 233–239, (1995)

Giombini A., Rossi F., Pettrone F.A. et al., 'Posterosuperior glenoid rim impingement as a cause of shoulder pain in top level water polo player', *J. Sports Med. Phys. Fitness* 37: 273–278, (1997)

Goodwin-Gerberich S.G., Luhmann S., Finke C. et al., 'Analysis of severe injuries associated with volleyball activities', *Phys. Sports Med.* 15: 75–79, (1987)

Gowan I.D., Jobe F.W., Tibone J.E. et al., 'A comparative electromyographic analysis of the shoulder during pitching. Professional versus amateur pitchers', *Am. J. Sports Med.* 15: 586–590, (1987)

Gregg J.R., Labosky D., Harthy M. et al., 'Serratus anterior paralysis in young athletes', *J. Bone Joint Surg.* (Am) 61: 825–832, (1979)

Gregg J.R., Torg J.R., 'Upper extremity injuries in adolescent tennis players', *Clin. Sports Med.* 7: 371–385, (1998)

Greipp J.F., 'Swimmer's shoulder: the influence of flexibility and weight training', *Phys. Sports Med.* 13: 92–105, (1985)

Hawkins R.J., Hobeika P.E., 'Impingement syndrome in the athletic shoulder', *Clin. Sports Med.* 2: 391–405, (1983)

Holzgraefe M., Kukowski B., Eggert S., 'Prevalence of latent and manifest suprascapular neuropathy in high-performance volleyball players', *Br. J. Sports Med.* 28: 177–179, (1994)

Hovis W.D., Dean M.T., Mallon W.J., Hawkins R.F., 'Posterior instability of the shoulder with secondary impingement in elite golfers', *Am. J. Sports Med.* 30: 886–890, (2002)

Jobe C.M., 'Posterior superior glenoid impingement. Expanded spectrum', *Arthroscopy* 11: 530–537, (1995)

Jobe F.W., Kivtne R.S., Giangarra C.E., 'Shoulder pain in the overhand or throwing athlete. The relationship of anterior instability and rotator cuff impingement', *Orthop. Rev.* 18: 963–975, (1989)

Jobe F.W., Moynes D.R., Tibone J.E. et al., 'EMG analysis of the shoulder in pitching', *Am. J. Sports Med.* 12: 218–220, (1984)

Kammer C.S., Young C.C., Niedfeld T M.W., 'Swimming injuries and illnesses', *Phys. Sports Med.* 27: 51–60, (1999)

Kenal K.A., Knapp L.D., 'Rehabilitation of injuries in competitive swimmers', *Sports Med.* 22: 337–347, (1996)

Kibler W.B., McQueen C., Uhl T., 'Fitness evaluation and fitness findings in competitive junior tennis players', *Clin. Sports Med.* 7: 403–416, (1988)

Lehman R.C., 'Shoulder pain in competitive tennis players', *Clin. Sports Med.* 7: 309–327, (1988)

Lombardo S., Jobe F.W., Kerlan R.K. et al., 'Posterior shoulder lesions in throwing athletes', *Am. J. Sports Med.* 5: 106–110, (1977)

Loosli A.R., Requa R.K., Garrick J.G. et al., 'Injuries to pitchers in women's collegiate fast-pitch softball', *Am. J. Sports Med.* 20: 35–37, (1992)

Lyman S., Fleming G.S., Andrews J.R., Osinski F.D., 'Effect of pitch type, pitch count, and pitching mechanics on risk of elbow and shoulder pain in youth baseball pitchers', *Am. J. Sports Med.* 30: 463–468, (2002)

McCarthy W.J., Yaos J.S., Schafer M.F. et al., 'Upper extremity arterial injury in athletes', *J. Vasc. Surg.* 9: 317–321, (1989)

McFarland E.G., Wasik M., 'Epidemiology of collegiate baseball injuries', *Clin. J. Sports Med.* 8: 10–13, (1998)

McLeod W.D., Andrews J.R., 'Mechanisms of shoulder injuries', *Phys. Ther.* 66: 1901–1904, (1986)

McMaster W.C., 'Painful shoulder in swimmers: a diagnostic challenge', *Phys. Sports Med.* 14: 108–122, (1986)

McMaster W.C., 'Swimming injuries: an overview', *Sports Med.* 22: 332–336, (1996)

McMaster W.C., Roberts A., Stoddard T., 'A correlation between shoulder laxity and interfering pain in competitive swimmers', *Am. J. Sports Med.* 26: 83–86, (1998)

McMaster W.C., Troup S., 'A survey of interfering shoulder pain in United States competitive swimmers', *Am. J. Sports Med.* 21: 67–70, (1993)

Meister K., Andrews J.R., Batts J.B. et al., 'Symptomatic thrower's exostosis. Arthroscopic evaluation and treatment', *Am. J. Sports Med.* 27: 133–136, (1999)

Morgan C.D., Burkhart S.S., Palmeri M. et al., 'Type II SLAP-lesions: three subtypes and their relationship to superior instability and rotator cuff tears', *Arthroscopy* 14: 553–565, (1998)

Moynes D.R., Perry J., Antonelli D.J. et al., 'Electromyograpy and motion analysis of the upper extremity in sports', *Phys. Ther.* 66: 1905–1911, (1986)

Neer C.S., 'Impingement lesions', *Clin. Orthop.* 173: 70–77, (1983)

Nuber G.W., McCarthy W.J., Yaos J.S. et al., 'Arterial abnormalities of the shoulder in athletes', *Am. J. Sports Med.* 18: 514–519, (1990)

Oberlander M.A., Chisar M.A., Campbell B., 'Epidemiology of shoulder injuries in throwing and overhead athletes', *Sports Med. Arthrosc. Rev.* 8: 115–123, (2000)

Otis J.C., Warren R.F., Backus S.I. et al., 'Torque production in the shoulder of the normal young adult male: the interaction of function, dominance, joint angle, and angular velocity', *Am. J. Sports Med.* 18: 119–123, (1990)

Paley K.J., Jobe F.W., Pink M.M. et al., 'Arthroscopic findings in the overhand throwing athlete: evidence for posterior or internal impingement of the rotator cuff', *Arthroscopy* 16: 35–40, (2000)

Pappas A.M., Goss T.P. 'Glenohumeral instability', In: Pappas A.M. (eds.), 'Upper Extremity Injuries in the Athlete', Churchill Livingston, New York, pp. 193–212, (1995)

Pappas A.M., Zawacki R.M., Sullivan J.J., 'Biomechanics of baseball pitching: a preliminary report', *Am. J. Sports Med.* 13: 216–222, (1985)

Epidemiology of shoulder lesions in sport

Powell J.W., Barber-Foss K.D., 'Injury patterns in selected high school sports: a review of the 1995–97 season', *J. Athletic Train* 34: 277–284, (1999)

Priest J.D., Nagel D.A., 'Tennis shoulder', *Am. J. Sports Med.* 4: 28–42, (1976)

Rettagliata F., Pisu G., 'Osservazioni cliniche e radiografiche sul rachide cervicale dei pallanuotisti', *Med. Sport* 21: 53–57, (1968)

Riand N., Boulahia A., Walch G., 'Posterosuperior impingement of the shoulder in the athlete: results of arthroscopic debridement in 75 patients', Rev. *Chir. Orthop. Reparatrice Appar. Mot.* 88: 19–27, (2002)

Richardson A.B., 'Overuse syndrome in baseball, tennis, gymnastics, and swimming', *Clin. Sports Med.* 2: 379–389, (1983)

Rollins J., Puffer J.C., Whiting W.C., 'Water polo injuries to the upper extremity', In: Zarins B., Andrews J.R., Carson W.G. (eds.), *Injuries to the throwing arm*, W.B. Saunders, Philadelphia, pp. 311–317, (1985)

Rossi F., Dragoni S., Giombini A., 'Painful gleno-humeral joint instability in athletes. Radiographic findings', *Radiol. Med.* 81: 813–817, (1991)

Roye R.P., Grana W.A., Yates C.K. Arthroscopic subacromial decompression: two-to-seven-year follow-up. Arthroscopy 11: 301–306, (1995)

Schafle M.D., Requa R.K., Patton W.L. et al., 'Injuries in the 1987 national amateur volleyball tournament', *Am. J. Sports Med.* 18: 624–631, (1990)

Sereni G., Reggiani E., Odaglia G., Chiodini G., 'Isolated paralysis of the anterior serratus muscle in an athlete. Some aspects of rehabilitation therapy', *J. Sports Traumatology* 4: 243–249, (1982)

Silliman J.F., Hawkins R.J., 'Current concepts and recent advances in the athlete's shoulder', *Clin. Sports Med.* 10: 693–705, (1991)

Sisto D.J., Jobe F.W., Moynes D.R. et al., 'An electromyographic analysis of the elbow in pitching', *Am. J. Sports Med.* 15: 206–263, (1987)

Stocker D., Pink M., Jobe F.W., 'Comparison of shoulder injuries in collegiate and master's level swimmers', *Clin. J. Sports Med.* 5: 4–8, (1995)

Takagishi K., Saitoh A., Tonegawa M. et al., 'Isolated paralysis of the supraspinatus muscle', *J. Bone Joint Surg.* (Br) 76: 584–587, (1994)

Tibone J.E., Elrod B., Jobe F.W. et al., 'Surgical treatment of tears of the rotator cuff in athletes', *J. Bone Joint Surg.* (Am) 68: 887–891, (1986)

Tullos H.S., Erwin W.D., Woods G.W. et al., 'Unusual lesions of the pitching arm', *Clin. Orthop.* 88: 169–182, (1972)

Vastamaki M., Kauppila L.I., 'Etiologic factors in isolated paralysis of the serratus anterior muscle: a report of 97 cases', *J. Shoulder Elbow Surg.* 2: 5–12, (1993)

Von Eisenhart-Rothe R., Jager A., Englmeier K., Vogl T., Graicher H., 'Relevance of arm position and muscle activity on three-dimensional glenohumeral translation in patients with traumatic and atraumatic shoulder instability', *Am. J. Sports Med.* 30: 514–522, (2002)

Walch G., Liotard J.P., Boileau J. et al., 'Postero-superior glenoid impingement. Another impingement of the shoulder', *J. Radiol.* 74: 47, (1993)

Weldon E.J. 3rd, Richardson A.B., 'Upper extremity overuse injuries in swimming. A discussion of swimmer's shoulder', *Clin. Sports Med.* 20: 423–438, (2001)

Zemek M.J., Magee D.J., 'Comparison of glenohumeral joint laxity in elite and recreational swimmers', *Clin. J. Sports Med.* 6: 40–47, (1996)

SPECIALIST EXAMINATION

CHAPTER 6

G. VILLANI

Pain is almost invariably the symptom, in shoulder disorders, that leads the patient to consult a doctor for a specialist examination.

A clinical examination should be carried out in order to diagnose whether the disorder the patient is suffering from actually originates in the shoulder joint complex and what the disease involved is, but an attempt should also be made to understand what type of patient is being examined.

The choice of the subsequent diagnostic and therapeutic strategy is determined by the age, limitations, requirements and expectations of the patient.

The evaluation of a rotator cuff lesion in an elderly patient with moderate functional requirements is different from that of a young patient with a manual occupation; similarly instability in a sedentary patient or in a high level competitive athlete should be viewed differently (Rockwood, 1999).

The instruments available for the precise classification of the patient and for an adequate diagnosis are a detailed case history and a correct objective examination, based on the careful application and interpretation of the many functional tests.

A careful clinical evaluation should not be neglected owing to the use nowadays of increasingly sophisticated imaging examinations; unfortunately this is increasingly the case. Imaging should be used merely to summarize and confirm a diagnosis, or at the least a suspected diagnosis, already obtained in both cases.

History

A careful clinical history of the patient can reveal whether pain reported in the shoulder actually originates there or whether it is attributable to a disorder of other anatomical structures.

Pain reported by patients in the shoulder frequently originates in the cervical spine. In this case the patient places a hand on the upper surface of the shoulder, in the region of the clavicle and trapezius, to indicate the exact location of the pain; pain spreading along the upper limb in radicular disease generally reaches the hand and fingers, whereas pain starting from the shoulder spreads up to and no further than the elbow.

Other disorders may also involve shoulder pain, though more rarely, as a related symptom, for example cardiological or lung diseases of the chest, and hepatic or gall bladder diseases of the abdomen (Porcellini, 2003).

Shoulder pain and functional loss of power may also be a corollary of systemic diseases such as rheumatoid arthritis or adhesive capsulitis, which occurs fairly frequently in diabetic patients; these possibilities should, therefore, also be carefully investigated.

The following parameters should be evaluated in patients with shoulder disorders:

- age;
- work and sports;
- traumas; and
- type of pain.

The patient's age can provide clues. Degenerative rotator cuff rupture generally occurs in patients over 40–45 years, while between the ages of 25 and 40 subacromial impingement syndrome is more common, and unstable painful shoulder is typical of young athletes (Porcellini, 2003).

The type of work or sport can often be the cause of a painful shoulder. It is necessary to know what type of work patients do or what sports they play, to be able to understand whether they involve lifting weights, overhead activity such as whitewashing, or an overhead sport such as volleyball or water polo, or whether there may be a high incidence of injury, such as in contact sports.

Patients frequently report the appearance of pain as a result of an injury, particularly for an insurance claim, but a careful examination may reveal that the reported injury is often not severe enough to justify the occurrence of the disorder alone. An injury which is the possible cause of the anatomical damage may, however, have preceded the appearance of the symptoms by a long way and the patient consequently neglected to mention this.

The type of pain reported by the patient is of vital importance in the differential diagnosis. The site, spread, association with certain movements or postures, possible exacerbation at night, and manner of appearance should consequently be evaluated.

Objective examination

The objective examination of the shoulder comprises the following:
- inspection;
- palpation;
- mobility; and
- specific functional tests.

Inspection

The inspection should evaluate the conformation of the shoulder and the status of the muscles.

A winged scapula can sometimes be detected, which is frequently a sign of long thoracic nerve deficit with secondary paralysis of the anterior serratus muscle.

A prominence on the scapular spine is generally due to hypotrophy of the muscles of the supraspinous or infraspinous fossa, typical of lesions of the rotator cuff tendon.

Atrophy of the deltoid is manifested by loss of the normal roundness of the shoulder, which takes on an 'epaulette shoulder' appearance. Distal displacement of the muscle belly of the biceps is indicative of rupture of the long head of the biceps, a lesion which almost never occurs in isolation, generally being associated with rotator cuff rupture.

A raised lateral end of the clavicle is a sign of acute or previous dislocation of the AC joint.

Palpation

Shoulder palpation is performed to identify the location of painful points which may be in the AC joint, if this joint is affected by osteoarthritis or instability, in the region of the trochanter of the humerus in rotator cuff disorder, or in the bicipital groove in tendinitis of the long head of the biceps.

Palpation can also demonstrate articular crepitus, which is frequent.

Symptomatic subacromial crepitus, i.e. crepitus associated with the symptoms the patient is complaining of, is often caused by subacromial impingement and can be perceived by placing the thumb and the other fingers on the anterior and posterior rims, respectively, of the acromion during movements of the humerus on the scapula.

Glenohumeral crepitus, which is generally louder than subacromial crepitus, is demonstrated more easily when elevating and lowering the limb against resistance, and it is often due to arthropathy secondary to massive rotator cuff rupture (Neer, 1997).

Mobility

The shoulder has the greatest mobility of all the body's joints in all the spatial planes and the four joints that form it contribute to this, i.e. the sternoclavicular, acromioclavicular and above all scapulothoracic and glenohumeral.

The ratio of contribution to movement between the glenohumeral and scapulothoracic varies from 2:1 to 5:4, with an increase in the scapulothoracic component as elevation progresses (Rockwood, 1999).

Diseases that cause stiffness, such as adhesive capsulitis or glenohumeral osteoarthritis, alter this ratio in favour of the scapulothoracic component.

It is therefore necessary, when evaluating the movement arc, to observe the lateral movement of the lower angle of the scapula, comparing it with the opposite side, and to examine the movement keeping the scapula down.

Passive joint function must always be distinguished from active joint function when evaluating shoulder mobility. A reduction in active joint function while the passive function is unaffected is a frequent characteristic of neurological deficit or rotator cuff lesion, although articular limitation related to the analgesic reaction could invalidate the evaluation.

Compensatory movements of the spinal column and pelvis may influence and mislead the examiner when measuring joint mobility. The effect of this can be limited by evaluating abduction and internal rotation with the patient seated, while the supine position allows a more accurate examination of elevation and external rotation (Rockwood, 1999).

An objective examination of the shoulder can be supplemented by functional tests specific to the type of disorder.

Specific functional tests

Functional tests are divided into the following:
- tests for impingement;
- tests for the rotator cuff;
- tests for the long head of the biceps;
- tests for the glenoid labrum; and
- tests for instability.

Tests for impingement

Tests for impingement should be considered positive when they trigger pain, demonstrating impingement between the rotator cuff and the coracoacromial arch.
- *Neer sign:* the examiner stands behind the patient and performs passive elevation of the internally rotated arm keeping the scapula down (Çalis, 2000; Murrel, 2001; Porcellini, 2003; Rockwood, 1999; Tennet, 2003; Vienne, 1998) (Fig. 6.1);

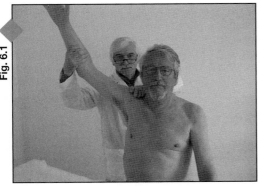

Fig. 6.1

Neer sign.

- *Hawkins test:* the arm is rapidly rotated internally keeping the shoulder and elbow flexed at 90° (Çalis, 2000; Murrel, 2001; Porcellini, 2003; Rockwood, 1999; Tennet, 2003; Vienne, 1998) (Fig. 6.2);

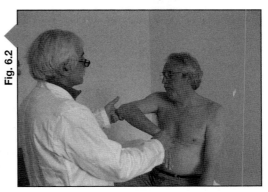

Fig. 6.2

Hawkins test.

- *Yocum's test:* this is performed by asking the patient to place a hand on the opposite shoulder and to push the elbow upwards against resistance provided by the examiner (Yergason, 1931) (Fig. 6.3);

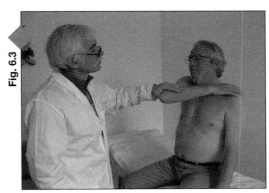

Fig. 6.3

Yocum's test.

- *Internal rotation resistance strength test (IRRST):* the examiner stands behind the patient and holds the arm at 90° abduction and approximately 80° external rotation. The patient is asked first to perform external rotation and then internal rotation against resistance. If the patient shows lower resistance to internal rotation than to external rotation, the test is considered to be positive for internal (non-outlet) impingement (Zaslav, 2001); and
- *Gerber's test:* this test is performed by carrying out passive adduction with the shoulder rotated internally and flexed at 90° and is positive in cases of coracoid impingement (Porcellini, 2003; Rockwood, 1999; Vienne, 1998).

Specialist examination

SECTION II

Tests for the rotator cuff

These may be tests against resistance or tests of holding position and they evaluate rotator cuff tendon integrity and muscle strength.

Tests against resistance

- *Jobe's test:* with the shoulder abducted at 90°, forwards by 30° and rotated internally (thumbs downwards), the patient is required to resist pressure exerted downwards by the examiner. This test is actually considered to be intermediate between the tests for impingement and for the rotator cuff. It is positive if pain appears and if resistance to the examiner's pressure is reduced. It evaluates the supraspinatus muscle, but muscle weakness may be difficult to assess owing to pain (Porcellini, 2003; Rockwood, 1999) (Fig. 6.4);

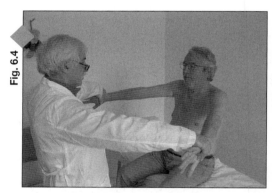

Jobe's test.

- *Test of external rotation against resistance in adduction:* the patient sits in front of the examiner with the shoulder adducted, in neutral rotation and with the elbow at 90°, and is asked to push in external rotation against resistance. This test assesses the infraspinatus muscle (Porcellini, 2003) (Fig. 6.5);
- *Patte's test:* the patient is asked to perform external rotation against resistance, with the shoulder abducted by 90° and the elbow flexed. This assesses the infraspinatus, like the previous test (Porcellini, 2003; Rockwood, 1999) (Fig. 6.6);
- *Lift-off test:* with a hand placed behind the back, the patient is required to push backwards against resistance. This evaluates the subscapularis muscle (Çalis, 2000; Hertel, 1996; Litaker, 2000; Murrel, 2001; Porcellini, 2003; Rockwood, 1999; Tennet, 2003; Vienne, 1998) (Fig. 6.7); and

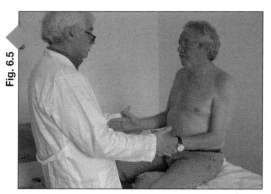

Test of external rotation against resistance in adduction.

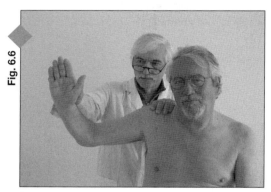

Patte's test.

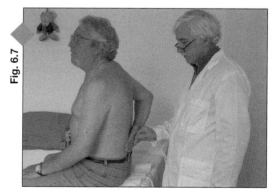

Lift-off test.

- *Napoleon test:* the patient has to push a hand against the abdomen against resistance. The test is positive when the patient does not succeed in exerting pressure comparable with that of the opposite arm or when the elbow tends to translate backwards while performing the test. It assesses the subscapularis and may be useful if the patient cannot perform the lift-off test or the IRLS owing to an inability to rotate the limb internally sufficiently because of pain or in overweight individuals (Rockwood, 1999) (Fig. 6.8).

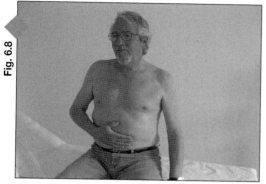

Fig. 6.8

Napoleon test.

Tests of holding position

- *External rotation lag sign (ERLS):* the examiner holds the shoulder in maximum external rotation and elevation at 20° with the elbow flexed at 90°, and lets go of the patient's hand; if the test is positive, there is a loss of external rotation of more than 5°, indicating superior cuff lesion (Rockwood, 1999);
- *Internal rotation lag sign (IRLS):* this is performed like the lift-off test, except it evaluates holding position. The examiner holds the patient's hand away from the back. The test is positive for a subscapularis lesion if, once the hand has been let go, the patient is unable to keep it in that position (Rockwood, 1999) (Fig. 6.9); and

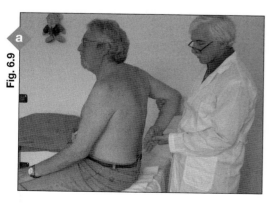

Fig. 6.9

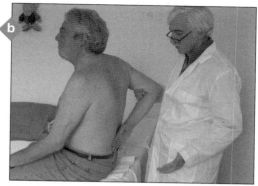

Internal rotation lag sign.

- *Drop sign:* this is a test of holding position: the shoulder is kept abducted at 90° in maximum external rotation with the elbow at 90°. If, when the hand is released, there is a loss of external rotation of more than 5°, this indicates a posterior cuff lesion (Murrel, 2001; Porcellini, 2003; Rockwood, 1999; Tennet, 2003) (Fig. 6.10).

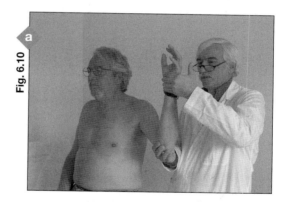

Fig. 6.10

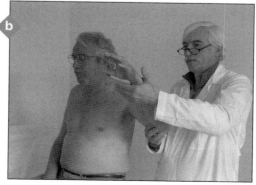

Drop sign.

Specialist examination

Tests for the long head of the biceps

- *Popeye or Ludington's sign:* this is performed by asking the patient to contract both biceps with the hands resting on the head: distal retraction of the muscle belly or lack of contraction is a sign of rupture of the long head of the biceps (Çalis, 2000; Porcellini, 2003; Rockwood, 1999);
- *Palm-up test (or Speed's or the Gilchrist test):* this is performed by asking the patient to elevate the arm against resistance keeping it tense, with the palm facing upwards. The test is considered positive if pain appears (Çalis, 2000; Porcellini, 2003; Rockwood, 1999) (Fig. 6.11); and

Fig. 6.12

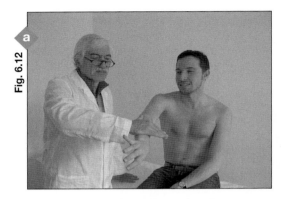

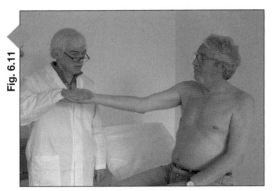

Fig. 6.11

Palm-up test (or Speed's or the Gilchrist test).

- *Yergason's test:* with the elbow flexed at 90° and next to the trunk, the patient is asked to perform external rotation against resistance in forced supination. The test is positive if pain appears in the bicipital groove, indicating subluxation of the tendon from the groove in which it slides (Burkhart, 2000; Porcellini, 2003; Rockwood, 1999, Yergason, 1931).

Tests for the glenoid labrum

- *O'Brien's test:* the patient sits with the shoulder flexed to 90° and in adduction by 10° and is asked to resist pressure exerted downwards by the examiner, first in maximum internal rotation and then in maximum external rotation. The test is considered positive if pain appears with the internally rotated limb (Fig. 6.12a) and the pain decreases with the limb externally rotated (Fig. 6.12b); this is a sign of glenoid labrum anomaly (SLAP lesion) (Kim, 1999, 2001; Lerat, 1994;

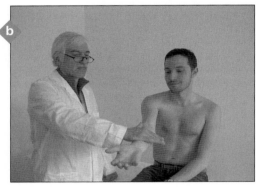

O'Brien's test.

Liu, 1996a, 1996b; Mc Farland, 1996; Mimori, 1999; O'Brien, 1998; Porcellini, 2003; Rockwood, 1999); and
- *Pain provocation test for SLAP:* the patient's limb is raised to 90–100° with the elbow flexed at 90° and the forearm in pronation; the forearm is then supinated and the patient is asked which of the two positions causes pain. If pain appears only or predominantly with the forearm in pronation, the test is considered positive for an upper labrum lesion (Mimori, 1999) (Fig. 6.13).

Tests for instability

- *Apprehension test:* the patient is seated with the shoulder abducted by 90° and the elbow flexed; the limb is externally rotated while the humeral head is gently pushed forwards by the other hand at the same time. This manoeuvre causes a patient with anterior shoulder instability to feel apprehension, which will be evident from the patient's face or words (the patient reports that the shoulder 'is

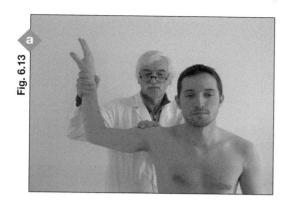

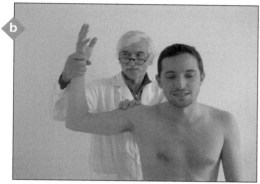

Pain provocation test for SLAP.

about to come out') (Henry, 1997; Liu, 1996b; Mc Farland, 1996; Porcellini, 2003; Rockwood, 1999, Vienne, 1998) (Fig. 6.14);

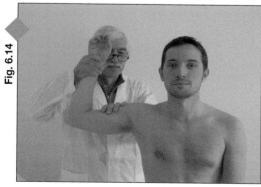

Apprehension test.

- *Fulcrum test:* the patient lies supine with the limb abducted and externally rotated by 90°. The examiner places a fist under the proximal humerus

to act as a fulcrum, while pushing the elbow downwards with the other hand. This manoeuvre causes anterior translation of the humeral head on the glenoid, prompting a similar reaction from the patient as the apprehension test (Burkhart, 2000; Liu, 1996b; Mimori, 1999; Porcellini, 2003; Rockwood, 1999, Vienne, 1998, Yocum, 1983) (Fig. 6.15);

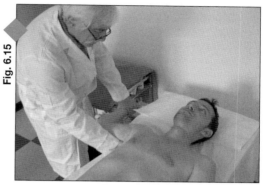

Fulcrum test.

- *Relocation test:* if the apprehension test and the fulcrum test are positive, the manoeuvre is repeated with the patient supine, using the edge of the bed as a fulcrum, but exerting pressure from the front to the back on the proximal end of the humerus. The test is positive if there is a reduction in apprehension and if it is possible to obtain greater external rotation (Henry, 1997; Porcellini, 2003; Rockwood, 1999, Vienne, 1998, Yocum, 1983); and
- *Load and shift test:* this test must be performed in either a seated position (with the arm in a neutral position) or a supine position (with the limb at 20° abduction and anterior flexion). Before performing the evaluation, the examiner should make sure that the humeral head is correctly centred in the glenoid, which may not be the case in patients with multidirectional instability or with scars from previous surgery. Once the humeral head has been pushed into the glenoid in a neutral position, it is grasped and translated in the anterior and posterior directions, by pushing with the thumb and index finger.

The quantification of humeral translation uses a grading scale recommended by the society of american shoulder and elbow surgeons (SASES):
- *Grade 0:* no translation;
- *Grade 1:* moderate translation (0–1 cm);

Specialist examination

- *Grade 2:* moderate translation towards the glenoid rim (1–2 cm);
- *Grade 3:* severe translation beyond the glenoid rim (2–3 cm):
  — with spontaneous reduction;
  — without spontaneous reduction (Fig. 6.16);
- *Sulcus sign:* the patient is seated with the limb in a neutral position and the examiner exerts pressure downwards on the elbow. The appearance of a groove immediately below the lateral rim of the acromion is observed in patients with multidirectional instability (Porcellini, 2003; Rockwood, 1999, Vienne, 1998, Yocum, 1983).

In order to be able to use the results obtained from specific functional tests correctly, the value of these tests for identifying the disorder must be known.

It is, therefore, important to clarify a number of fundamental principles to be applied to clinical tests.

Sensitivity is the ability of a test to identify individuals affected by the disorder. A high sensitivity (measured as a percentage) means that there is a high probability that the patient will have a positive test result, i.e. that the test yields few false negatives, but it gives no information about false positives or about how many healthy individuals will have a positive result.

This information is provided by the specificity, which is the ability of the test to identify healthy individuals.

A high specificity of a test indicates a high probability that a healthy individual will have a negative test result; the test thus yields few false positives but tells us nothing about false negatives, i.e. about how many patients will have negative results.

Accordingly, if a test with high sensitivity is positive, we will have no information on the disorder because it might be a false positive; if, however, it is negative, we will have a very high probability that the patient is not affected by the disorder tested for.

The opposite is the case with a test with high specificity, which, if positive, would indicate that the disorder is present with a high degree of probability, whereas if it is negative, it could not be ruled out with a sufficient degree of probability.

By putting the two test results together, we can obtain:

- the positive predictive value (PPV), i.e. the probability that an individual with a positive test result really has the disorder, and the negative predictive value (NPV), i.e. the probability that an individual with a negative test result is really healthy;

Fig. 6.16

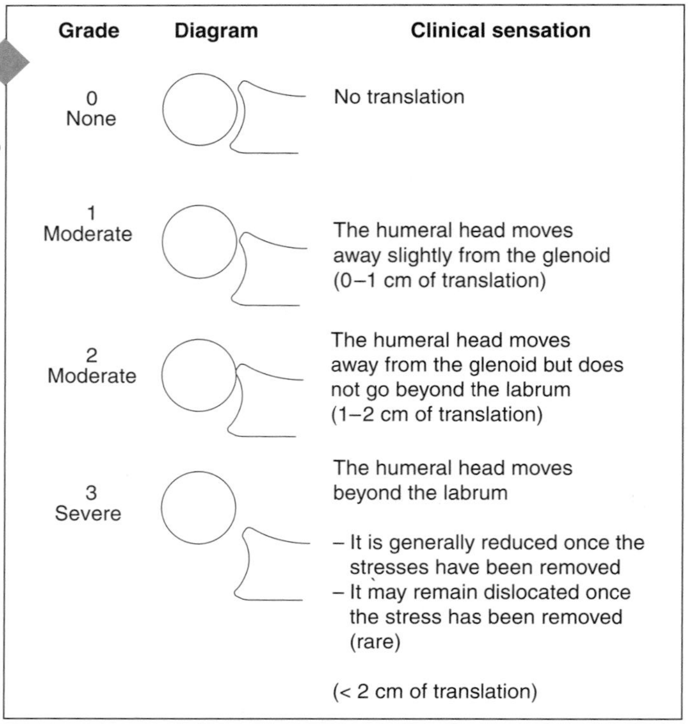

Grade	Diagram	Clinical sensation
0 None		No translation
1 Moderate		The humeral head moves away slightly from the glenoid (0–1 cm of translation)
2 Moderate		The humeral head moves away from the glenoid but does not go beyond the labrum (1–2 cm of translation)
3 Severe		The humeral head moves beyond the labrum – It is generally reduced once the stresses have been removed – It may remain dislocated once the stress has been removed (rare) (< 2 cm of translation)

Quantification of humeral translation (modified from Rockwood, 1999).

Table 6.1

Sensitivity, specificity, PPV, NPV, accuracy of the various specific shoulder tests

	Sensitivity %	Specificity %	Accuracy %	PPV %	NPV %
Tests for impingement					
• Neer test	88	30	72	75	52
• Hawkins test	92.1	25	72.8	75.2	56.2
• Yocum's test	78	—	—	—	—
• IRRST	88	96	—	—	—
Tests for the rotator cuff					
• Jobe's test for pain	63	55	57	31	82
• Jobe's test for weakness	77	68	70	44	90
• Jobe's test for pain + weakness	89	50	59	36	93
• Patte's test	92	30	—	29	93
• Lift-off test	100	100	—	—	—
• Drop sign	100	100	—	—	—
Test for the LHB					
• Palm-up test	68	55	64.8	79.2	41.6
Tests for the glenoid labrum					
• O'Brien's test	100	98.5	—	94	100
• PPT for SLAP	100	90	97	—	—
Tests for instability					
• Apprehension test	89	47	83	—	—
• Relocation test	73	71	73	—	—
• Sulcus sign	97	99	98	—	—

• the accuracy, which shows the validity of the test (total percentage of true positives and true negatives).

These values are also determined by the prevalence, i.e. by how rare the disorder examined is among the test population.

A rotator cuff lesion is fairly common in the elderly and far less common in the young, consequently the predictive value of a test for this disorder will be far higher in the first group than in the second.

Several tests are used during the clinical examination to reach a sufficiently certain diagnosis.

The various tests can be performed in parallel (the patient is considered to be affected if a positive result is obtained in one of the tests performed) or in series (the individual is regarded as suffering from the disorder if all the tests yield positive results, and in this case the next test is performed only if the previous one has been positive). Testing in parallel increases the sensitivity, while testing in series increases the specificity (Table 6.1).

Discussion

An accurate clinical evaluation of a shoulder disorder should be based on a detailed case history, to understand the clinical background and type of patient, and a careful objective examination.

An objective examination uses the conventional parameters for examining joints, such as inspection, palpation and evaluation of active and passive joint function, but above all it involves the performance of tests specific to the type of disorder.

Specific functional tests comprise manoeuvres performed by the examiner to reproduce the conditions that trigger the patient's symptoms.

Since tests cannot be absolutely specific in themselves, it is only by carefully performing tests in series or in parallel and interpreting the results on the basis of a full knowledge of their predictive values that a sufficiently accurate diagnosis can be reached.

Confirmation of the diagnostic conclusions reached by clinical examination must then be subjected to

Specialist examination

further investigation by means of instrumental diagnostic imaging examinations; these examinations, by means of either traditional radiology with standard radiological projections and particular, increasingly specific, projections for the type of disorder, or ultrasonography, owing to the advent of apparatus with increasingly high resolution and to the ever-increasing experience acquired by specialists, and finally owing to MR, with and without contrast media, allow an accurate diagnosis to be made, and this diagnosis is essential for establishing a therapeutic programme suited to the treatment of the disorder and the type of patient.

Bibliography

Burkhart S.S., Morgan C.D., Kibler W.B., 'Shoulder injuries in overhead athletes. The "dead arm" revisited', *Clinics in Sports Medicine* 19 (1): 125–158, (2000)

Çalis M. et al., 'Diagnostic Values of Clinical Diagnostic Tests in Subacromial Impingement Syndrome', *Ann. Rheum. Disease* 59: 44–47, (2000)

Henry M.H. et al., 'Accuracy of inferior sulcus, apprehension and relocation test compared to intraoperative findings', AOSSM Special Day, February, (1997)

Hertel R., Ballmer F.T., Lombert S.M., Gerber C. et al., 'Lag sign in the diagnosis of rotator cuff rupture', *J. Shoulder Elbow Surg.* 5: 307–313, (1996)

Itoi E. et al., 'Which is more useful, the full can test or the empty can test, in detecting the torn supraspinatus tendon?' *Am J Sports Med* 27(1): 65–68, (1999)

Jobe C.M., 'Superior glenoid impingement', *Orthop. Clin. of North Am.* 28(2): 137–143, (1997)

Kibler W.B., 'Specificity and sensitivity of anterior slide test in throwing athletes with superior glenoid labral tears', *Arthroscopy* 11: 296–300, (1995)

Kim S.H. et al., 'Biceps Load Test II: a clinical test for SLAP-lesions of the shoulder', *Arthroscopy: Arthroscopic Related Surg.* 17(2): 160–164, (2001)

Kim S.H. et al., 'Biceps load test. A clinical test for SLAP-lesions in the shoulders with recurrent anterior dislocation', *Am. J. Sports Med.* 27: 300–303, (1999)

Lerat J.L. et al., 'Dynamic anterior jerk of the shoulder. A new clinical test for shoulder instability. Preliminary study', *Rev. Chir. Orthop. Rep. Appar. Mot.* 80: 461–467, (1994)

Litaker D. et al., 'Returning to the bedside: using history and physical examination to identify rotator cuff tears'. *J. Am. Geriatrics So.* 48(12): 1633–1637, (2000)

Liu S.H. et al., 'Diagnosis of glenoid labral tears. A comparison between magnetic resonance imaging and clinical examination', *Am. J. Sport Med.* 24: 149–154, (1996a)

Liu S.H. et al., 'A prospective evaluation of a new physical examination in predicting glenoid labra tears', *Am. J. Sport Med.* 24: 721–725, (1996b)

McFarland E.G. et al., 'Evaluation of shoulder laxity', *Sport Med.* 22: 264–272, (1996)

Mimori K. et al., 'A new pain provocation test for labral tears of shoulder', *Am. J. Sports Med.* 27: 137–142, (1999)

Murrel G.A.G., Walton J.R., 'Diagnosis of rotator cuff tears', *The Lancet* 357: 769–770, (2001)

Neer C.S. et al., 'The shoulder in sports', *Orthop. Clin. North Am.* 8: 583–591, (1997)

O'Brien S.J. et al., 'The Active Compression Test for Diagnosing Labral Tears and Acromioclavicular Joint Abnormality', *Am. J. Sports Med.* 26: 610–613, (1998)

Porcellini G., Castagna A., Campi F., Paladini P., 'La spalla: patologia, tecnica chirurgica, riabilitazione', Verduci Ed., Rome (2003)

Rockwood C.A., Matsen F.A., *La spalla*, Verduci Ed., Rome (1999)

Tasto J.P., 'Shoulder instability testing using the lateral decubitus position', *Phis. Sports Med.* 26: 12–13 (1998)

Tennet T.D., Beach W.R., Meyers J.F., 'Clinical sport medicine update. A review of special tests associated with shoulder examination. Part I: the rotator cuff tests', AM. J. SPORT MED. 31(1): 154–160, (2003)

Vienne P., Gerber C., 'Clinical examination of the shoulder' *Ther. Umsch.* 55: 161–68, (1998)

Walch G. et al., 'The dropping and Hornblower's sign in evaluation of rotor cuff tears', *J. Bone Joint Surg. Br.* 80: 624–628, (1998)

Yergason R.M., 'Supination sign', *J. Bone Joint Surg.* 13: 160, (1931)

Yocum L.A., 'Assessing the shoulder. History, physical examination, differential diagnosis, and special test used', *Clin. Sport Med.* 2: 281–289, (1983)

Zaslav K.R., 'Internal rotation resistance strength test. A new diagnostic test to differentiate intra-articular pathology from outlet (Neer) impingement syndrome in the shoulder', *J. Shoulder Elbow Surg.* 10: 23–27, (2001)

DIAGNOSTIC IMAGING

CHAPTER 7

N. Gandolfo
G. Serafini

The diagnostic imaging techniques employed in evaluation of the rotator cuff (RC) can be non-invasive (conventional radiology, ultrasound, and magnetic resonance) or invasive (arthrographic techniques: conventional arthrography, arthro-CT and arthro-MR).

The individual examinations complement rather than compete with one another for an anatomical and clinical evaluation of the rotator cuff.

Conventional radiology (Rx) is always the first-line examination. Standard projections (internal rotation, external rotation and outlet view as per Neer) are used for an accurate evaluation of bone structures, the acromioclavicular and glenohumeral joints, the morphology of the coracoacromial arch and the acromion, the acromiohumeral space, and the presence and exact topography of calcific enthesopathy of the rotator cuff. Although it cannot evaluate tendon structures, Rx can often accurately identify indirect signs of tendinopathy of the RC.

Ultrasound (US), using high-frequency surface probes, can be used for an accurate evaluation of the whole RC. The advantages of US are its higher spatial resolution, its demonstration of capillary diffusion in the area, its non-invasive nature, and its relative speed and low cost. It nevertheless remains an operator-dependent technique. Compared to MR, it can assess partial tendon ruptures (e.g. a lesion of the supraspinatus, on the bursa surface) with greater diagnostic confidence, allowing early identification of fine structural intratendon fibril alterations. Dynamic US can be used to evaluate possible reducible subluxations of the long head of the biceps in relation to the bicipital groove. The subacromiosubdeltoid bursa is clearly identified, as is muscle trophism. US does not allow

evaluation of the glenoid labra, the capsuloligamentous complex or the osteochondral structures.

MR is the most accurate technique for a general evaluation and overview of the soft tissues (musculotendon, ligamentous and osteochondral structures).

The accurate identification of RC lesions (traumatic versus degenerative; partial versus complete), the degree of muscle atrophy and the fibrocartilaginous structures will enable the correct therapeutic approach to be planned. It is the most discerning technique for evaluating the bone marrow, and can provide early identification of contusion oedema of spongy tissue not detectable on Rx, which is often the cause of pain. It can also identify possible expansive neoformations of the soft tissues, which may cause pain and functional limitation. Owing to the multiplanar nature of the examination, it can evaluate the morphology of the coracoacromial arch and the acromiohumeral space. The high contrast resolution, which is an intrinsic feature of the technique, increases the diagnostic confidence of evaluation of the RC.

Computed tomography (CT) is indicated for the evaluation of bone cortex, and for detection of small detached osteochondral fragments with the formation of free endoarticular fragments; it is often a second-line examination, to complement diagnosis by Rx and MR.

Owing to the ability to identify the calcific matrix, free osteochondromatous fragments can be evaluated accurately or the progress of a bony callus monitored.

Arthrographic techniques, in particular arthro-MR and arthro-CT, are electively indicated for the evaluation of unstable shoulder. By introducing paramagnetic contrast medium (gadolinium chelates) or non-ionic iodinated contrast medium into the glenohumeral

Diagnostic imaging

joint, the capsuloligamentous complex (in particular the IGHLs), small lesions of the glenoid labra and partial ruptures of the joint surface of tendons (e.g. the supraspinatus) can be evaluated. Arthro-MR increasingly has an integral and complementary role in conventional MR of painful shoulder.

Technical principles and radiological anatomy

The individual diagnostic imaging techniques (Rx, US, MR, CT and arthrographic techniques) will be discussed below, with a brief mention of physical principles, with particular emphasis on signs and the radiological anatomy for each method. The aim of this chapter is to provide practical information on each of the methods so as to allow normal findings to be distinguished from pathological findings in RC disorder, and to discuss differential diagnoses in the clinical context of 'painful shoulder'.

Conventional radiology

A correct radiological study is carried out in various projections: two anteroposterior (AP) projections with the humerus in internal and external rotation, a caudal tilt projection, a Neer or outlet view projection, and an axillary projection.

The first examination to be performed, regardless of the clinical request made, is a true AP projection of the scapulohumeral joint. This projection must be carried out in internal and external rotation to examine the whole tuberosity.

The projection is technically correct when the glenoid cavity appears on the radiological image to have a curvilinear rather than an oval morphology, and the humeral head projects in isolation. The clavicle and the acromion may overlap (Fig. 7.1a).

A true AP projection is indicated in the following disorders:
— impingement syndrome;
— scapulohumeral osteoarthritis;
— instability (habitual or acute scapulohumeral dislocation); and
— fractures of the proximal end of the humerus (head or surgical neck).

An AP projection can demonstrate the following:
— tendon calcification (calcific enthesopathy of the RC) or calcification of the subacromial space (an expression of associated calcific tendinitis), resulting from precipitation of calcium salts in

necrotic tendons with areas of hyaline degeneration of collagen. The calcification is generally the outcome of small post-traumatic haematomas which tend to merge and may develop into osseo-calcific metaplastic processes; and
— sclerotic or cystic focal areas of the greater tuberosity or degenerative alterations of the acromioclavicular or glenohumeral joint.

The ascent of the humeral head, which reduces the acromiohumeral space as a result, is a sign of a massive RC lesion. Under normal conditions, the acromiohumeral distance is usually between 7 and 14 mm, in radiographs performed in AP, in neutral rotation.

A caudal tilt projection (AP projection with the X-ray tube inclined at 30° in the craniocaudal direction and the X-ray beam tangential to the acromion) can evaluate osteostructural alterations of the acromion (acromial osteophyte).

The technical criterion for a correct image is similar to that for a true AP projection. This projection is indicated in impingement syndrome.

The Neer projection, recommended by English-speaking authors for the supraspinatus outlet view, provides an evaluation of the morphology and deformity of the acromion and the acromioclavicular arch, under which the supraspinatus tendon travels (Fig. 7.1b, c). This projection is capable of identifying topographically the expected course of the tendons of the RC and the long head of the biceps brachii, and can separate the anterior plane from the posterior plane.

The projection is technically correct when the base of the coracoid process, the base of the acromial process and the lateral and medial rims of the scapula join to form a Y on the X-ray image, and the humeral head projects at the centre of this Y.

It is indicated in the following:
— impingement syndrome;
— scapulohumeral osteoarthritis; and
— topographical identification of calcific enthesopathies.

Bigliani (1991) defined three types of acromial morphology: type I: a flat acromion; type II: a curved acromion with an inferior surface parallel to the humeral profile; and type III: a hooked acromion. Edelson (1995) subsequently described a fourth type: a curved acromion with a convex inferior surface (Fig. 7.2).

Types III and IV are associated with subacromial impingement of the supraspinatus; type III is found in 70–80% of patients with RC lesion (Kaplan, 2001).

Axillary projection is useful for evaluating the profile of the acromion in the axial plane and identifying a possible acromial bone.

Fig. 7.1

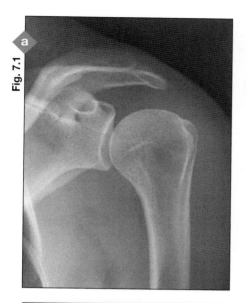

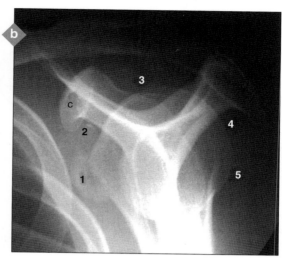

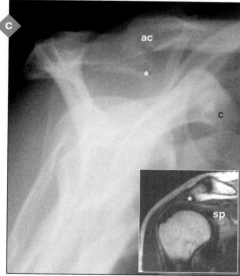

(a) Standard AP shoulder projection in a normal individual. Digital technique. Overview of the glenohumeral joint, the AC joint, the bicipital groove and the acromiohumeral space. The digital technique can assess bone structures and periarticular soft tissues at the same time. (b, c) Outlet view or Neer projection or scapula Y-view (b) in a normal individual and in an individual with a hooked acromion at an inferolateral angle (c). Patient erect, rotated by approximately 30° in relation to the radiological table, with the shoulder under examination supported in the sensitive plane. Incident ray inclined in a craniocaudal direction by about 10–15°. The radiograph is technically correct if the humeral head projects to the centre of the triangle formed by the coracoid, spine and scapula, and is concentric with respect to the glenoid. The coracoid process identifies the anterior plane of the projection. Calcific enthesopathy of the subscapularis is demonstrated (1). The image in (c) shows uneven morphostructural alteration of the acromion (asterisk), responsible for a reduction in the acromiohumeral space and subacromial impingement of the supraspinatus, as confirmed by MR.

1: subscapularis tendon; 2: long head of the biceps brachii; 3: supraspinatus tendon; 4: infraspinatus tendon; 5: teres minor tendon; sp: supraspinatus; c: coracoid; ac: acromioclavicular.

The projection is technically correct when the acromion and the surrounding space are visible in axial projection in the radiological image.

It is indicated in the following disorders:
— glenohumeral instability; and
— fractures of the proximal end of the humerus.

The modified (West Point) axillary projection is indicated in glenohumeral instability.

The projection is technically correct when the glenohumeral joint is visible in axial projection in the radiological image, showing in particular the inferior rim of the glenoid labrum, the site of Bankart lesions (Lagalla, 2000).

If a radiological study is performed using digital technology, very high quality images can be obtained, benefiting from the inherent advantages of the technique,

Diagnostic imaging

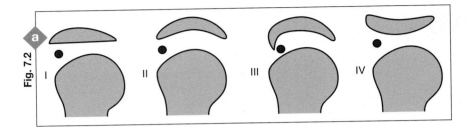

Fig. 7.2

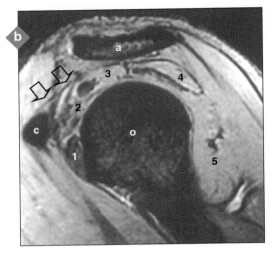

Drawing of the various types of acromial morphology **(a)**. The black dot represents the supraspinatus tendon in its anterior position to the shoulder. T2-weighted MR sequence **(b)**, sagittal plane. Type III (hooked acromion) and type IV (convex inferior acromial surface) are more frequently associated with impingement of the supraspinatus. The MR **(b)** clearly shows an acromion with type IV morphology, and the relative topography of the RC, the bone structures and the acromiohumeral ligament (outline arrows).

1: subscapularis tendon; 2: long head of the biceps brachii; 3: supraspinatus tendon; 4: infraspinatus tendon; 5: teres minor tendon; o: humerus; a: acromion; c: coracoid.

such as modifications of the windows, inversion of the tone scale, very wide latitude of exposure, edge effect and selective use of filters.

The reduction of up to 20% in the radiation dose with the digital technique should not be underestimated.

Ultrasound

The study of the shoulder uses linear probes with a frequency varying from 7.5 MHz to 10 MHz (Lagalla, 2000).

Leaving aside the method of carrying out the examination, US allows an evaluation of the echostructure, morphology and thickness of the tendon. The incidence of the ultrasound beam is important as regards the echostructure of the tendon; the tendon is hyperechoic when the incident beam is perpendicular to its fibres (fibrillar structure). Technically, the supraspinatus tendon is examined in coronal scans (frontal plane), when the tendon emerges from the acoustic shadow of the acromion and continues towards the trochanter.

The most important scan is performed with the arm in abduction and flexed at 90°. A normal tendon varies in thickness from 4 to 8 mm (Lagalla, 2000).

The option to examine the tendon during dynamic manoeuvres, in abduction and active and passive external rotation of the arm, can allow a more accurate identification of the tendon and its 'critical zone'. The deltoid muscle is separated from the supraspinatus by a hyperechoic band, represented by the subacromiosubdeltoid bursa (Fig. 7.3).

The bicipital groove can be easily detected by anterior axial scanning; the tendon of the long head of the biceps brachii (LHBB) can be seen inside it, as a hyperechoic oval image. Slight fluid distensions of its sheath can be regarded as physiological. A longitudinal view (along the long axis of the tendon) shows the medioproximal diaphyseal course in the bicipital groove, and then in the intra-articular segment.

The infraspinatus muscle covers the posterior surface of the glenohumeral joint and the posterior glenoid labrum. The tendon is easily identifiable along the length of its course.

The subscapularis muscle cannot be visualized in its proximal section, since it is hidden by the acoustic shadow of the ribs, but it can be visualized in its distal section. The landmark is the bicipital groove scanned transversely.

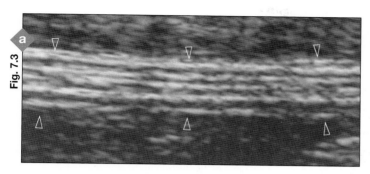

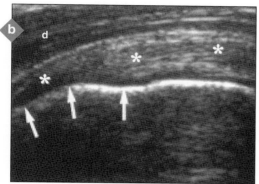

Fig. 7.3

Basic fibrillar echostructure of the tendon (**a**); echostructure of the supraspinatus tendon (**b**). The normal tendon (arrow tips) is characterized by a fibrillar structure, with alternating hyperechoic (white) linear structures and hypoechoic (black) structures. US accurately identifies the path of the supraspinatus tendon (asterisks), and can evaluate the 'critical zone' and the segment inserted in the humerus. The humeral cortex appears to be a hyperechoic structure (arrows). A thin hyperechoic linear structure separates the supraspinatus from the deltoid (d).

Magnetic resonance

MR has the advantage of being non-invasive, having a high intrinsic contrast resolution (it can distinguish skeletal from extraskeletal structures) and a high spatial resolution (2–3 mm), and it is multiplanar (it can examine a given body structure in the three orthogonal spatial planes: sagittal, transverse, and coronal) (Kaplan, 2001). Leaving aside the technical data, the MR signal is formed by a number of physical tissue parameters (T1, T2) or by the intrinsic structure (proton density, PD). For information, sequences defined as T1-weighted provide a morphological evaluation, anatomical detail and a high signal intensity of fatty tissue, which is hyperintense (white). In T1-weighted sequences, water is hypointense (black). Sequences defined as T2-weighted, however, intensify the signal of water which will be hyperintense (white). All pathological processes (traumas, infections, inflammation, or neoplasias) contain a variable quantity of water, which can be identified, and often typified, by T2 sequences.

In practical terms, the ability to distinguish between fat and water is electively indicated in the evaluation of musculoskeletal disorders. The ability to intensify the pathological signal of water (e.g. in oedema of the spongy tissue, tendon oedema, or intrabursal or intra-articular fluid effusion) can be enhanced by the use of sequences that cancel out the signal from fatty tissue, known as fat suppression techniques. These include STIR which increases diagnostic confidence when identifying osteomedullary and extraskeletal soft tissue disease. The damaged tendon always exhibits contusion and haemorrhage which can be identified by using these sequences (Kaplan, 2001).

Proton density (PD) is an expression of the quantity of protons contained, for example, fat is rich in protons. Integration of the type of MR signal (T1, T2, PD, or STIR) with the multiplanar aspect makes MR particularly suitable for the study of musculoskeletal disease. Remember that not all patients can have MR owing to absolute contraindications (pacemakers) and relative contraindications (devices inside the body with ferromagnetic properties, capable of being orientated in the MR static magnetic field).

The normal tendon appears to be a structure of homogeneously low T1 and T2 signal intensity; the glenoid labra exhibit a triangular or oval morphology, characterized by low T1 and T2 signal intensity; the muscles exhibit an intermediate signal in T1 and T2.

Medullary spongy tissue, rich in fat, displays typical signal hyperintensity in T1 and DP, and moderate hyperintensity in T2.

T1-weighted sequences generally provide morphological and anatomical detail; STIR and T2-weighted sequences identify oedema and RC lesion.

Computed tomography

The CT image depends physically on the different attenuation of the X-ray beam; it is, therefore, a function of the structural density (atomic number) of what is being studied. Since bone has a very compact structure (high atomic number), it causes a high level of absorption of the X-ray beam, resulting in a reduction in the energy of the Rx beam which will produce an impression on the radiographic film. In practical terms, in CT cortical bone is white (hyperdense), and medullary spongy tissue which is less dense than compact bone will be off-white. Anatomical structures with medium density (e.g. muscles) will appear an intermediate grey (medium hypodensity), and fat as a dark grey (hypodensity). Air which absorbs the Rx photon only very slightly will be plain black. The essential difference from MR is that CT provides information based on structural density, while MR yields biochemical information. CT images, acquired in transverse planes, can subsequently be reconstructed, since they are digital images, in three orthogonal planes (multiplanar technique, MPR or three-dimensional mode (3D)).

CT accurately identifies the glenohumeral and AC joints and is indicated in mechanical trauma and in the morphological evaluation of joint fissures; it can identify small osteophyte formations, fracture fissures, and traumatic detached fragments better than MR. CT is often used to complement and succeed conventional radiology. It is also indicated for the evaluation of bone cortex, to detect small detached osteochondral fragments with the formation of free endoarticular fragments (Helms, 1998; Raby, 1995; Schwartz, 2000). The fact that the calcific matrix can be identified means that free osteochondromatous fragments can be evaluated accurately (Helms, 1998).

Arthrographic techniques

The option of administering iodinated contrast media (conventional arthrography and arthro-CT of the shoulder) or paramagnetic contrast media, such as gadolinium chelates (arthro-MR), inside the glenohumeral joint offers a more accurate evaluation of the glenoid labra and the capsuloligamentous complex.

If a partial rupture of the glenoid labrum is present, the contrast medium will diffuse from the joint into the defect in the fibrocartilaginous structure. Similarly, if there are partial ruptures of the articular side of the tendon (supraspinatus, subscapularis), arthrographic techniques increase diagnostic confidence (Helms, 1998; Kaplan, 2001).

Rotator cuff

The concept of impingement was proposed in 1972; any cause of a reduction in the amplitude of the coracoacromial arch may potentially predispose to impingement of a tendon, predominantly the supraspinatus.

Morphological alteration of the coracoacromial arch may result in the following (Helms, 1998; Kaplan, 2001):
- *acromial morphology:*
  — *Type III:* bone irregularity of the inferior profile (oblique sagittal). The 'hooked' morphology of the anteroinferior surface of the acromion causes recurrent microtrauma in the critical (hypovascular) zone of the supraspinatus. Acromial osteoarthritis with inferior articular osteophytosis is a very common cause of subacromial impingement in adults. MR accurately distinguishes acromial osteophytosis affecting the tendon insertion of the deltoid from that affecting the insertion of the coracoacromial ligament;
- *acromial orientation:*
  — anteroinferior sliding (oblique sagittal);
  — inferolateral angulation (oblique coronal);
- degeneration of the AC joint;
- *acromial bone:*
  — accessory ossification centre, which does not fuse in 15% of the adult population. The bone is mobile and, therefore, reduces the space in the coracoacromial arch;
- *thickened coracoacromial ligament:*
  — chronic anterior instability may predispose towards an increase in ligament thickness, responsible for impingement;
- post-traumatic bone deformity;
- instability;
- *muscle hypertrophy:*
  — in athletes, hypertrophy of the supraspinatus reduces the coracoacromial arch and acromiohumeral space. MR alone is able to identify focal compression of the cranial surface of the muscle by the AC joint.

Macroscopically, the morphostructural alterations of tendons vary from oedema to complete rupture.

The potential consequences and subsequent course are as follows (Kaplan, 2001):
- *Supraspinatus:* degeneration, partial rupture, complete rupture;
- *Proximal long head, biceps brachii tendon:* degeneration, partial rupture, complete rupture;
- *Bone:* degenerative cysts, sclerosis of the greater tuberosity and the humeral head; and
- *Bursa:* subacromiosubdeltoid (SASD) bursitis.

Rx and MR can accurately identify morphological alteration of the coracoacromial arch and the acromion (Figs. 7.4, 7.5).

Identification of the type (traumatic versus degenerative), dimensions, degree of tendon rupture (partial versus complete) and degree of retraction of the tendon is easy with US and MR (Helms, 1998).

Supraspinatus

In impingement, MR identifies variations in the signal (degeneration, partial ruptures) and thickness (thin, thickened, irregular, defect) of the tendon; reactive effusion of the SASD bursa.

The sensitivity and specificity of MR in complete ruptures of the supraspinatus is 90% (Kaplan, 2001).

MR can also accurately identify the degree of fatty degeneration of the muscle belly, and can distinguish between hypotrophy that is still reversible, and, therefore, eligible for surgery, and irreversible atrophy in the presence of complete, established tendon rupture (Fig. 7.6).

Partial rupture of the tendon shows focal alteration or the presence of fluid effusion in the subacromial bursa; complete rupture shows structural dyshomogeneity throughout the thickness, the presence of fluid inside the tendon, and retraction of the myotendinous junction, i.e. direct signs; reactive fluid effusion in the SASD bursa and muscle atrophy, i.e. associated signs (Helms, 1998).

Long head of the biceps

Seven per cent of patients with a supraspinatus lesion also have LHBB damage (Kaplan, 2001).

Complete proximal humeral rupture of the LHBB causes a distal retraction of the tendon fragment and the muscle, leaving the bicipital groove empty, and this can be clearly demonstrated by US and MR performed in transverse planes.

The LHBB lesion may occur at its insertion in the superior glenoid labrum (associated with a SLAP lesion) or proximally to the bicipital groove, in impingement associated with a supraspinatus lesion.

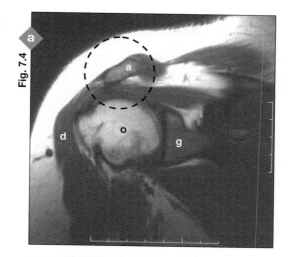

Fig. 7.4

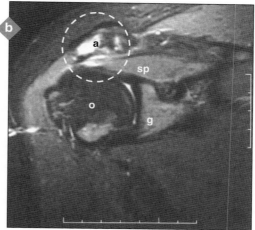

T1-weighted **(a)** and STIR **(b)** MR sequences, anterior coronal plane. Inferolateral angulation of the acromion. The normal spongy tissue of the humerus (o) and of the scapular glenoid (g), since it consists mainly of fatty tissue ('yellow bone marrow'), shows a characteristic signal hyperintensity in T1 (see Fig. 7.3a) and signal decay in STIR (see Fig. 7.3b). The pathological acromion (a) shows lateral and caudal angulation, with a reduction in the acromiohumeral space and tendon impingement of the supraspinatus (sp), which shows high signal intensity in STIR (see Fig. 7.3b), indicating diffuse intratendon and acromial oedema of the spongy tissue. Muscle trophism is normal.
d: deltoid muscle.

A lesion of the myotendinous junction is usually traumatic and acute in young individuals.

An acute trauma can cause avulsion, subluxation or dislocation of the LHBB. Lesion of the humeral transverse ligament (it forms a bridge between the

Diagnostic imaging

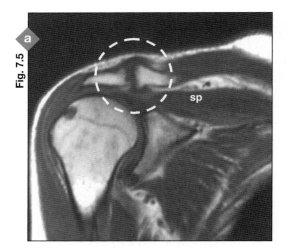

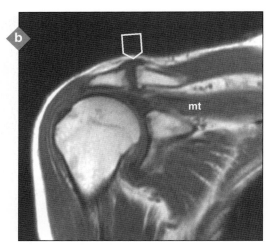

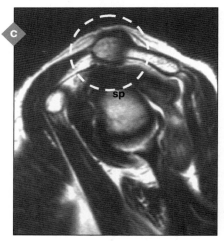

T1-weighted MR sequences **(a, b)**, anterior coronal plane, and T2-weighted **(c)**, sagittal plane. Type III acromion, with subacromial impingement of the supraspinatus. Alteration of the morphology of the coracoacromial arch by the presence of small osteophyte formations on the inferior joint surface (circle), with subsequent subacromial impingement of the supraspinatus (sp), corresponding to its critical zone. The tendon is ruptured, with medial retraction of the myotendinous junction (mt). This is associated with fibrous hypertrophy of the joint capsule of the AC (outline arrow).

The oblique sagittal plane **(c)** confirms the subacromial impingement of the myotendinous junction of the supraspinatus, with an impression in its cranial surface (loss of the physiological cranial convexity). The acromiohumeral space is reduced in amplitude.

lesser and the greater tuberosity) and the subscapularis tendon may cause anteromedial dislocation of the LHBB (Gandolfo, 1998), leaving the bicipital groove empty (Fig. 7.7).

Infraspinatus and teres minor

Lesions of the infraspinatus and teres minor may be isolated, in the context of an acute trauma, or associated with a massive lesion of the supraspinatus or with posterosuperior impingement of the shoulder, occurring during maximum abduction and external rotation (Kaplan, 2001). Impingement of the supraspinatus and infraspinatus tendons occurs between the humeral head and the posterosuperior labrum.

This is reflected clinically in posterosuperior pain and anterior instability. Diagnostic imaging can demonstrate humeral cysts adjacent to the infraspinatus, lesions of the supraspinatus and infraspinatus, and lesion of the posterosuperior labrum (Fig. 7.8).

Subscapularis

Lesion of the subscapularis is relatively common, occurring during acute trauma with the arm adducted and in hyperextension or in internal rotation. This type of injury may result in anterior dislocation of the shoulder, associated with massive RC damage, lesion involving anteromedial dislocation of the LHBB or subcoracoid impingement. Subcoracoid impingement

Fig. 7.6

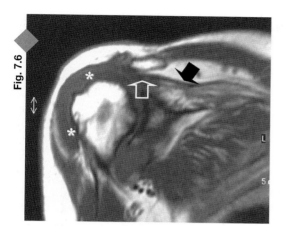

T1-weighted MR sequences, anterior coronal plane. Complete rupture of the supraspinatus tendon. Complete lesion of the supraspinatus segment inserted in the humerus, with disinsertion of the tendon (outline arrow) and medial retraction of the myotendinous junction (solid arrow). Atrophy of the muscle is associated with fatty infiltration and reduction in the amplitude of the acromiohumeral space. Osteoarthritic degeneration of the acromion and the glenohumeral rim, with fluid effusion in the subacromiodeltoid bursa (*).

Fig. 7.8

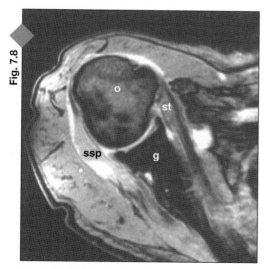

T2-weighted MR sequences, transverse plane. Traumatic lesion of the infraspinatus tendon. Diffuse structural dyshomogeneity with contusion oedema of the humeral insertion of the infraspinatus tendon. The thickness of the tendon is generally increased.

o: humerus; g: scapular glenoid; st: subscapularis tendon; ssp: infraspinatus tendon.

Fig. 7.7

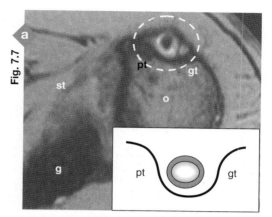

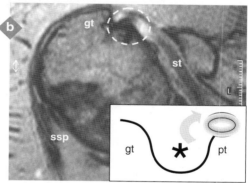

T2-weighted MR sequences, transverse plane. LHBB normal **(a)** and subluxated medially **(b)**. The LHBB is physiologically located in the bicipital groove, in its extra-articular segment, delimited by the greater tuberosity (laterally) and the lesser tuberosity (medially). It appears to be an oval structure, with low signal intensity, surrounded by a very small quantity of physiological fluid in the sheath **(a)**. The LHBB lies over the lesser humeral tuberosity (circle), and is subluxated medially **(b)**. pt: lesser tuberosity; gt: greater tuberosity; o: humerus; g: scapular glenoid; st: subscapularis tendon; ssp: infraspinatus tendon.

causes a reduction in the space between the humerus and the end of the coracoid, which may be congenital or secondary to a coracoid fracture or surgery (Kaplan, 2001).

The tendon lesion can be clearly demonstrated by US and MR in transverse planes. The clinical picture is characterized by direct signs (focal or full thickness intratendon deficit, significant reduction or increase in tendon thickness, insertion avulsion with detachment of the lesser tuberosity of the humerus) and indirect signs (retraction of the myotendinous junction, muscle atrophy, and associated dislocation or medial subluxation of the LHBB) (Fig. 7.9).

Fig. 7.9

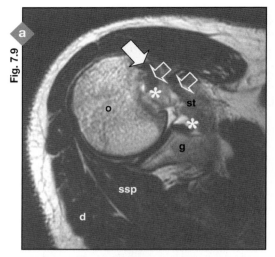

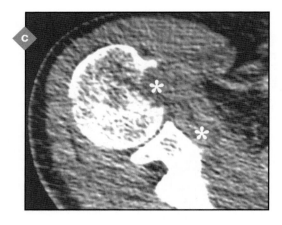

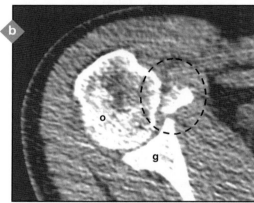

T2-weighted MR sequences, transverse plane **(a)**; CT of right shoulder, contiguous planes **(b)** with soft tissue window. Acute and complete traumatic rupture of the subscapularis tendon, with associated glenohumeral fracture. MR shows **(a)** evidence of an insertion lesion of the subscapularis tendon (st), which has a serpiginous morphology and is medially retracted (outline arrows). This is associated with avulsion of the lesser tuberosity of the humerus and a comminuted fracture of the anterior glenoid (asterisks) **(c)**. The LHBB (arrow) is medially subluxated. CT gives a better view **(b)** of the uneven free osteochondral fragment (circle).
d: deltoid; o: humerus; g: scapular glenoid; ssp: infraspinatus tendon.

Massive RC lesion

Massive RC lesions are generally found in elderly patients with chronic degenerative tendinopathy or associated predisposing factors, such as inflammatory arthritis, diabetes, or long-term corticosteroid therapy (Kaplan, 2001). They generally involve tendons, with complete full thickness ruptures, musculotendon retraction and muscle atrophy. A large full thickness tendon defect places the glenohumeral joint in direct communication with the SASD bursa; it is not uncommon for a large synovial fluid cyst to form, which develops cranially through the AC joint, simulating neoformation of the soft tissues on objective examination. The cranial ascent of the humeral head increases the bone microtrauma, resulting in new osteophytosis in the joint and a further increase in subacromial tendon and subcoracoid impingement.

Massive RC lesions are less frequently found in major trauma (Fig. 7.10).

Osteomedullary trauma

Conventional radiology is the first-line examination to evaluate clinically suspected dislocation of the shoulder or fractures.

X-rays can often be normal, even in the presence of extensive contusion and haemorrhagic oedema of the spongy tissue. MR with dedicated sequences for the study of the bone marrow can help to identify bone contusion and evaluate its severity and exact topography (Fig. 7.11).

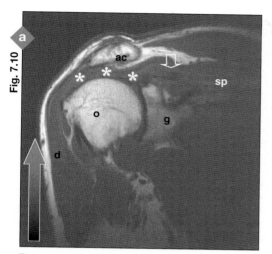
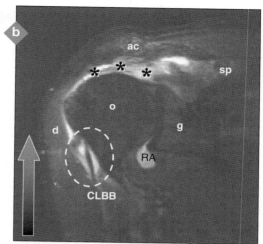

Fig. 7.10

T1-weighted **(a)** and STIR **(b)** MR sequences, anterior coronal planes. Acute and complete traumatic rupture of the suprapinatus tendon, with associated traumatic sequelae affecting the extra-articular LHBB. MR shows diffuse structural dyshomogeneity of the supraspinatus tendon (asterisks), characterized by haemorrhagic oedema, reactive fluid sequelae affecting the SASD bursa and glenohumeral haemarthrosis, with elective distribution in the axillary recess (RA) owing to a supine position. The myotendinous junction (outline arrow) is significantly retracted medially; the muscle trophism of the supraspinatus (sp) is normal. The LHBB shows moderate fluid effusion in its sheath in the extra-articular segment (circle). The humeral head has ascended cranially (large arrow), with a subsequent reduction in the acromiohumeral space. No osteomedullary contusion visible.
d: deltoid; o: humerus; g: scapular glenoid; ac: acromioclavicular.

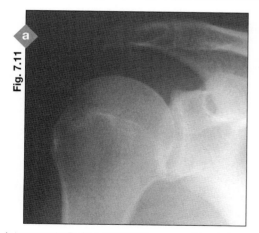
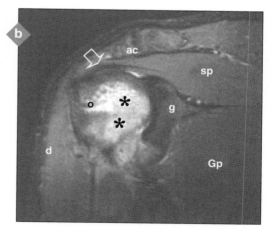

Fig. 7.11

Anteroposterior Rx **(a)** and STIR MR sequence **(b)**, anterior coronal plane. Bone contusion. The X-ray **(a)** does not show any traumatic osteostructural alterations. MR **(b)** shows diffuse, extensive oedema of the medullary spongy tissue (asterisks) with proximal epiphyseal and metadiaphyseal distribution of the humerus, without involvement of the scapular glenoid. The humeral insertion (outline arrow) of the supraspinatus (sp) is intact.
d: deltoid; o: humerus; g: scapular glenoid; ac: acromioclavicular; Gp: greater pectoralis.

Instability

Instability is the next most frequent disorder, after impingement, affecting the shoulder. Shoulder impingement and instability often occur together (Kaplan, 2001; Helms, 1998).

Shoulder instability is understood to mean subluxation or dislocation of the glenohumeral joint, which may be traumatic or non-traumatic.

Anatomical factors predisposing to instability are: glenoid labrum anomalies, joint capsule lesion or

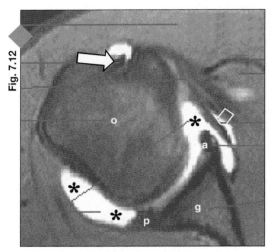

Fig. 7.12

T1-weighted arthro-MR sequence with fat suppression, transverse plane. Glenoid labra normal. Both the anterior (a) and posterior (p) glenoid labra have a triangular morphology. The glenohumeral joint cavity is distended by the paramagnetic contrast medium (gadolinium chelates) which creates high contrast and spatial resolution between the joint cavity distended by the contrast medium (asterisks), the glenoid labra (a, p) and the middle glenohumeral ligament (outline arrow). The extra-articular LHBB (arrow) is in place, physiologically located in the bicipital groove.
g: scapular glenoid; o: humerus.

laxity, glenohumeral ligament lesion or laxity, hypoplasia of the scapular glenoid and traumatic lesions due to impact, such as Hill-Sachs and Bankart lesions, complications of previous dislocations.

Instability can be divided clinically into two types:

— functional: subjective instability, with a joint that is clinically stable on objective examination. It is often associated with glenoid labrum lesions; and

— anatomical: objective instability on clinical evaluation.

Instability can be either anterior (95%), posterior, superior or multidirectional (5%). Superior instability generally occurs with multidirectional instability, resulting in cranial subluxation of the humeral head, and recurrent microtraumas against the supraspinatus tendon which is interposed between the coracoacromial arch and the humeral head.

Instability, regardless of its type, will naturally progress to hypertrophy with sclerosis of the greater tuberosity, subacromial osteophytosis, and thickening of the acromiohumeral ligament with glenohumeral osteophytosis and subsequent secondary impingement.

Destruction of the capsuloligamentous complex is considered a traumatic aetiology. In athletes, repeated functional stresses can cause laxity of the anterior capsuloligamentous complex, to allow the maximum degree of external rotation (tennis, swimming, and baseball).

Regardless of the type of instability, MR with intra-articular administration of paramagnetic contrast medium (arthro-MR) is the most accurate diagnostic method of evaluating the anatomical structures involved or affected (Kaplan, 2001). Percutaneous introduction of contrast medium into the glenohumeral joint, with posterior or anterior access depending on the suspected diagnosis, can distend the capsuloligamentous complex, creating a natural contrast between the joint cavity distended by the contrast medium, the glenohumeral ligaments (superior, middle and inferior), the glenoid labra and the joint surface of the RC tendons (Fig. 7.12).

When a shoulder dislocation is suspected clinically, an X-ray can identify any traumatic osteostructural lesions due to impact affecting the humerus and scapular glenoid, as well as confirming the type of dislocation. MR and arthro-MR offer a supplementary diagnostic tool in these cases for the evaluation of the glenoid labra, in order to rule out osteochondral lesions of the capsuloligamentous complex and the RC (Figs. 7.13, 7.14).

As a brief reminder, the principal anatomical morphostructural alterations after shoulder instability are given below (Kaplan, 2001).

- *Bone:*
  — glenohumeral dislocation;
  — *Hill-Sachs fracture:* lesion due to impact on the posterolateral surface of the humeral head. Anterior dislocation;
  — *Bankart fracture:* lesion due to impact on the anteroinferior surface of the scapular glenoid. Anterior dislocation;
  — lesion due to impact on the anteromedial surface of the humeral head. Posterior dislocation; and
  — *Reverse Bankart fracture:* lesion of the posterior surface of the scapular glenoid. Posterior dislocation.

- *Capsule:*
  — *type III* capsular adhesion to the humeral neck (>1 cm medially to the labrum);
  — irregular, thickened capsule; and
  — progressive ossification or mineralization of the posterior extra-articular capsule (Bennett lesion).

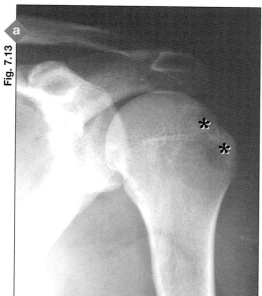

Fig. 7.13 a

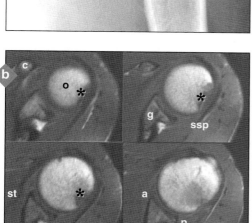

b

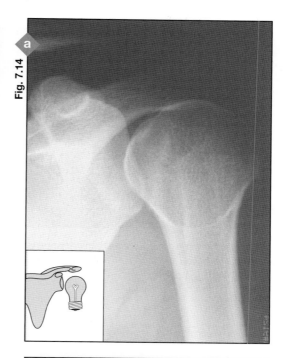

Fig. 7.14 a

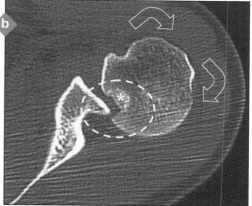

b

Anteroposterior Rx (**a**) and T1-weighted MR sequence, contiguous transverse planes (**b**), in the craniocaudal direction (clockwise). Hill-Sachs lesion. Conventional radiography (**a**) shows a focal osteostructural alteration of the posterolateral surface of the humeral head (asterisks), characterized by focal pitting of the posterior bone cortex. The alteration is confirmed by MR (**b**). The morphostructural characteristics and the clinical context (previous anterior dislocation) are compatible with a Hill-Sachs impact lesion.
No traumatic lesions of the anterior and posterior (a, p) glenoid labra, or scapular glenoid (g) are visible, particularly in an anteroinferior location. The subscapular (st) and infraspinatus tendons (ssp) are normal.
c: coracoid.

Anteroposterior Rx (**a**) and CT of shoulder, transverse plane with bone window (**b**). Reverse Hill-Sachs lesion. Conventional radiography (**a**) shows a posterior dislocation of the humeral head, with loss of the normal oval morphology. On X-ray, in frontal projection, the humeral head resembles a light bulb. CT (**b**) confirms the posterior dislocation of the head in relation to the glenoid (curved arrows) and shows an impact fracture with pitting of the cortex of the head in a posteromedial location (circle). This is described as a reverse Hill-Sachs lesion. CT can identify initial subcortical perifocal reparative osteosclerosis (asterisk), reflecting the initial formation of a bony callus with a calcific matrix.

Diagnostic imaging

Fig. 7.15

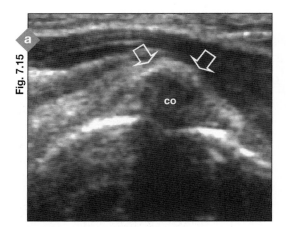

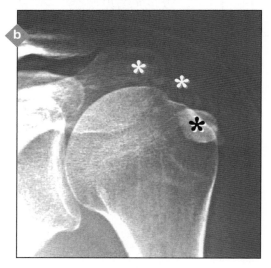

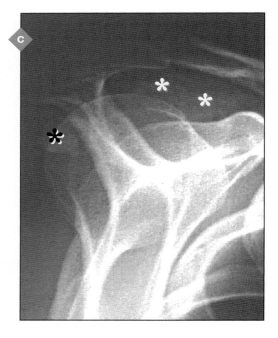

US, transverse plane **(a)** and Rx in anteroposterior projection **(b)** and outlet-view **(c)**. Calcific enthesopathy of the RC. US **(a)** shows extensive calcification of the rotator cuff arch (outline arrows), with the characteristic posterior shadow cone (co). Digital X-ray in standard projection **(b)** shows numerous calcifications of the arch, characterized by the different morphology and density. The Neer projection **(c)** distinguishes microcalcifications on the supraspinatus (white asterisks) from the denser, homogeneous calcification on the infraspinatus (black asterisks).

- *Glenohumeral ligaments:*
  — rupture, avulsion, thickening;
  — the inferior glenohumeral ligament is the most important; ligament avulsion from the humerus and from the labrum may occur.
- *Labrum:*
  — rupture, avulsion from the glenoid;
  — *Bankart lesion:* detachment of the anteroinferior labrum with fracture of the anterior scapular periosteum, sometimes with fracture of the glenoid rim; and
  — *ALPSA lesion:* variant of Bankart lesion, but with the anterior scapular periosteum intact.

- *Tendons:*
  — *subscapularis:* rupture or avulsion of the lesser tuberosity;
  — *LHBB:* medial dislocation.

Calcific enthesopathy, tendinitis and bursitis

The vague and obsolete term of scapulohumeral peri-arthritis covers a range of often calcific degenerative capsule and tendon lesions of the shoulder (calcific enthesopathy). They result from the precipitation of calcium salts in necrotic tendons with areas of hyaline degeneration of collagen.

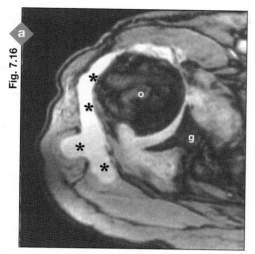
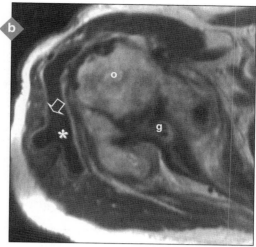

T2-weighted **(a)** and T1-weighted MR sequence after the iv administration of paramagnetic contrast medium **(b)**, transverse plane. SASD bursitis. The T2-weighted sequence **(a)** shows abundant fluid effusion distending the SASD bursa (asterisks), with glenohumeral intra-articular communication. Contrastographic synovial hyperaemia (arrow) is confirmed after iv contrast **(b)**.
o: humerus; g: glenoid.

The calcification is generally the outcome of small post-traumatic haematomas which tend to merge and may develop into osseo-calcific metaplastic processes.

The supraspinatus is the tendon most affected. Clinically the patient reports pain at rest, during movement and at night. The calcification may secondarily involve the glenohumeral joint and the SASD bursa.

Rx can accurately identify calcific enthesopathy, particularly when it is small (Kaplan, 1986). MR, where it is performed, always in relation to Rx, is capable of providing information on the status of the RC. US accurately identifies calcific enthesopathy as a hyperechoic structure, with the classic posterior shadow cone owing to the reflection of the ultrasound beam, corresponding to the acoustic interface between the calcification and the deeper soft tissues (Fig. 7.15).

US and MR accurately identify SASD bursitis (Fig. 7.16); the subcoracoid bursa, which is located anterior to the subscapularis muscle, does not communicate with the glenohumeral joint or with the articular recess of the subscapularis.

In approximately 20% of cases it communicates with the SASD bursa. If subcoracoid bursitis is present, the patient complains of anterior pain.

The radiological diagnosis of adhesive capsulitis can be considered during arthro-MR if the intra-articular administration of contrast medium is reduced (<7 ml). Intracapsular adhesions do not allow adequate distension of the capsule by the contrast medium. The volume of the intra-articular administration of contrast medium is usually 10 ml (Kaplan, 2001).

Nerve entrapment syndromes

Muscle atrophy may be found in lesions intrinsic or extrinsic to the nerves responsible for the motor component of the muscles of the shoulder girdle.

The suprascapular nerve runs superior to the scapula in an anteroposterior direction. It has sensory branches for the acromioclavicular and glenohumeral joints; it provides motor branches for the supraspinatus and infraspinatus tendons when it travels in the suprascapular notch; it provides motor innervation for the infraspinatus only when it takes a more posterior course, in the spinoglenoid notch.

MR can accurately identify the suprascapular nerve along its anterior course (suprascapular notch) in a coronal scan plane, and its posterior course (spinoglenoid notch), in the transverse plane (Kaplan, 2001).

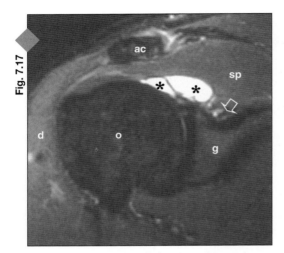

Fig. 7.17

T2-weighted MR sequence with fat suppression, anterior coronal plane. Cystic ganglion in an athlete (weight-lifter). MR shows an extensive expansive neoformation (asterisks), with an oval, partitioned morphology, containing fluid, developing anteriorly in the suprascapular notch, becoming contiguous with the suprascapular nerve (outline arrow). The anterior view of the coronal plane shows a normal supraspinatus, with normal muscle trophism.

o: humerus; g: glenoid; ac: acromioclavicular; d: deltoid; sp: supraspinatus.

The commonest cause of suprascapular nerve entrapment is a mucous cyst (cystic ganglion), generally associated with a lesion of the superior glenoid labrum (Fig. 7.17). US-guided percutaneous drainage is a therapeutic alternative to surgical excision, although surgery is required in the presence of a glenoid labrum lesion.

Venous ectasia, soft tissue neoplasia and scapular fracture, conditions which can cause extrinsic compression or infiltration of the suprascapular notch, are less common.

The axillary nerve runs anatomically in the quadrilateral space which is delimited by the humerus (laterally), the long head of the triceps (medially), the teres minor (superiorly) and the teres major (inferiorly). The axillary nerve is compressed clinically by fibrous bands, neoplasia or humeral fractures, and atrophy of the deltoid or teres minor muscle is evident (Kaplan, 2001).

In Parsonage-Turner syndrome, pain and functional limitation can be caused by acute brachial neuritis, generally of viral aetiology. The muscles involved are the supraspinatus, the infraspinatus and the deltoid. MR identifies the damage initially as diffuse intramuscular oedema, with the eventual development of atrophy (Kaplan, 2001).

Osteolysis of the clavicle

Post-traumatic osteolysis of the distal end of the clavicle is a known cause of painful shoulder, and is known to take two aetiological forms: direct trauma (post-traumatic osteolysis in the strict sense) and repeated microtrauma (stress-induced or atraumatic osteolysis).

Post-traumatic osteolysis of the distal clavicle has long been known and described in the literature; it appears after an acute traumatic episode, after an interval ranging from two weeks to several years. The traumatic event is often a minor injury, generally not associated with a fracture; acromioclavicular subluxation and dislocation are not uncommon. Osteolysis of the distal clavicle induced by repeated microtrauma or stress has been described more recently in individuals carrying out heavy manual work and in athletes involved in weight lifting or throwing (Kaplan, 1986). Both activities can reduce shoulder mobility, decreasing muscle strength. Swelling of the soft tissues around the AC joint may also be present, accompanied in some cases by crepitus. The lytic process may persist for approximately 12–18 months and, if not properly treated, progressive reabsorption of the lateral end of the clavicle along with erosion with 'cup' reshaping of the acromion, and dystrophic calcification or intra-articular bone fragments may be observed.

A differential diagnosis includes septic arthritis, rheumatoid arthritis, hyperparathyroidism, scleroderma, gout, primary and secondary tumours, massive Gorham osteolysis and joint diseases secondary to corticosteroids (Kaplan, 1986, 2001). The main MR feature (Gandolfo, 2000) has proved to be an increase in signal intensity in the distal clavicle in T2-weighted images, a finding indicative of medullary oedema. Medullary oedema of the distal clavicle is thus considered to be the commonest manifestation of the disease (Fig. 7.18).

Soft tissues

MR and US are particularly indicated in the diagnosis and local staging of solid neoformations of the soft tissues, and can accurately evaluate the extent of the process and consequently guide biopsies.

The most frequent histotypes are lipoma (Fig. 7.19), benign fibrous histiocytoma and elastofibroma of the back.

The most frequent malignant variant is liposarcoma (Helms, 1998; Kaplan, 2001).

Fig. 7.18

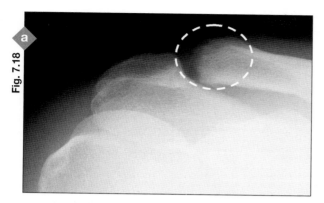

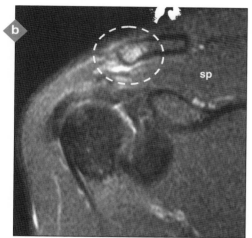

AP X-ray centred on the AC joint with the beam at an angle of 25°
(a) and T2-weighted MR sequence with fat suppression, anterior
coronal plane. Osteolysis of the clavicle. Focal areas of erosion of
the cortex of the distal end of the clavicle can be seen (circle). MR
(b) shows oedema of the spongy tissue in the distal third of the
clavicle (circle), with slight reactive oedema of the subclavian soft
tissues.
sp: supraspinatus.

Fig. 7.19

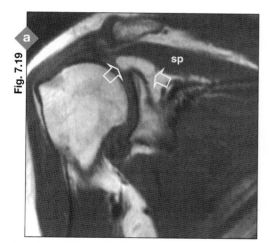

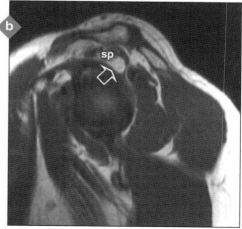

T1-weighted MR sequences, anterior coronal **(a)** and sagittal plane **(b)**. Lipoma. A small lipoma (outline arrows), located deep in the
supraspinatus muscle (sp), is dislocating the myotendinous junction cranially against the bone surface of the AC joint, reducing the
acromiohumeral space and probably causing tendon impingement. The tendon is normal.

Diagnostic imaging

Bibliography

Bigliani L.U., Ticker J.B., Flatlow E.L. et al., 'The relationship of the acromial architecture to rotator cuff disease', *Clin. Sports Med.* 10: 823–838, (1991)

Edelson J.C., 'The "hooked" acromion revisited', *J. Bone Joint Surg.* 77: 284–287, (1995)

Gandolfo N. et al., 'Instabilità del tendine del capo lungo del muscolo bicipite brachiale. Ruolo dell'ecografia', *Radiol. Med.* 96: 18–22, (1998)

Gandolfo N. et al., 'Osteolisi post-traumatica e da stress dell'estremo distale della clavicola', Proceedings of the 39th National Congress of the SIRM, Milan, p. 288, (2000)

Helms C.A., 'Fundamentals of skeletal radiology', Saunders, Philadelphia (1998)

Kaplan P.A. et al., 'Musculoskeletal MRI', Saunders, Philadelphia (2001)

Kaplan P.A. et al., 'Stress induced osteolysis of the clavicle', *Radiology* 158: 139–140, (1986)

Lagalla R., 'Radiology. Diploma universitario per tecnici sanitari di radiologia medica', vol. III. Idelson-Gnocchi, Naples (2000)

Raby N. et al., 'Accident and emergency radiology. A survival guide', Saunders, Philadelphia (1995)

Schwartz D.T., 'Emergency radiology', McGraw Hill, New York (2000)

FUNCTIONAL EXAMINATION AS PART OF MANUAL THERAPY

A. FOGLIA

The evaluation and clinical management of the shoulder have traditionally been considered problematic, probably firstly because of the degree of functional overlap between the many structures necessary for normal activity, and secondly because of each person's unique 'experience of illness or pain', due to which everyone describes their own sensation of pain differently (Jones, 2000, 2002).

Pain in the shoulder region is a symptom common to many disorders. Effective treatment requires a precise medical diagnosis and the physiotherapist must be able to conduct an accurate and appropriate functional evaluation (FE). The process of acquiring 'proof' and 'clues' to the functional state of the shoulder complex is, nevertheless, a subjective 'product', based on the reasoning and experience of the person conducting the process. The evaluation, which is the responsibility of the rehabilitation specialist, essentially needs to verify the nature and extent of impairments (pain, movement restriction, impaired proprioception, etc.), to ascertain the degree of the resulting disability (difficulty throwing, tennis service impaired or impossible, inability to perform a freestyle stroke in swimming, etc.) and to gather any significant information about the patient (level of motivation, expectations, occupation and sport activities, etc.).

The physiotherapist will use the information obtained from the FE, along with the specialist's recommendations, to draw up a health profile for the patient (see Chapter 12).

The medical diagnosis, the treatment guidelines which the doctor should provide and the best interpretation of the data acquired from the FE will all help to plan the therapeutic approach and to correctly identify a starting point against which to judge progress.

The current scientific literature, and in particular evidence based medicine (EBM), recognizes its own limits in terms of evaluation and acknowledges that acceptable standards are still far from being achieved (Cartabellotta, 2000). Although it is reasonable to assume that a thorough evaluation conducted by the therapist, a clear treatment plan and detailed clinical documentation will yield better therapeutic results, a recent study has nevertheless shown that evaluation methodologies still show significant differences in completeness and specificity in relation to the type of examiner. The documentation produced during the initial examination shows weak associations with the clinical results subsequently obtained and does not, therefore, appear to be particularly indicative of the quality of the healing process itself (Solomon, 2000).

Diagnostic prejudice regarding pain of the shoulder complex, which can sometimes be attributed to clinical specialties and trends, is frequently correlated with inadequate physical examination of the neuromusculoskeletal system (Donatelli, 1997); it should include an evaluation of all the joints of the shoulder complex (glenohumeral, acromioclavicular, sternoclavicular and scapulothoracic) and very often of the cervical and dorsal spine, and of other structures not belonging to the shoulder girdle.

This chapter will attempt to provide a manual approach to the FE of shoulder pain in the athlete, while bearing in mind, however, that it is precisely by constantly and critically performing evaluation procedures that the physiotherapist will be able to acquire the

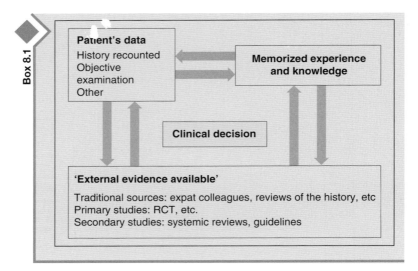

Box 8.1

Patient's data
History recounted
Objective
examination
Other

**Memorized experience
and knowledge**

Clinical decision

'External evidence available'
Traditional sources: expat colleagues, reviews of the history, etc
Primary studies: RCT, etc.
Secondary studies: systemic reviews, guidelines

level of experience necessary to take advantage of its great potential.

In the process of clinical decision making, the knowledge and experience memorized by the examiner are known to be the primary and often the most decisive source of information in support of clinical and therapeutic decisions (Box. 8.1).

History and objective examination

Before starting a physical examination, the patient's clinical history should be reconstructed in meticulous detail. There are many factors which have a key role in defining the clinical condition, something that is particularly problematic owing to the anatomic and functional complexity of the shoulder (Bigliani, 1997).

An important part of the subjective examination is the formulation of an initial hypothesis (clinical presentation) which takes into consideration various aspects such as the observation of the patient's physical and psychosocial 'discomfort' (international classification of functioning, disability and health (ICFDH), WHO), precautions and contraindications to physical examination (Gifford, 2000; Jones, 2000).

An understanding of clinical models of the shoulder complex will help to interpret the information received and will allow the therapist to direct the conversation in order to establish information which will support or refute specific clinical models (Table 8.1).

Lesions of the shoulder, as we have seen in previous chapters, often affect several structures and the medical literature has increasingly frequently in recent years demonstrated and described 'combinations' of

The steps in a functional evaluation

Table 8.1

Measurement of subjective variables
• Interview
• Self-assessment questionnaires
Measurement of objective variables
• Physical (or functional) examination

lesions (Jobe, 1997), with an aetiology which can in many cases be defined as multifactorial.

The differential diagnosis, which we can define as secondary (after the diagnosis by the doctor) and functional, and in which generic shoulder pain can be representative of conditions such as cervical root syndrome, acromioclavicular osteoarthritis, nerve compression syndrome, thoracic outlet syndrome (TOS) or degenerative joint disorders, should not overlook the fact that many of these disorders may jointly cause pain.

The primary aim of the interview between the therapist and the patient is to guide the therapist and to form an initial impression (Box 8.2).

A rapport is established with the patient at the beginning of the interview, in order to gain the patient's confidence so that the physical examination can take place with the patient as relaxed as possible. The first details that the examiner will obtain will be personal data, such as age, handedness, occupation, and sport and leisure activities which are frequently predisposing factors for certain disorders. During the

Box 8.2

Recognition of clinical presentations and generation of a prognostic health profile (modified from *Evidence Based Medicine* 1999)

If the examiner is not experienced in either unusual or more complex cases, the clinical reasoning is based on a process of hypothesis and deduction, involving one or more hypotheses and a search for further data which should be present or absent.

If the rehabilitation specialist is expert or the clinical case is familiar to the specialist, the problem may be recognized immediately by matching it with the memorized characteristics of patients seen in the past.

interview, the physiotherapist should select the activities generally associated with shoulder disorders, such as overhead sports, and the conditions most and least likely to be responsible for the symptoms described.

It is more likely that a young patient will be suffering from instability than an older patient, who is more likely to be affected by degenerative or mechanical disorders (Tytherleigh-Strong, 2001). Many examiners, guided by their experience, base their initial diagnostic hypotheses on these factors (Box 8.2).

The next step in the data-gathering relates to recording symptoms and reconstructing the patient's history. It is necessary, above all, to establish which is the principal disturbance and to ask the patient precise questions, such as: 'Why are you here today? When did your problem begin? How did it begin?' (Wilk, 1997). Similar questions are useful for understanding the

patient's request for help and for understanding the onset and progression of the disturbance in question, for example: 'Did it start gradually or was there a specific traumatic event?'. The distinction between an acute problem and a chronic one is fundamental, not only from the diagnostic point of view (Woodward, 2000), but also as regards therapy; an acute problem will most likely be attributable to a macrotrauma, and a chronic problem to a microtrauma. A macrotrauma is a lesion deriving from a specific traumatic event, while a microtrauma is a lesion resulting from repeated tissue stress, characterized by the gradual onset of the symptoms.

If the principal cause of the damage is an acute trauma, it will be necessary to reconstruct the lesion mechanism to identify the body structures that may be damaged and any contraindications to the examination; forcing a limb in abduction and external rotation beyond the normal amplitude of natural movement will suggest to the therapist a hypothesis of subluxation or dislocation of the shoulder, and of possible glenoid labrum damage.

If the patient has not yet been diagnosed in these cases, an investigation of subjective variables should be carried out, with no physical examination (or a limited one), and the patient referred to a specialist.

If, however, the patient has been given a specific diagnosis following an acute traumatic event, the therapist may proceed with the evaluation, while following the specialist's instructions (Box 8.3).

If a microtrauma, due to overuse, for example, is suspected, the therapist will direct the investigation at intrinsic or extrinsic factors which may have contributed to the lesion and thus to the clinical picture

Box 8.3

Orthopedic specialist and physiotherapist: two health workers at the patient's service

The orthopaedic specialist proposes the following:

The rehabilitation of the shoulder is more difficult than that of any other joint, owing to its unique anatomical and functional structure. It, therefore, requires greater cooperation between the orthopaedic specialist, rehabilitation specialist and physiotherapist than any other situation, directed at an eventual target identified from objectives planned at the start of the therapeutic journey.

Since the rehabilitation programme is critical in both non-surgical and postoperative treatment, the orthopaedic specialist needs not only to understand this type of rehabilitation, but to be actively involved in it.

It is also essential for the rehabilitation specialist to know the orthopaedic specialist's clinical diagnosis and the outcome of any surgery.

It is, furthermore, absolutely vital that the patient is given precise information about the situation, the therapeutic journey to be undertaken and the obstacles to be overcome.

This demonstrates the need to work as a team where everyone shares a common objective, though with different roles and professional specialties (see diagram).

Patient

Orthopaedic specialist

Physiotherapist

exhibited by the patient. Intrinsic factors are functional anomalies of the shoulder region and of the musculoskeletal structures predisposing to damage; extrinsic factors, by contrast, are external causes, such as participation in sports and repetitive activities or certain postures at work (Frost, 1999).

The symptoms associated with shoulder lesions may be very varied and the patient should, therefore, be asked in detail about pain experienced, weakness, instability of the limb, fear of movement, stiffness, locking, clicking, crepitus and noises perceived in relation to certain movements, swelling, paraesthesia, tingling, etc.

Despite an incomplete pathophysiological and clinical understanding of pain, and although many individual factors may interfere with it, pain nevertheless remains a key aspect of the clinical picture in individuals who take part in sport.

Pain is clearly the commonest symptom that can be associated with the lesion, and the other symptoms, such as weakness, stiffness, and reduction in or loss of movement, are often secondary to it and resolve when it disappears. It is, therefore, very important to distinguish a genuine state of weakness from a state of pain inhibition. If weakness persists beyond the pain, the evaluation should tend towards rupture of the cuff or a neurological problem secondary to cervical radiculopathy or entrapment of the suprascapular nerve. If stiffness persists, conditions which may be associated with inert structures, i.e. capsular conditions, should be considered.

The pain may present in various locations and it may, therefore, be very difficult to establish its origin.

For example, in rotator cuff disorder and in subacromial impingement syndrome, the pain tends to be located in the anterolateral area of the shoulder, and if rupture has occurred, it may be reported at the insertion of the deltoid. If a concomitant disorder of the long head of the biceps brachii is present, the pain may be reported in the arm and elbow; more distal pain is rarely associated with a rotator cuff disorder (Jobe, 1997). Patients with anterior traumatic instability frequently describe posterior shoulder pain, secondary to impingement against the posterior rim of the glenoid. Patients with multidirectional shoulder instability, however, report diffuse, rather widespread pain, which may result from secondary tendinopathy in an overused rotator cuff.

In order to establish the origin of the pain (Table 8.2), it will also be necessary to ask questions about its nature, quality, intensity and depth. It is important to identify the position in which the patient experiences the maximum pain or discomfort. For example, pain

Table 8.2

Definition of the pain

Symptom reported	Probable location
Deep, dull pain, difficult to pinpoint	Visceral, ligamentous, deep muscle and bone structures
Superficial, sharp, biting pain	Skin, tendons and bursal tissue
Pulsating pain	Vascular lesion
Paraesthesia, torpor	Nerve damage or irritation

with the limb above the head in abduction and external rotation suggests anterior shoulder instability; a sensation of discomfort with the limb flexed forward and rotated internally (such as when you push a door to open it) suggests posterior instability. Patients with multidirectional instability often complain of pain, weakness or paraesthesia while carrying heavy objects, owing to the traction exerted on the brachial plexus; these patients have inferior laxity with concomitant anterior or posterior instability, or both.

The behaviour of the symptoms, the course of the pain over a 24-hour period, its duration and the association between pain and activity, i.e. the presence or absence of pain at rest or during movement, should also be determined. This will provide information about the patient's level of activity and, therefore, about the relative loss of functional power.

Patients with acute rotator cuff disorder have mild, intermittent pain during movements above the head; patients with a chronic disorder have persistent, moderate pain during overhead activities and pain may also be present at rest. Patients with partial or total rupture of the cuff have persistent pain, and those with complete rupture typically present with pain at night (Wolin, 1997).

Further differential signs are factors that aggravate or alleviate the pain. Musculoskeletal pain during the day is generally subject to variations associated with activity and posture.

Having identified the characteristics of the pain or the symptoms, the possibility of referred somatic, visceral or radicular pain should be excluded. Warning signs noted during history-taking may suggest other disorders (Table 8.3). Many diseases of the cardiovascular, pulmonary or gastrointestinal systems, such as angina pectoris, peptic ulcer, hiatus hernia, and neoplasias, for example, cause referred shoulder pain. Neck pain which spreads below the elbow is, however,

Characteristics of visceral pain

Table 8.3

The pain is constant

The appearance of the pain is unrelated to trauma or excessive use

The pain is pulsating, acute, deep, lancing or colic

The symptoms are not alleviated by resting

The symptoms are bilateral

Constitutional symptoms (fever, nausea, instability, unexplained weight loss) are present

The pain worsens at night

The pain does not change with body position or activity

The pain is dramatically lessened by aspirin (bone tumour)

The pain changes in relation to organ function (eating, intestinal activity, coughing, breathing deeply)

Indigestion, constipation, diarrhoea or rectal bleeding are present

The shoulder pain increases with effort in which it is not involved (walking or climbing stairs)

Gathering information

Table 8.4

Personal information
- Reference data provided by the doctor
- Personal details
- Co-morbidity
- Patient's expectations

Information on the course of the disease
- Inventory of disorders
- Development of the disease over time
- Course of impairments
- Course of disabilities
- Course of participation in sports

Information on links between different areas
- Inventory of links between: impairment and disability and between impairment-disability and participation

Present status of the disease
- Current disturbances
- Current level of activity and participation
- Evaluation of the link between load and load ability
- Evaluation of local and general capacity for adaptation (reaction to the load)
- Evaluation of current coping strategies
- Use of drugs

often a subtle sign of cervical disorder, which may be confused with a shoulder problem. It should also be kept in mind that almost all the structures of the shoulder arise from segment C5, and the pain is consequently perceived inside this dermatome, with the exception of the AC joint which refers pain to the C4 dermatome.

In a patient with muscle atrophy and deficit, with no pain and an atraumatic disorder, the evaluation should rather suggest neuropathy, particularly if the problem is bilateral.

Part of the proposed examination is aimed at establishing the level of reactivity of the lesion (and thus the stage of the clinical condition) in order to predict how the patient will tolerate the evaluation and to decide on the most appropriate treatment.

It should be noted, in this respect, that both the pain threshold and the pain tolerance threshold are higher in athletes, and that the pain sensitivity range (the difference between the pain threshold and the pain tolerance threshold) of individuals who perform more intense motor activities is significantly wider than in normal individuals.

The therapist should finally ask about the patient's general health, past and present, and document all factors including any social or lifestyle changes, pharmacological therapies used, previous corticosteroid injections, surgical procedures, physiotherapy received and the outcome of these with regard to the disorder (Table 8.4).

Self-assessment questionnaires

A patient suffering from shoulder pain provides the therapist with an opportunity to evaluate the subjectivity of the pain. In order to quantify the data observed, it will, therefore, be necessary to measure the pain.

It is useful, in this respect, to make an initial distinction, suggested by McGuire (1992), between measurement and assessment.

Measurement is a process which defines the quantity, degree or level of something, using a measuring tool or a standard unit of measurement.

Functional examination as part of manual therapy

Assessment comprises analysis of the nature, significance or status of something; in this specific case it includes, for example, the cognitive-affective correlates of pain, the relational aspects, the impact on the lifestyle and athletic performance of the patient, etc. Assessment thus involves a descriptive component and an evaluation component. When applied to pain, it refers to the experience as a whole.

It is still difficult, with current tools, to quantify precisely such a subjective phenomenon as pain. Furthermore, it is not possible to rely exclusively on the patient's verbal description, although this remains indispensable, since the experience of pain depends qualitatively and quantitatively on cognitive, emotional and other factors. This means that in the arduous task of drawing as close as possible to a measurement of pain, we must bear in mind the 'multidimensionality of the experience', so as to avoid ending up with a flat, distorted image of the reality we intend to measure.

Pain measurement scales

The absolute variable most studied in relation to pain is intensity. Numerous methods have been developed to date to measure pain intensity; besides verbal numeric scales (Jensen, 1989), the visual analogue scale (VAS) as per Huskisson (1983), is perhaps one of the most widely used tools.

Visual Analogue Scale

This consists of a straight line, usually 10 cms long, the ends of which correspond to the extremes of pain intensity. The patient is asked to make a pen stroke at the point on the line which corresponds to the severity of the pain. The distance between the left end, which indicates that pain is absent, and the mark made by the patient, measured in millimetres, provides a measure of intensity. The VAS is usually horizontal, and more rarely vertical. Intensity is regarded as increasing from left to right in the former case and from the bottom to the top in the latter case. The VAS is simple to administer: the task can be understood even by 5-year-old children (Scott, 1976).

Tools for the assessment of pain

These tools are used if the measurement obtained with the VAS is poor and insufficient for an evaluation of the quality, as well as of the quantity, of the pain experienced.

An Italian tool is available, developed by Benedittis et al., called the Italian pain questionnaire (IPQ) (De Benedittis, 1988).

Italian pain questionnaire

Dissatisfaction with the Italian versions of the McGill pain questionnaire (MPQ) (Villamira, 1983; Majani, 1985; De Benedittis, 1988) recently prompted the development of an Italian alternative called the Italian pain questionnaire (De Benedittis, 1993) (IPQ).

This is the first semantic questionnaire in Italian based on the original method of Melzack and Torgerson and reconstructed strictly in parallel with the original MPQ.

In its final formulation, it uses 42 descriptors of pain divided into 4 classes:
— sensory;
— affective;
— evaluative;
— miscellaneous;
and 16 subclasses:
— sensory (8);
— affective (4);
— evaluative (2);
— miscellaneous (2).

The last part of the questionnaire contains the scale measuring present pain intensity (PPI), consisting of 5 points: mild, moderate, severe, very severe and excruciating.

This is followed by the section for the examiner's use. This contains the following:
— clinical diagnosis of the patient;
— pain rating index rank (PRIr) for each class (PRIr-S; PRIr-A; PRIr-E; PRIr-M), and for the total (PRIr-T);
— number of words chosen (NWC);
— pain rating index rank coefficient (PRIrc), i.e. the ordinal (or rank) coefficient of use of the individual descriptors for each subclass;
— PPI;
— verbal analogue (VA); and
— VAS.

The IPQ may be given to the patient to complete or preferably be administered by the examiner reading the descriptors directly to the patient.

The second method is preferable for an initial evaluation, while the first is recommended during therapeutic monitoring.

There are two ways in which patients can select the descriptors (putting a cross next to the chosen option): free selection, i.e. patients can select as many descriptors for each subclass as they want; limited selection, i.e. the patient can select no more than one term for each subclass.

In general, free selection is preferable since the individual descriptors are not mutually exclusive, but represent discrete qualities of the pain experienced.

The patient is asked to choose, without any restrictions, the descriptors in each subclass as they are offered. The patient is free to choose one, more than one, all or none, depending on the case, of the descriptors that best represent current experience of pain (for the calculation of the score, see De Benedettis, 1993).

The principal uses of the IPQ are the following:
— quantitative and qualitative measurements of the perception of pain;
— differential diagnosis between states of chronic pain;
— differential diagnosis between 'somatic' and 'psychogenic', 'acute' and 'chronic' pain; and
— for therapeutic monitoring, and for the prediction and evaluation of analgesic methods.

Choice of tool for evaluating pain

The choice of the level of evaluation, and consequently of the tool, is a crucial part of clinical work. There must be a high level of coherence between the type of evaluation and its purpose, for example, during FE it is advisable to use specific assessment tools for contextualizing the pain reported by the patient; if the outcome is inexplicably negative, the use of assessment tools for identifying why the therapeutic objectives have not been met may be considered.

The first decision to be taken is whether to give preference to direct observation of the patient or whether to administer scales or tools for the assessment of pain.

McGuire (1992) has laid down useful criteria for making this choice, as reported in Table 8.5.

Using pain assessment tools means creating a context around the simple quantitative description expressed by the patient.

Although the VAS is simple to apply, more sophisticated tools, such as the IPQ, may be more appropriate, owing to two facts observed in the outcome of therapy (Lamberto, 1999):
— many patients exhibit a high level of anxiety and depression; and
— sometimes the outcome is inexplicably negative, even with equivalent technical, methodological and procedural conditions applied by the operators.

Table 8.5

Criteria for choosing pain evaluation tools (modified by McGuire, 1992)

Use of the questionnaire
- The patient does not have cognitive deficits
- The patient is able to complete questionnaires
- The patient is willing to complete questionnaires
- The aim is to measure the quality of the pain
- The aim is to carry out a multidimensional evaluation of the pain

Direct observation
- The patient is cognitively impaired
- The patient has an acute illness
- The patient has very intense pain
- The aim is to evaluate behaviour connected with the pain
- The aim is to measure the frequency of individual behavioural units

Pain has a frequent association with anxiety and depression, since these are the ultimate manifestations of intense or prolonged stress.

A fundamental consideration is the subjective impact of pain on the life of the individual, since according to what we currently know, events are not stressful in absolute terms but only in relation to how they are viewed by the individual.

The characteristics of the patient's personality and psychological state prior to the onset of the pain are also fundamental.

Although they take different forms, both anxiety and depression take energy from the body, which is already under stress, and this increases asthenia and impairs the patient's commitment to planned therapeutic rehabilitation activities.

Physical problems of various types, such as dizziness, diffuse paraesthesia, tachycardia and tachypnoea, increased muscle tension, headache, and chest or abdominal pain, are signs of a state of anxiety. Observation of the patient will reveal restlessness, difficulty keeping still, disorganized thoughts and remarks, hyperhidrosis, tachycardia, hypertension and increased muscle tone. Phobias may also be present.

Depression requires an affective component (depressed mood, anhedonia, apathy, guilty feelings, loss of hope, lack of initiative), a cognitive component (lack of concentration and general interest in

Fig. 8.1

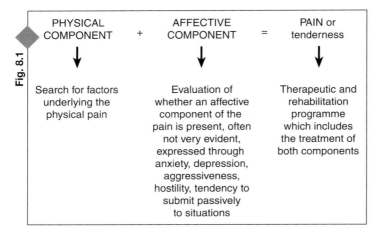

PHYSICAL COMPONENT	+	AFFECTIVE COMPONENT	=	PAIN or tenderness
Search for factors underlying the physical pain		Evaluation of whether an affective component of the pain is present, often not very evident, expressed through anxiety, depression, aggressiveness, hostility, tendency to submit passively to situations		Therapeutic and rehabilitation programme which includes the treatment of both components

Components of pain.

the various aspects of life, poverty and redundancy of thought) and a physical component (insomnia, too much or too little appetite, dry mouth and constipation). Furthermore, a depressed patient often moves and talks slowly, has a lethargic, sad expression on his or her face, and has a generally neglected appearance.

Figure 8.1 highlights the need to consider possible emotional as well as physical factors of the pain expressed by the patient.

The need to identify a possible anxious or depressive component is particularly important since these two factors, if present, have a heavy influence on the perception of both acute and chronic pain, and, therefore, on the type of therapy; the patient may be asked to deal with both in order to obtain a better therapeutic result.

It is vital that the patient is aware, along with the anxiety and depression, of any personal tendency to submit passively to situations and to adopt a hostile, aggressive attitude to others; the patient must also be capable of facing stressful situations.

The need to consider both the physical component of pain, as has always been the case, and its affective component is consequently clear.

From the physical point of view, we shall, therefore, seek the factors causing the pain.

From the affective point of view, the assessment should be carried out by a psychologist, if the case requires it, who will investigate the presence of anxiety, depression, hostility or aggressiveness, which can adversely influence whether therapeutic objectives are met. Since not only the disorder but also the therapeutic programme is a source of stress for the individual, helping patients to improve their strategies for dealing with it is a useful means of achieving the therapeutic objectives.

A therapeutic rehabilitation programme will, therefore, be based on this procedural model which includes the treatment of both components, provided the patient consents to it.

Subjective shoulder rating scale

The subjective shoulder rating scale (SSRS) was proposed by Kohn for any type of shoulder disorder.

This system of measurement is based on the patient's own estimate of the condition of their own shoulder.

It places more emphasis on articular structures (35 points), than on function (10 + 5), or instability (15 points). Pain is evaluated as a score based not on intensity, but on frequency, duration and circumstances.

The maximum possible score for a shoulder without any problems is 100 points.

Functional examination

After the patient's history has been taken, a physical examination of the painful shoulder is performed; this allows the therapist to ascertain the patient's health profile in detail. Examination of the shoulder should be undertaken systematically and, although there is no standardized procedure, it should, according to the majority of authors (Scheibel, 2005) always comprise an inspection, a thorough palpation (in manual therapy palpation is performed at the end of the physical examination), an evaluation of movement, an evaluation of strength and specific tests. When the clinical presentation requires it, the physical examination should also include a detailed evaluation of other joints (lower limbs, spine and elbow) because of the possible effects that these joints, if dysfunctional, can have on the shoulder. The cervicothoracic area seems to have a decisive role in shoulder function. It is a generator of force capable of accelerating the arm, and a limiter of force capable of attenuating the forces acting on the glenohumeral joint during throwing; cervicothoracic tilt and rotation also facilitate the visual acquisition of the target aimed at by the athlete. Reduced extendibility of the hip muscles and weakness of the muscles forming the insertion of the thoracolumbar fascia have significant effects on spinal function, and increase stress on the glenohumeral joint and rotator cuff (Young, 1996).

The physiotherapist will identify the physical tests that reproduce the symptoms complained of by the patient; positive tests are then used to monitor the treatment phases periodically (Petty, 1998).

The physical examination is based on the examination procedures described by several authors, including Maitland (1991), and supported by data from other sources (from the subjective examination and from information provided by the doctor). Specific aspects which have proved to be particularly useful in the functional diagnosis and, as clinical indicators, in the diagnosis of disorders will now be implemented to assess and define the patient's state of health. The focus on the aspects mentioned below should not, however, exclude consideration of other structures of the shoulder complex.

Inspection

The inspection begins with the observation, first overall and then in detail, of the undressed patient, under both static and dynamic conditions. The therapist observes how the patient moves and uses the arm; the therapist may often encounter a 'traumatized attitude', in which the patient uses the opposite hand to support the forearm of the affected limb (Grimberg, 1999), i.e. the affected side is lifted protectively by the patient.

The therapist can, therefore, assess fluidity and quality of movement, the possible presence of impaired motor patterns or 'defective positions', representing specific disorders such as, for example, irreducible internal humeral rotation caused by posterior glenohumeral dislocation.

The observation then continues with an examination of static posture with the patient standing upright, conducted from various perspectives (anterior, lateral, and posterior).

Cervicothoracic posture has a considerable influence on the position and mobility of the scapula

(Crawford, 1991; Culham, 2000; Solem-Bertoft, 1993).

In anterior view, for example, we should observe the following:
— the height of the acromion and the morphology of the clavicle (hyperostosis, deformity);
— asymmetrical or abnormal muscle hypotrophy and atrophy;
— whether the upper limb is in internal or external rotation;
— the space between the arm and trunk;
— the piano key sign: if the acromion is raised in relation to the clavicle, determine whether pressing on the acromion will lower it, and whether releasing the pressure makes the acromion spring back. This phenomenon is known to occur in 'structural' instability of the joint, in which the acromial portion of the clavicle is positioned more cranially to the acromion;
— whether the shoulder is protracted: this is observed when the glenoid cavity is orientated forwards and down; in this case slight internal rotation and adduction of the upper limb are noted. Observation may reveal a more developed deltopectoral groove on the opposite side (Fig. 8.2); and

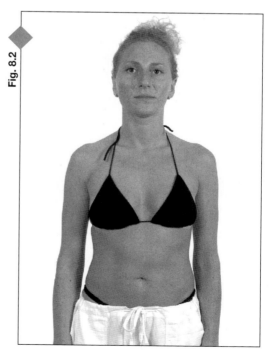

Fig. 8.2

Anterior view.

— the morphology of the sternoclavicular joint.
  A lateral view should show the following:
— cervicodorsal junction;
— dorsal kyphosis;
— anteposition of the head: there is a link between shoulder problems and anteposition of the head, but there is no link between the degree of anteposition and shoulder problems;
— protraction of the shoulder; and
— winged scapula.

A posterior view should show the following (Fig. 8.3):
— the morphology of the trapezius muscles and symmetry of the shoulders;

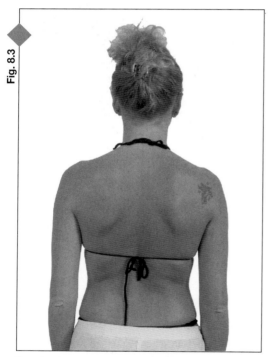

Fig. 8.3

Posterior view.

— the space between the trunk and arm (waist triangle);
— the trophism of certain muscles: deltoid, supraspinatus, infraspinatus, teres minor;
— the position of the scapula in relation to the trunk. Reference position: the medial rim positioned approximately 5 cm from the vertebral column; the inferior angle located at T7-T8; the

superior angle at T2; the scapular spine at T3. Scapula rotated by 30° in the frontal plane. The acromion should be higher than the vertebral angle of the scapula;
— winged scapula: observe whether only the inferior angle or the whole medial rim of the scapula is raised in relation to the chest;
— anterior tilt: inferior angle lifted by the chest and raised scapula; and
— caudal or inferior rotation: superior angle positioned higher than the acromion.

The presence or absence of scapulothoracic dyskinesis will then be evaluated during active movement.

Various clinical proposals have been made, suggesting that certain changes in the resting position of the scapula are associated with a number of shoulder disorders, including subacromial impingement and glenohumeral instability (Solem-Bertoft, 1992; Kibler, 2003; Myers, 2005).

Although there is little evidence for these assertions, the position of the scapula is considered an essential part of the clinical examination of the shoulder.

Some authors (Lewis, 2002) suggest studying scapular position by skin surface palpation of bony landmarks (if there are doubts about inter-rater and intrarater reliability and the validity of measurements):
— thoracic spinous process corresponding to the root of the scapular spine (T2-T3);
— thoracic spinous process corresponding to the inferior angle of the scapula (T7-T8);
— root of the scapular spine (Fig. 8.4);
— acromial angle (Fig. 8.5); and
— inferior angle of the scapula (Fig. 8.6).

DiVeta (1990) proposed a procedure for measuring scapular protraction in this phase, based on the ratio between scapular width (measured from the root of the spine to the inferior acromial angle) and the distance between T3 and the inferior acromial angle; the reliability of this procedure is controversial, however.

The inspection of the outlines of the anatomical structures is completed by examination for any signs of current or previous tissue changes, indicating scars, dyschromia, swelling, deformity, ecchymosis, venous distension, asymmetry, muscle atrophy, prominence of the AC joint and biceps rupture. The simplest way of detecting an abnormality is comparison with the opposite side. The comparative method is one of the keys to a good objective examination and is essential not only for inspection, but for all other diagnostic tests.

Atrophy of the supraspinatus or infraspinatus suggests that the physiotherapist should conduct a further

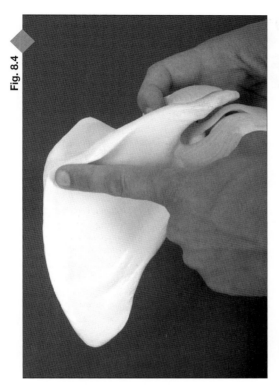

Fig. 8.4

Root of the scapular spine.

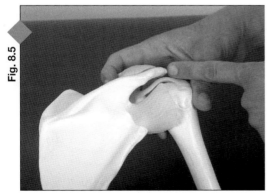

Fig. 8.5

Acromial angle.

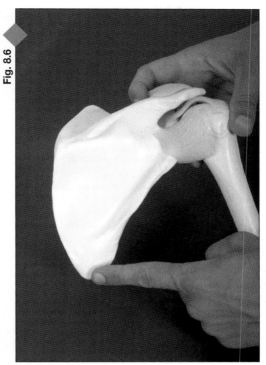

Fig. 8.6

Inferior angle of the scapula.

The normally rounded outline of the deltoid may appear square as a result of inferior subluxation of the humeral head, thus revealing the square morphology of the acromion. The sometimes late discovery of a haematoma on the medial part of the arm, in the axillary region and at the side of the chest (Hennequin or brachiothoracic ecchymosis), is often a sign of proximal fracture of the humerus. If the inspection finds no significant lesions, the examiner will ask the patient to move the limb.

Evaluation of movement

Evaluation of physiological joint movement is based on a knowledge of the functional and mechanical anatomy of the scapulohumeral complex and of osteokinematic and arthrokinematic movement. The examination is carried out by performing active, passive, and accessory movements, tests for strength and, if necessary, specific tests.

Active and passive tests and tests for evaluating strength should be regarded as screening tests and are

direct investigation to identify disorders, such as cuff rupture, entrapment of the suprascapular nerve or radiculopathy. Bone deformities are generally the result of a trauma (acromioclavicular separation, dislocation of the shoulder, or clavicular fractures) and are often rapidly masked by post-traumatic oedema.

performed in each case, whereas specific tests are chosen according to clinical reasoning and the hypotheses formulated.

Active movement

The function of a joint is considered normal if it is capable of performing movement throughout its whole amplitude, without causing pain.

The active arc of movement allows the examiner to evaluate not only the quantity (amplitude) of movement in the various spatial planes, but also its quality. Active movement also provides information about the contractile and inert structures (capsule and related structures) of the joint and shows the examiner whether the patient is willing and able to move the shoulder, allowing an assessment of the patient's limits.

The examiner identifies the limitations or excesses of mobility and any deviation from the normal motor patterns. During these operations, the affected limb is compared with the opposite one, bearing in mind that the dominant side often shows less mobility than the non-dominant side.

The patient is asked to reproduce the painful movement and shows the examiner the movement or actions that principally cause the pain; the examiner should observe the movement being performed, the muscle activation pattern and timing, and any compensation (Kelly, 2005).

Ask the patient in detail about the pain, i.e. the site, the intensity, and whether the arc of pain is present, etc.

The patient is then asked to perform a complete movement of the limb while standing, sitting and lying supine; at the same time, the examiner asks the patient what they feel while performing the movement. The shoulder movements in the cardinal planes are the following:

— flexion (160–180°);
— extension (45–60°);
— abduction (170–180°);
— adduction (65–75°);
— external rotation (80–90°);
— internal rotation (70–80°);
— horizontal abduction (30–45°);
— horizontal adduction (135–140°); and
— elevation (160–180°) in the scapular plane (30–45° anterior to the frontal plane).

The SASES recommend documenting only four, functionally important, arcs of movement; these are complete or possible abduction (Fig. 8.7), external rotation at 0° (Fig. 8.8) and 90° of abduction (Fig. 8.9), and internal rotation (Fig. 8.10).

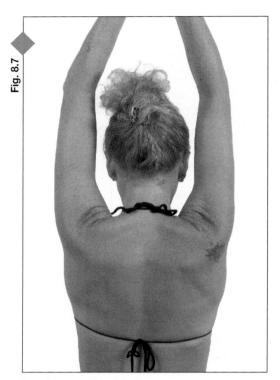

Fig. 8.7

Complete or possible abduction.

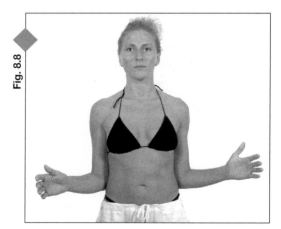

Fig. 8.8

External rotation at 0° abduction.

Observing the raising, lowering, protraction and retraction of the shoulder provides additional information for the evaluation. During active abduction (Fig. 8.11), the scapulohumeral rhythm is closely

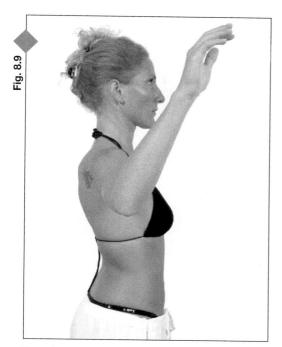

External rotation at 90° abduction.

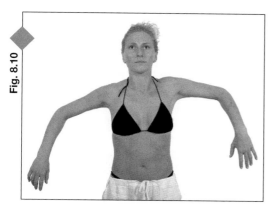

Internal rotation.

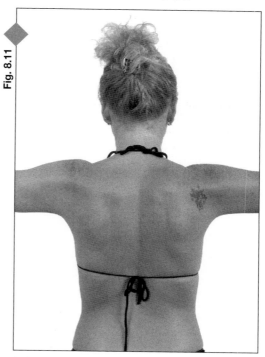

Active abduction.

— movement of the scapula (the scapula starts to move at about 60–70° of abduction);
— whether the arc of pain can be relieved by an abduction movement performed in a more anterior plane.

Pain and muscle weakness may cause loss of joint movement, and the appearance of compensation, which is demonstrated, for example, in the scapulothoracic contribution to glenohumeral rotations and in the extension of the trunk during elevation of the arm.

In active abduction or elevation, the presence of an arc of pain between 70° and 120° could indicate impingement.

At this point the examiner will ask the patient to perform the following functional movements:
— *hand behind the head:* patients are asked to bring their hand above their head and to reach the backbone, if possible, with their thumb (glenohumeral elevation and external rotation and scapular rotation); the functional limitation consists in this case of an inability to perform actions above the head, such as combing the hair or throwing (Fig. 8.12);
— *hand behind the back:* patients are asked to bring their hand behind their back and to touch the backbone

observed; if neuromuscular control of the scapulothoracic joint is inadequate, there will be no stable base to support the glenohumeral joint (Davies, 1993).

During active abduction, observe the following:
— compensation in the sagittal plane, such as an increase in lumbar lordosis, and assess whether the patient is able to correct compensatory movements;
— quality of movement in abduction and in the return phase;

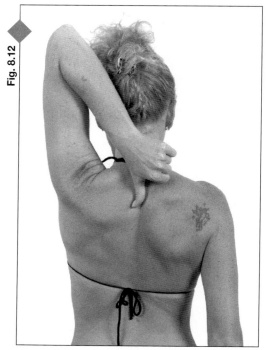

Fig. 8.12

Hand behind the head test.

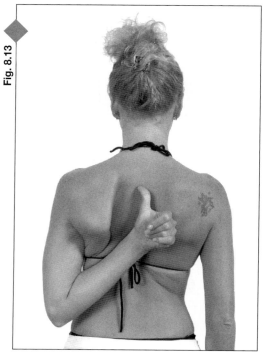

Fig. 8.13

Hand behind the back.

Fig. 8.14

with the thumb (extension, adduction and internal rotation and scapular distraction); this limitation prevents movements such as fastening a brassiere or reaching back pockets (Fig. 8.13);

— *hand on the opposite shoulder:* patients are asked to bring their hand in front of face and to touch the backbone with the thumb (flexion and horizontal adduction); it involves limitations in various athletic movements and towards the opposite side of the body (Fig. 8.14).

Raising, lowering, protraction and retraction of the shoulders conclude the general muscle examination of the scapulothoracic complex. Kibler (1991) described the lateral slide scapular test as an objective means of quantifying scapular stability. The examiner measures the bilateral distance between the inferior apex of the scapula and the T7 spinous process of the patient in three progressive positions: with the arms by the sides, supported on the hips with the thumbs pointing backwards, and abducted at 90°. The presence of asymmetry of more than 1.5 cm is correlated with reduced functionality of the affected shoulder (Morrison, 2000) (Fig. 8.15).

The same author (Kibler, 1998) proposed the scapular squeeze test to assess scapular retraction

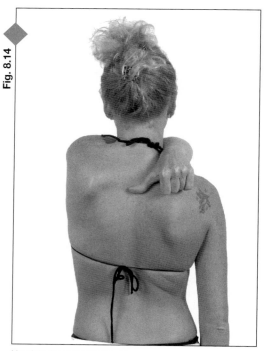

Hand on the opposite shoulder.

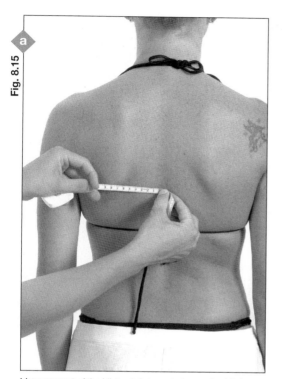

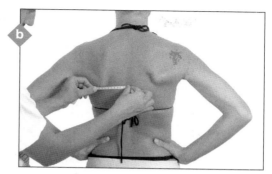

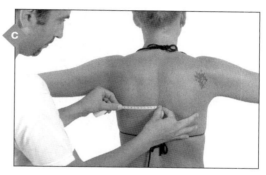

Fig. 8.15

Measurement of the bilateral distance between the inferior apex of the scapula and the T7 spinous process in three progressive positions: (a) arms by the sides; (b) arms supported on the hips with the thumbs pointing backwards; (c) arms abducted a 90°.

strength: the inability to maintain scapular retraction (pinch) for more than 15 seconds, without feeling a significant burning sensation, may indicate scapular weakness (Meister 2000) (Fig. 8.16).

Other functional tests, such as pushing against a wall (Fig. 8.17) or lifting from a sitting position, evaluate the integrity of the stabilizer muscles of the scapula.

To conclude the study of the scapulothoracic joint, we suggest the following active tests:

— *Scapular retraction test:* the examiner performs the test comparatively for the external rotators (adduction and external rotation) and Jobe's test for the supraspinatus.

The patient is asked to raise, retract and lower the shoulder blades, and then to perform the two strength tests described above again; the test is considered positive if an improvement is noted in the patient's ability in the second sets of tests. This test determines whether even a temporary repositioning of the scapulothoracic joint (retraction) can improve the muscle action of the shoulder activators;

— *Scapular assistance test:* this test identifies a deficit in the active elevation of the acromion, to

determine whether subacromial impingement depends on an impaired scapulothoracic rhythm. The examiner pushes the medial rim of the scapula at the side and top, to substitute for the action of the anterior serratus and the inferior portion of the trapezius (Fig. 8.18). The patient's clinical manifestations (pain) will thus be reduced or relieved completely. The therapist stabilizes the scapula at the top with the other hand.

Passive osteokinematic movement

Examination of passive movement excludes the component dependent on muscle strength and allows inert joint structures to be tested. This examination may be conducted sitting or lying supine, and the patient needs to be completely relaxed and must not participate in the movement. The examiner should, therefore, start the evaluation on the unaffected limb.

It is important that the tests are always performed in the same basic position and these tests must be compared bilaterally. If one of the shoulder blades is more protracted or in adduction, this plane must be

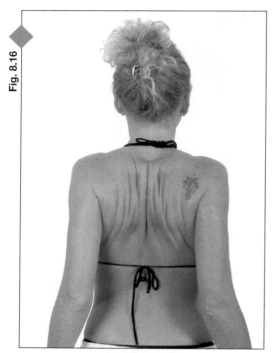

Fig. 8.16

Scapular squeeze test.

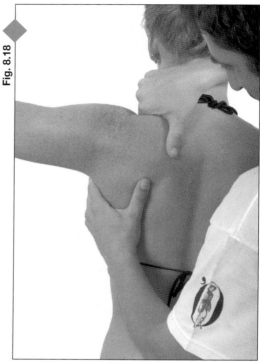

Fig. 8.18

Scapular assistance test.

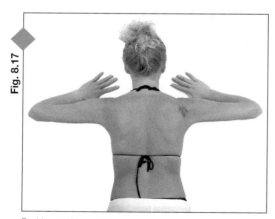

Fig. 8.17

Pushing against a wall.

respected to obtain a correct evaluation of the gleno-humeral joint.

The following are evaluated during the tests:
— pain (where, when, what type);
— range of motion (limited, normal or hypermobile);
— quality of movement (any resistance during the test);

— crepitus; and
— end of range sensation.

Three limits of excursion can normally be identified in an evaluation of the ROM: an active limit, up to the point the movement can be made with muscle activity; a physiological limit, which is the passive excursion of the movement, and an anatomical limit, which also stresses the plastic and elastic components of the capsule tissue. A further movement would necessarily involve damage to the anatomical structures. The anatomical limit takes its name from the anatomical stop of the movement. Where a disorder is present, two further limits can be found: a pain limit and a non-physiological excursion limit.

There are two different methods of evaluating passive joint movement:
— a procedure targeted at the osteokinematic or angular component; and
— a procedure targeted at the arthrokinematic or accessory component.

Osteokinematic evaluation focuses essentially on angular movement, i.e. flexion, extension, abduction, adduction, and external or internal rotation.

During angular movements, the bone segments move in the space around an articular rotation axis and in a plane perpendicular to the axis.

It is vital that the therapist works extremely carefully and precisely during the passive movements typically tested, i.e.:

— in complete abduction;
— in glenohumeral abduction at 90° (120°);
— clavicle rhythm (Stenvers Test);
— in flexion;
— in external rotation in the scapular plane;
— in external rotation at 0° abduction;
— in external rotation at 90° abduction;
— in internal rotation at 0° abduction (Fig. 8.19); and
— in internal rotation at 90° abduction.

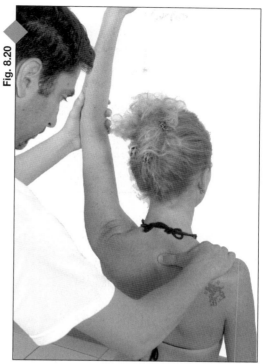

Fig. 8.20

Complete elevation/abduction.

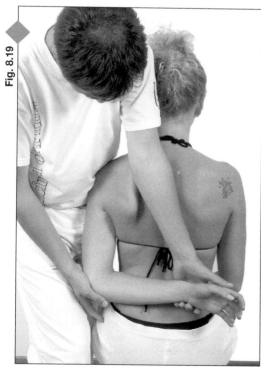

Fig. 8.19

Internal rotation at 0° of abduction.

Complete elevation/abduction

This test is useful for determining whether the arc of pain observed during active functional tests is also present during passive movement. It is also useful for obtaining information on the severity and location of the problem. It may also be defined as a provocation

test for the AC and SC joints. It additionally allows an evaluation of the movement of the cervicodorsal junction (Fig. 8.20).

Abduction should occur in line with the orientation of the glenoid (30° in an anterior direction), bearing in mind that in patients with kyphosis, the scapular plane could be even more anterior.

Clavicle rhythm

This test evaluates the behaviour of the clavicle during anteflexion (Fig. 8.21).

The clavicle rotates around the examiner's finger during anterior flexion, during the test: at about 120° the therapist notices the finger being pushed (by a cranial and dorsal movement of the clavicle). If the movement of the clavicle is abnormal (owing to scapular protraction or restriction of movement), the finger will be pushed out of the supraclavicular space before the shoulder has achieved 120° of anterior flexion.

The following can be suspected if the clavicle rotates early during the test:
— glenohumeral stiffness;
— acromioclavicular stiffness; and
— a sternoclavicular problem.

Functional examination as part of manual therapy

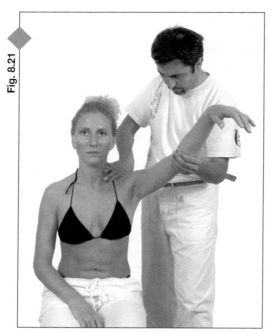

Fig. 8.21

Clavicle rhythm.

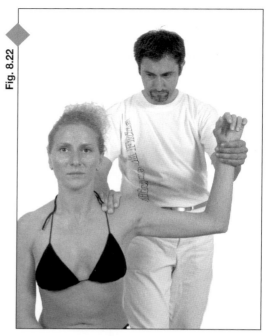

Fig. 8.22

Example of excessive external rotation with soft end feel.

By comparing the weakness, stiffness or pain found in the active examination and in the passive examination, the therapist can determine whether the structure responsible for the limitation or symptoms is contractile (extra-articular: muscles or tendons) or non-contractile (articular: ligaments, capsule, etc.).

A reduction in passive internal rotation, for example, if isolated, is indicative of posterior capsular retraction and suggests secondary impingement. For a better distinction between intra-articular and extra-articular stiffness, attention should also be paid to the quality and type of joint movement stop by evaluating the 'end feel'. Cyriax (1982) described six types of end feel, three of which were normal and three abnormal. Kaltenborn (1989) described four types, three normal and one abnormal; and Paris and Loubert (1990) described fifteen types, five normal and ten abnormal.

Although the exact diagnostic significance and interpretation of end feel are controversial, the presence of abnormal or pathological types should, in any case, suggest dysfunction (Petersen, 2000). Patients with shoulder instability frequently exhibit an end range with muscle spasm or empty end feel (there is no resistance owing to pain or apprehension). Excessive external rotation with a soft end feel suggests hypermobility and thus excessive anterior humeral movement on clinical examination (Fig. 8.22).

Passive arthrokinematic movement

Accessory movements occur naturally and involuntarily during physiological joint movements of the shoulder complex and consist of rolling, translation and rotation. Arthrokinematic evaluation takes into account the movement of a joint surface in relation to another joint surface (e.g. the humeral head on the glenoid); it takes into consideration the geometry of the joint profiles and the arrangement of the periarticular tissues. It is thus possible to test the reciprocal movement of the joint surfaces, the migration of the contact areas, and the position and orientation of the instantaneous centre of rotation (ICR). An evaluation of accessory movements will guide the therapist in identifying the structures responsible for restriction or excess movement, and in specifying which areas of the capsule are involved.

Mennell (1964), who coined the phrase 'articular play', mentions seven accessory movements of the glenohumeral joint:
— anterior slide;
— posterior slide;
— lateral slide;

— inferoposterior slide;
— lateroposterior slide;
— external rotation of the humeral head inside the glenoid cavity; and
— posterior slide of the humeral head in the glenoid cavity with the shoulder flexed at 90°.

According to Maitland (1986), accessory movements can be performed on the patient and comprise slide, traction/compression and rotation of the joint; six are described:
— anteroposterior;
— posteroanterior;
— caudal longitudinal;
— cephalic longitudinal;
— lateral; and
— medial.

Examination of accessory movements, which can be performed with the patient seated or lying supine or prone, should respect the orientation of the gleno-humeral joint surfaces. The evaluation should also involve the AC, SC and scapulothoracic joints (scapular distraction and slide along the chest) and should assess end feel or any abnormal reactions (spasm, pain or apprehension).

Translation tests are used for the diagnosis of shoulder instability, and as provocation tests. In instability, humeral slides are very large in contrast with the situation in frozen shoulder, in which there is involvement of mainly capsular connective tissue or subacromial impingement, where ascent of the humeral head is noted, along with a reduction in the joint space.

The quantification of these movements using graduated scales, such as that proposed by Altchek and Dines (1993), is still under investigation and is controversial owing to the subjective nature of performing (position of the tests, strength used) and interpreting them, and inter-rater reliability is moderate (Ellenbecker, 2002).

The tests are described in detail in Chapter 14 (Manual therapy in rehabilitation); these are tests and treatment techniques at the same time and will not, therefore, be addressed here.

Passive 'accessory' tests are essentially intended to test two indicators: joint play and end feel (Tables 8.6 and 8.7).

Evaluation of strength

The efficiency of shoulder muscle activity depends on many factors, including the optimal position of the scapula, and the relation between the tension and length of the stabilizers of the scapula (anterior serratus,

Table 8.6 **Passive accessory tests**

Joint play
• Characterized by a segment in which movement occurs without any resistance from the soft tissues
• Beyond this range, the tissues are under tension, they distend and begin to to offer initial mild resistance

End feel
• Articular end feel

Table 8.7 **End feel**

Physiological quality of end feel
• Elastic sensation
Pathological quality of end feel
• Hard: low reactivity/marked PROM limitation
• Spastic resistance: to reactivity/muscle defence contractions
• Empty: resistance to movement – 'pain limit'

trapezius and rhomboids) and the rotator cuff (supraspinatus, infraspinatus, teres minor and subscapularis). These muscles must be examined carefully using the manual isometric muscle test.

Manual isometric muscle test

Strength is examined by means of the manual muscle test (MMT); this provides information on the degree of resistance that a musculotendon unit is capable of offering. Several electromyographic studies are currently being conducted to identify positions that can isolate the muscles to be examined more precisely (Lyons, 1998), and this might result in modifying how some tests are performed.

A general examination of the shoulder muscles comprises the following:
— flexion of the elbow at 0° abduction, with the elbow flexed and with the forearm in a neutral position (Fig. 8.23);
— extension of the elbow at 0° abduction, with the elbow flexed and with the forearm in a neutral position (Fig. 8.24);
— abduction at 30° abduction (starting position);

Functional examination as part of manual therapy

— adduction at 30° abduction (starting position) (Fig. 8.25);
— external rotation at 0° abduction (starting position) (Fig. 8.26); and
— internal rotation at 0° abduction (starting position) (Fig. 8.27).

Evaluation is carried out by means of maximum isometric contraction. When the patient performs the movement, the therapist applies pressure to the arm, opposing the action until an equal and opposite resistance is produced. The examination is then compared with the opposite limb to quantify the findings according to the medical research council (MRC) scale (grade 0–5).

The tenomuscular component of the rotator cuff and of other structures responsible for the dynamic stabilization of the scapulohumeral joint is conventionally taken into consideration by means of a maximal isometric test in a neutral position. The pain and weakness associated with resistance to the movement probably involve a single component of the cuff, although the discriminatory value of these tests remains limited when the resistance to multiple movements is positive, as a consequence of the interdigitation of the rotator cuff fibres (Clark, 1992). Significant weakness, during both resisted adduction and external rotation, is, however, a sign of a severe lesion of the rotator cuff (Clark, 1990).

Fig. 8.24

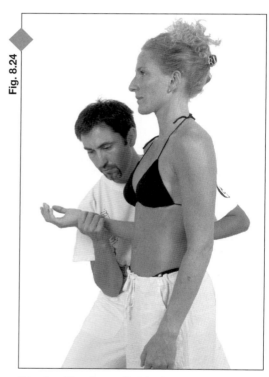

Extension of the elbow at 0° abduction, with the elbow flexed and the forearm in a neutral position.

Fig. 8.23

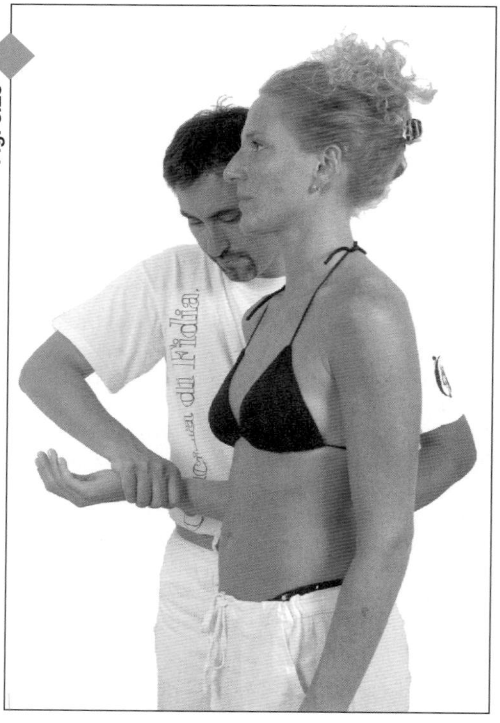

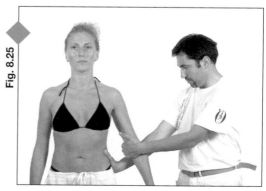

Flexion of the elbow at 0° abduction, with the elbow flexed and the forearm in a neutral position.

Fig. 8.25

Adduction at 30° abduction (starting position).

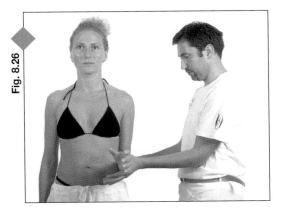

External rotation at 0° abduction (starting position).

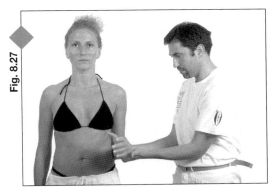

Internal rotation at 0° abduction (starting position).

Of the many tests proposed in the literature, we suggest the six tests against resistance mentioned above to assess shoulder strength and pain.

According to the author, debility or effort limiting pain during isometric testing is considered a positive tendon sign. According to other authors, tests against resistance trigger selective pain, which is the diagnostic key, provided the test is performed at different levels of muscle tension and several levels of muscle amplitude (Danowski, 2000).

Pain accompanied by weakness is a common finding, in particular in rotator cuff problems. As already mentioned, true hyposthenia should be distinguished from weakness caused by the pain. A patient with subacromial bursitis and cuff lesion often has objective muscle weakness caused by pain when the limb is positioned in the impingement arc. If the arm is not tested in abduction, a patient with bursitis will have normal strength.

The supraspinatus tendon is often involved in rotator cuff lesions. The function of this muscle is easily isolated with the limb at 90° elevation in the scapular plane and in complete internal rotation (empty can position). Muscle evaluation against resistance in this position may reveal weakness, secondary to a tendon lesion, or pain associated with cuff impingement. A positive result in this test is, therefore, difficult to interpret. Some clinicians consider the test to be positive for supraspinatus tendon rupture if weakness or pain is present, while others regard this test purely as a method of evaluating muscle strength.

An electromyographic study conducted by Malanga (1996) confirms that the same test, performed with the thumbs pointing upwards (full can position), does not isolate the supraspinatus muscle better. A comparative study recently found that, if the only criterion chosen for interpreting the two tests is muscle weakness, both the tests are more accurate in indicating a tendon lesion. According to other authors, the full can test causes less pain and is, therefore, preferable in a clinical environment (Itoi, 1999). The strength of the subscapularis can be evaluated by means of the lift-off test.

The lift-off test is used, as for testing the supraspinatus, both to evaluate muscle strength and to demonstrate the lesion. This examination, described by Gerber and Krushell in 1991, is performed with the affected limb extended and rotated internally behind the back, and the elbow flexed. The inability of patients to move the back of the hand away from the body, with subsequent internal rotation, indicates lesion of the subscapularis.

The test is very accurate (Hertel, 1996); however Deutsch noted in a 1997 study that only a small number of patients with confirmed rupture of the subscapularis showed a positive test result; the remaining patients were unable to complete the test owing to pain.

A modified version of this examination has been studied for patients with limitations in internal rotation of the limb, since these patients are unable to position their right hands behind their backs. For this version, the patient places an open hand on the abdomen and keeps the elbow in front of the body. If the patient is capable of resisting the external rotation applied by the therapist, maintaining the anterior position of the elbow, the function of the subscapularis is normal. If, however, the elbow gives way in a posterior direction and touches the side, the subscapularis is defective (belly test).

A diagnosis of complete rupture of the long head of the biceps tendon is clear in the presence of distal descent of the muscle belly. Partial rupture and tenosynovitis may be more difficult or impossible to confirm, because the specific tests for these disorders are not very reliable. A stable dislocation of the biceps tendon is difficult to recognize on clinical examination, unlike a reducible dislocation, in which the protrusion and relocation of the tendon can be observed in the bicipital groove in abduction and external and internal rotation (Abbott-Saunders test) (Postacchini, 2001).

Patients with rotator cuff tendinitis frequently present with concomitant inflammation of the bicipital tendon. The therapist can use Yergason's test to evaluate instability or inflammation of this tendon: the patient's elbow is flexed at 90° with the thumbs pointing upwards, and the examiner holds the patient's wrist to offer resistance to the patient's attempt to supinate the forearm and flex the elbow.

Speed's manoeuvre, which is more sensitive than Yergason's test, evaluates the proximal part of the biceps tendon, by flexing the patient's elbow by 20–30°, with the forearm supinated and the humerus flexed by about 60°. The examiner resists flexion of the arm and at the same time palpates the bicipital tendon on the anterior side of the shoulder. Speed's test has demonstrated diagnostic sensitivity of 90%, specificity of 14%, a positive predictive value of 23% and a negative predictive value of 83%. Both tests are considered positive for instability and inflammation if they cause pain.

The drop arm sign is performed when an extensive rotator cuff lesion is suspected. The test is performed by passively abducting the patient's limb and then observing its slow descent to the side, performed actively. If there is a cuff rupture or supraspinatus dysfunction, the arm will fall along the patient's side as soon as it reaches abduction of slightly less than 90°. If the patient is capable of lowering the limb slowly to 90° (since this function is performed to a greater extent by the deltoid muscle), a gentle tap on the forearm will make the limb fall along the trunk. Owing to its high specificity (98%), the drop arm sign has specific predictive power for cuff lesions, but its sensitivity is only 10% (Murrell, 2001). A positive test result may also indicate paralysis of the axillary nerve.

It should also be noted that features of the history such as age (Frost, 1999), shoulder trauma and night pain are relevant when diagnosing rotator cuff rupture. Indeed it has been found that the combination of factors most closely associated with a cuff lesion was age over 65 years, night pain and loss of strength in external rotation (Litaker, 2000).

Palpation

Palpation is the last phase of the physical examination of the patient. The physiotherapist assesses skin temperature, swelling, neurovegetative changes (increased sweating), crepitus and the patient's reaction to contact (pain, anxiety, muscle spasm) by applying firm but gentle contact. This phase includes palpation of the bony prominences, accessible joints and tendon insertions to detect painful areas (including trigger points), deformities or evident changes associated with them.

Any swelling or painful area should be located as accurately as possible. The supraspinatus tendon can be located by placing the fingertips under the anterior rim of the acromial process. The long head of the biceps tendon is adjacent, but just under the supraspinatus tendon, in the bicipital groove. It can be easily identified by holding the patient's elbow in one hand and moving the limb alternately in internal and external rotation. The examiner can feel it sliding under the fingers.

A good test for detecting a possible deficit of the long head of the biceps is to palpate the tendon using the index or middle finger below the anterior rim of the acromion, first with the shoulder in extension (the tendon is thus pushed forwards against the examiner's finger and the patient feels pain) and then with the shoulder slightly flexed (in this position the tendon disappears under the acromion and palpation, therefore, becomes difficult).

Particular attention should, therefore, be paid to examination of the AC and SC joints, the clavicle, the acromion, the joint lines, the bicipital groove, the coracoid apophysis and the humeral tuberosities. The soft tissues that can be assessed are the tendons of the supraspinatus, infraspinatus, teres minor, subscapularis and greater pectoral muscles and of the long head of the biceps, the serous bursae and the neurovascular structures.

Caution is nevertheless required when interpreting palpation findings. According to various authors, this is the least reliable diagnostic method for soft tissue lesions, since it yields little information and often irritates the affected structures. Comparison with the unaffected side is, therefore, essential.

Many disorders can be associated with pain caused by direct pressure, for example, fracture of the clavicle or acromioclavicular separation, acromioclavicular arthritis, supraspinatus or bicipital tendinitis and entrapment of the suprascapular nerve (suprascapular fossa) or axillary nerve (quadrangular space).

Disorder-targeted tests

Tests targeted at disorders (instability or impingement) form part of the specialist examination and have already been described (see Chapter 6). The doctor or physiotherapist should be able to carry out a sufficient number to be able to guide the patient in making the best therapeutic choice or to further diagnostic tests. These tests may be supplemented by an evaluation of the neurovascular structures of the upper quadrant; they include neural tension tests or upper limb tension tests (ULTT), which seem to be of particular interest for physiotherapists.

Neurovascular tests

The physiotherapist should consider TOS in the differential diagnosis of shoulder pain. This is a controversial clinical condition, in which the neurovascular structures are compressed where they leave the thorax, above the first rib (Fig. 8.28). It has many causes and its symptoms may be confused with those of far commoner disorders, such as rotator cuff disorders. The symptoms reported by the patient may include paraesthesia, pain, and sensory and motor loss. Incessant pain is recorded as the commonest symptom.

Standard clinical tests used to evaluate areas that might cause the compression of the neurovascular structures are sometimes ambiguous; neural tension tests have, therefore, been used very recently to assess and treat abnormal nerve dynamics of the brachial plexus. Each of the standard tests includes an upper limb tension test component, nowadays borrowed almost exclusively from physiotherapists. The commonest conventional tests are listed below.

Adson's test

Adson's test evaluates the role of the anterior scalene in abolishing the radial pulse when the muscle is tense.

The therapist holds the patient's wrist so as to detect the radial pulse, then abducts the affected limb by 30° and extends it, asking the patient to turn their head to the same side, to breathe in deeply and to hold it. The quality of the radial pulse is then compared with that measured with the limb by the side, to identify changes in amplitude, or its disappearance. The test is positive if these changes are detected and the patient's symptoms reproduced (see Fig. 8.29). If the radial pulse is diminished or absent, this indicates possible compression of the vascular component of the

Fig. 8.29

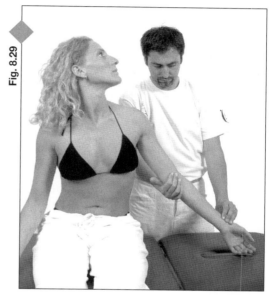

Adson's test.

Fig. 8.28

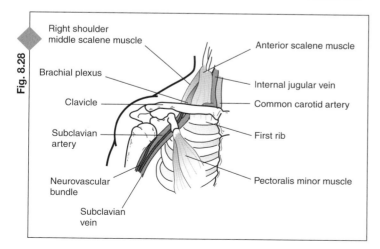

Right shoulder
middle scalene muscle

Brachial plexus

Clavicle

Subclavian
artery

Neurovascular
bundle

Subclavian
vein

Anterior scalene muscle

Internal jugular vein

Common carotid artery

First rib

Pectoralis minor muscle

The neurovascular bundle of the upper limb. Relations with clinically relevant musculoskeletal structures are illustrated.

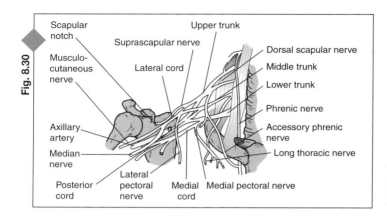

Fig. 8.30

Scapular notch
Suprascapular nerve
Musculo-cutaneous nerve
Lateral cord
Axillary artery
Median nerve
Posterior cord
Lateral pectoral nerve
Medial cord
Medial pectoral nerve
Upper trunk
Dorsal scapular nerve
Middle trunk
Lower trunk
Phrenic nerve
Accessory phrenic nerve
Long thoracic nerve

The brachial plexus: divisions into the upper, middle, and lower trunks and subsequent division into the peripheral nerves are shown.

neurovascular bundle by the anterior scalene muscle or by a cervical rib. Paraesthesia or radiculopathy of the upper limbs indicates compression of the nerve component of the neurovascular bundle (C8-T1 dermatomeres) (Figs. 8.29, 8.30).

Roos test

The test is performed on the patient with the limb abducted and rotated externally at 90° and with the elbow flexed at 90°, by repeatedly opening and closing the hand about 15 times. This posture assesses compression of the neurovascular structures between the clavicle and the first rib, adding an element of stress caused by the exercise. The progression of the symptoms during the test (fatigue, cramps, torpor) is a positive sign of thoracic syndrome.

If the sign considered during these tests is abolition of the radial pulse, their reliability is poor, since many asymptomatic individuals demonstrate changes in pulse during these manoeuvres. Reproduction of the neurological symptoms is, therefore, the most reliable guide for the physiotherapist (Fig. 8.31).

Test on the costoclavicular joint

With the patient seated, palpate the radial pulse and ask him or her to push his or her shoulders strongly backwards, with the chin flexed towards the chest (see Fig. 8.32).

If the radial pulse diminishes or disappears, this indicates compression of the vascular component of the neurovascular bundle. This is often due to a reduction in the space between the clavicle and the first rib. Paraesthesia and radiculopathy in the upper limbs

Fig. 8.31

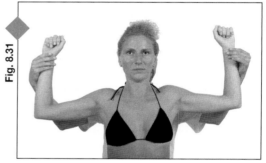

Roos test.

suggest compression of the nerve component of the neurovascular bundle (Figs. 8.32, 8.33).

Tension test

The ULTT, otherwise known as the brachial plexus tension test, or Elvey test, was introduced by Elvey in 1979 and has become popular in recent years.

Butler proposed four tests based on powerful tension manoeuvres of the nervous system, each test being specific to a prevalent nerve trunk:
— *ULTT 1:* for the median nerve and the C5 and C6 segments of the nerve roots, using abduction of the shoulder;
— *ULTT 2a/b:* for the median/radial nerve and the C5, C6 and C7 nerve roots, using the lowering of the shoulder and external-internal rotation;
— *ULTT 3:* for the ulnar nerve and the C8 and T1 nerve roots, using abduction of the shoulder and flexion of the elbow.

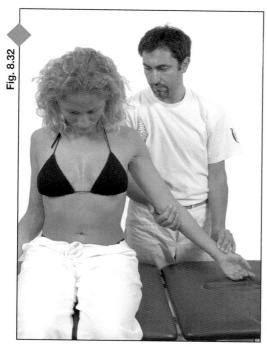

Fig. 8.32

Costoclavicular joint test.

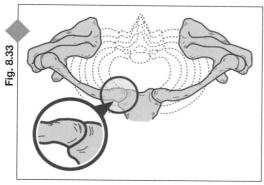

Fig. 8.33

Costoclavicular joint.

that it is easy to aggravate the symptoms of an upper limb with an 'irritated' nervous structure (Butler, 1991). For this reason, when the nerve tissue is examined, this should be done at the point of muscle tension or of defensive contraction of the muscle. Examining patients in the arc of movement in which the symptoms are stimulated is excessive, often causing their re-exacerbation.

The test is performed with the patient supine, with the limb to be examined off the couch; the therapist stabilizes the patient's shoulder with their own hip, and supports the elbow laterally with the proximal hand while extending it with the other hand. The therapist then depresses the shoulder with their own hip; and assists the extension and external rotation of the scapulohumeral with their proximal hand; the therapist then holds the elbow in extension and supination and the wrist in extension. The limb is finally abducted (Fig. 8.34).

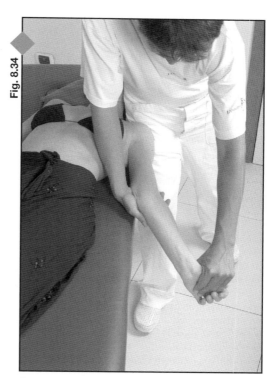

Fig. 8.34

Upper limb tension test.

ULTT 2 is recommended for all patients with diffuse symptoms affecting the arm, head, neck and thoracic spine and who have shoulder disorders. It should be performed during the initial evaluation, if the subjective and physical examinations suggest that damaged mechanics of the nervous system is a component of the patient's disorder.

The test should not be performed initially in severe disorders, since the physiotherapist should remember

Once one phase of the test has been performed, the position should be held firmly before adding the next

Functional examination as part of manual therapy

component. The symptoms and symptomatic changes should be identified and interpreted after each phase.

Notes on the functional examination of athletes

A patient who is an athlete, whether professional or amateur, young or no longer young, has unique features which require the functional examination to take into account factors associated with the individuality of the athlete and the characteristics of the sport involved.

These factors can be divided into internal or intrinsic, which can be influenced little if at all, and external or extrinsic factors, which can be modified at least partly.

Examples of internal factors are age, sex, race, the type of movement required, the limits imposed by the rule, and the perceptive and motor qualities of the athlete.

Examples of external factors are role in the sport, body and movement symmetry, and movement automatism.

Health workers should identify, take account of and explain the influence of intrinsic and extrinsic factors during the functional examination, as well as whether it will be possible to modify them by means of specific measures.

The aspects to be addressed form part of the measures to prevent disorders, and they will consequently be dealt with in Chapter 17.

Conclusions

A preliminary correct FE, or more precisely a 'rehabilitative' evaluation, is essential to identify suitable rehabilitation measures. This is entirely unrelated to the diagnosis of the disorder (provided by the doctor) which is vital, as already mentioned, for recognizing the biological damage, its severity, location and nature, and whether the damage will progress.

Carrying out an FE means:
— identifying and evaluating the various types of impairment and disability presented by the patient as a result of the damage caused by pathological conditions;
— identifying the corresponding 'modifiability gradient' of the patient's biopsychosocial status;
— identifying and evaluating the shoulder resources available and the patient's own resources (biological, psychological, etc.);
— identifying the most useful methods of intervention;

Table 8.8

The functional examination of athletes (sport-specific)

Points 1–6 are essential components of a basic functional evaluation: some of the aspects related to athletic technique are external factors of influence, which can be modified at least in part. Points 7–9 are internal factors of influence which are difficult to modify; they can be evaluated according to the biopsychosocial model (Unpublished A. Fusco, C. Grillet, 2003).

1 Identify the dysfunctions present: ask the patient to perform movements bilaterally and compare the movements performed unilaterally

2 Observe body alignment and posture: observe cervicothoracic movement in the sagittal plane, and symmetry and the presence of dorsal rotation in the frontal plane

3 Carry out an overall analysis of movement: observe the relationship between the position of the feet, the pelvis, the spine, the action of the shoulder, the role of the chest, and the role of cervicothoracic movement

4 Carry out an analysis of shoulder movement: observe direction, amplitude, speed and strength

5 Carry out an analysis of automatism in movement: observe changes in the parameters of automatism during subsequent repetitions

6 Evaluate adaptation to movement and any compensation (normal and pathological): ability and perception of compensation should be evaluated

7 Evaluate the individual level of the athlete and his or her competence: the technical and behavioural level of the patient, possibly in a multidisciplinary session

8 Evaluate physical, mental and social awareness: the patient's inter-awareness can be observed

9 Evaluate the person's identity and role in the group: the patient's interaction with the group and his or her relations with significant persons (friends, technicians and health workers) should be evaluated

— identifying the therapeutic tools which, based on the scientific evidence and personal experience of the team, are most likely to prove effective in modifying the various types of disability in the desired direction; arranging the method of administration, including the 'dosage'; and
— estimating the time required to achieve the various objectives.

The FE of the patient, carried out by the rehabilitation therapist to confirm the physical examination conducted by the doctor, is one of the most decisive and key components for a rehabilitation therapist; manual therapies and therapeutic exercise are, in fact, based on a specifically functional examination of the neuromuscular and joint system. This examination serves to define dysfunctions of the joint, muscle and nervous system, in physical terms. The examination also serves to distinguish conditions in which manual therapy or therapeutic training is contraindicated, and all the other anomalies or pathological processes which limit the direct use of manual therapy and manipulative procedures.

There can consequently be no rehabilitation without evaluation and this occurs not only when the patient is taken on, but is a continuous, constant procedure going hand in hand with the treatment.

The initial evaluation has three essential aims: detecting possible contraindications, deciding on a functional diagnosis, as we have already seen (and not a medical diagnosis), and implementing the treatment.

As regards possible contraindications, we should look for warning signs or symptoms, abnormal or inconsistent behaviour of the symptoms, and any factors defined as unfavourable in the current phase.

The initial evaluation also allows us to decide on a functional diagnosis, i.e. to demonstrate the unique characteristics of the patient's disorder. The various structures respond uniquely to passive and active tests, and tests against resistance, and these responses help us to formulate hypotheses about the anatomical components of the disorder.

Finally, the initial evaluation is a factor in implementing the treatment; logical conclusions can be drawn from the information gathered, therapeutic objectives can be identified and the most appropriate procedures or techniques chosen.

The changes caused by each procedure are thus monitored and recorded, for example, whether the symptoms improve, worsen or do not change, and in each of these cases whether the change is subjective (according to the patient), objective (according to the therapist's clinical examination) or both. A deterioration should always be seen as a warning and should prompt an investigation of whether this is due to a diagnostic error, choice of treatment (type of exercise used) or how the treatment is conducted (frequency, intensity, or amplitude of the exercise). A decision can then be taken on whether to continue with the same procedure or to alter it. The effects of any exercise should thus be monitored extremely rigorously.

Retrospective evaluation is used to compare the patient's current condition with that before the start of the treatment and with that before the last session.

This, therefore, provides an objective measure of the result obtained and the limits demonstrated using appropriate, reliable evaluation tools.

The aim of a conclusive evaluation is to compare the patient's initial condition, demonstrated at the first session, with that at the end of the treatment; the result (the progress achieved and any deficits as regards the patient's full functional recovery) can thus be measured, a functional prognosis made, and preventive instructions, which should always accompany any manual therapy, given to the patient.

Whatever method is chosen to manage musculoskeletal disorders of the shoulder, it will be effective only if supported by a thorough clinical evaluation and a reliable knowledge of the clinical models associated with shoulder dysfunction (Jones, 2000).

Acknowledgements

I am indebted to my wife and colleague, Arianna Marcucci, Dr Sabrina Tosi, psychologist, psychotherapist, and student and teacher at the European Institute of Training, Systemic Consultancy and Relational Therapy (IEFCoSTRe), Dr. Tommaso Vetrugno and Christine Grillet, Lecturer at the Università degli Studi di Genova on the Master's course in Rehabilitation of Musculoskeletal Disorders, for their help in this venture.

Bibliography

Andrews J.R. et al., 'La Spalla dell'Atleta. Delfino', Rome (1998)

Apley A.G., Solomon L., 'L'Esame Obiettivo in Ortopedia', Delfino, Rome (1999)

Aprill C., Dwyer A., Bogduk N., 'Cervical zygapophyseal joint pain patterns II: A clinical evaluation', Spine 15(6): 458–461, (1990)

Baker C.L., Liu SH., 'Neurovascular injuries to the shoulder', J. Orthop. Sports Phys. Ther. 18(1): 360–364, (1993)

Bigliani L.U., Levine W.N., 'Subacromial Impingement Syndrome', J. Bone Joint. Surg. Am. 79(12): 1854–1868, (1997)

Burkhart S.S., Morgan C.D., Kibler W.B., 'Shoulder injuries in overhead athletes. The "dead arm" revisited', Clin. Sports Med. 19(1): 125–158, (2000)

Butler D.M., 'Mobilisation of the Nervous System', Churchill Livingstone, Melbourne (1991)

Çalis M. et al., 'Diagnostic Values of Clinical Diagnostic Tests in Subacromial Impingement Syndrome', Ann.Rheum.Dis. 59: 44–47, (2000)

Functional examination as part of manual therapy

Cartabellotta A., 'Ebm e Ragionamento diagnostico: un matrimonio impossibile?', *Ricerca e Sanità* 1(3): 77–79, (2000)

Clark J.M., Harryman D.T. 2ND,. 'Tendons, ligaments, and capsule of the rotator cuff. Gross and microscopic anatomy', *J. Bone Joint. Surg. Am.* 74(5): 713–725, (1992)

Clark J., Sidles J.A., Matsen F.A., 'The relationship of the glenohumeral joint capsule to the rotator cuff', *Clin. Orthop. Relat. Res.* 254: 29–34, (1990)

Danowski R.G. et al., 'Traumatologia dello Sport. Edizioni Masson', Milan, p. 6., (2000)

Davies G.J. et al., 'Neuromuscular Testing and Rehabilitation of the Shoulder Complex', *JOSP* 18(2): 449–458, (1993)

De Benedittis G., *La cartella clinica del Dolor*, (II Rev.), Ospedale Maggiore di Milano, Milan (1988)

DE BENEDITTIS G., CORLI O., MASSEI R., NOBILI R., PIERI A., Questionario italiano del dolore. Organizzazioni Speciali, Florence 1993.

De Benedittis G., Massei R., Nobili R., Pieri A., 'The Italian Pain Questionnaire', *Pain* 33: 53–62, (1988)

Deutsch A., Altchek D.W., Veltri D.M., Potter H.G., Warren R.F., 'Traumatic tears of the subscapularis tendon. Clinical diagnosis, magnetic resonance imaging findings, and operative treatment', *Am. J. Sports Med.* 25(1): 13–22, (1997)

Di Giacomo G., Di Giacomo S., Silvestrini M.G., Costantini A., *L'artroscopia di spalla*, Verduci Editore, Rome (2003)

Diveta J., Walker M.L., Skibinski B., 'Relationship between performance of selected scapular muscles and scapular abduction in standing subjects', *Phys. Ther.* 70(8): 470–476, (1990)

Donatelli R.A., *Terapia Fisica della Spalla*, UTET, Milan, p. 91, (1999)

Ellenbecker T.S., Bailie D.S., Mattalino A.J., Carfagno D.G., Wolff M.W., Brown S.W., Kulikowich J.M., 'Intrarater and interrater reliability of a manual technique to assess anterior humeral head translation of the glenohumeral joint', *J. Shoulder Elbow Surg.* 11(5): 470–475, (2002)

Hertel R., Ballmer F.T., Lombert S.M., Gerber C., 'Lag signs in the diagnosis of rotator cuff rupture', *J. Shoulder Elbow Surg.* 5(4): 307–313, (1996)

Flegel K.M., 'Does the physical examination have a future?', *CMAJ* 161: 1117–1118, (1999)

Frosi G., Sulli A., Testa M., Cutolo M., 'The sterno-clavicular joint: anatomy, biomechanics, clinical features and aspects of manual therapy', *Reumatismo* 56(2): 82–88, (2004)

Frost P., Andersen J.H., 'Shoulder impingement syndrome in relation to shoulder intensive work', *Occup. Environ Med.* 56(7): 494–498, (1999)

Frost P., Andersen J.H, Lundorf E., 'Is Supraspinatus Pathology as Defined by Magnetic Resonance Imaging Associated with Clinical Signs of Shoulder Impingement?' *J. Shoulder Elbow Surg.* 8(6): 565–568, (1999)

Gerber C, Krushell R.J., 'Isolated rupture of the tendon of the subscapularis muscle. Clinical features in 16 cases', *J. Bone Joint Surg. Br.* 73(3): 389–394, (1991)

Gifford LS, 'Topical issues in pain 2. Biopsychosocial assessment. Relationships and pain', CNS Press, Falmouth (2000)

Grimberg J., Augereau B., 'Shoulder injury. Diagnostic orientation and management of emergency situations', *Rev. Prat.* 49(20): 2285–2292, (1999)

Hammer D.L. et al., 'A Modification of the Relocation Test: Arthroscopic Findings Associated with a Positive Test', *J. Shoulder Elbow Surg.* 9: 263–267, (2000)

Hoppenfeld S., *L'Esame Obbiettivo in Ortopedia*. A. Gaggi Editore, Bologna, p.15, (1978)

Huskisson E.C., 'Visual Analogue Scale' In. Melzack R. (by), *Pain measurement and assessment*, Raven Press, New York, pp. 33–37, (1983)

Itoi E., Kido T., Sano A., Urayama M., Sato K., 'Which is more useful, the "full can test" or the "empty can test," in detecting the torn supraspinatus tendon?', *Am. J. Sports Med.* 27(1): 65–68, (1999)

Jensen M.P., Karoly P., O'Riordan E.F., Bland F.JR., Burns R.S., 'The subjective experience of acute pain: an assessment of the utility of 10 indices', *Clin J Pain* 5(2): 153–159, (1989)

Jobe C.M., 'Superior Glenoid Impingement', *Orthop. Clin. North Am.* 28(2): 137–143, (1997)

Jones M., 'Clinical reasoning and pain', *Man. Ther.* 1(1): 17–24, (2000)

Jones M.A., Edwards I., Gifford L., 'Conceptual models for implementing biopsychosocial theory in clinical practice', Invited Masterclass article – *Manual Therapy* 7(1): 2–9, (2002)

Jones M.A., Jensen G., Edwards I., 'Clinical reasoning in physiotherapy', In: Higgs J., Jones M.A., 2nd, (eds):, *Clinical Reasoning in the Health Professions*, Butterworth Heinemann, Oxford, p. 117, (2000)

Jones M.A., Magarey M.E., 'Clinical reasoning in the use of manual therapy techniques for the shoulder girdle', In: Tovin B., Greenfield B.H. (eds): *Evaluation and rehabilitation of the shoulder*, FA Davis, Philadelphia, p. 317, (2001)

Kelly B.T., Williams R.J., Cordasco F.A., Backus S.I., Otis j.C., Weiland D.E., Altchek D.W., Craig E.V., Wickiewicz T.L., Warren R.F., 'Differential patterns of muscle activation in patients with symptomatic and asymptomatic rotator cuff tears', *J. Shoulder Elbow Surg.* 14(2): 165–171, (2005)

Kibler W.B., McMullen J., 'Scapular dyskinesis and its relation to shoulder pain', *J. Am. Acad. Orthop. Surg.* 11(2): 142–151, (2003)

Kim S.H., Ha K.I., Ahn J.H., Kim S.H., Choi H.J., 'Biceps Load Test II: A Clinical Test for SLAP-Lesions of the Shoulder', *Arthroscopy*, 17(2): 160–164, (2001)

Kim SH, Ha KI, Han KY., 'Biceps load test: a clinical test for superior labrum anterior and posterior lesions in shoulders with recurrent anterior dislocations', *Am. J. Sports Med.* 27(3): 300–303, (1999)

Lewis J., Green A., Reichard Z., Wright C., 'Scapular position: the validity of skin surface palpation', *Man. Ther.* 7(1): 26–30, (2002)

Litaker D., Pioro M., El Bilbeisi H., Brems J., 'Returning to the bedside: using the history and physical examination to identify rotator cuff tears', *J. Am. Geriatr. Soc.* 48(12): 1633–1637, (2000)

Lyons PM, Orwin JF., 'Rotator Cuff Tendinopathy and Subacromial Impingement Syndrome', *Med. Sci Sports Exerc.* 30(4 Suppl): 12–17, (1998)

MacDonald P.B., Clark P., Sutherland K., 'An analysis of the diagnostic accuracy of the Hawkins and Neer subacromial impingement signs', *J. Shoulder Elbow Surg.* 9(4): 299–301, (2000)

Magarey M.E., Jones M.A., 'Dynamic evaluation and early management of altered motor control around the shoulder complex', *Man. Ther.* 8(4): 195–206, (2003)

Majani G., Sanavio E., 'Semantic of Pain in Italy: the Italian version of the McGill Pain Questionnaire', *Pain* 22: 399–405, (1985)

Malanga G.A., Jenp Y.N., Growney E.S., An K.N., 'EMG analysis of shoulder positioning in testing and strengthening the supraspinatus', *Med. Sci Sports Exerc.* 28(6): 661–664, (1996)

Matsen III FA. et.al., 'Manuale Pratico di Valutazione e Trattamento della Spalla', Verduci Editore, p. 126, Rome (1996)

McGuire DB., 'Comprehensive and multidimensional assessment and measurement of pain', *J Pain Symp. Manag.* 7(5): 312–319, (1992)

Meister K., 'Injuries to the shoulder in the Throwing Athlete – Part Two: Evaluation/Treatment', *Am. J. Sports Med.* 28(4): 587–601, (2000)

Morrison D.S., Greenbaum B.S., Einhorn A., 'Shoulder Impingement', *Orthop. Clin. North Am.* 31(2): 285–293, (2000)

Mottram S.L., 'Dynamic stability of the scapula', *Man. Ther.* 2(3): 123–132, (1997)

Murrell G.A., Walton J.R., 'Diagnosis of Rotator Cuff Tears', *The Lancet* 357(9258): 769–770, (2001)

Myers J.B., Laudner K.G., Pasquale M.R., Bradley J.P., Lephart S.M., 'Scapular position and orientation in throwing athletes', *Am. J. Sports Med.* 33(2): 263–271, (2005)

O'Brien S.J., Pagnani M.J., Fealy S., McGlynn S.R., Wilson J.B., 'The Active Compression Test: A New and Effective Test for Diagnosing Labral Tears and Acromioclavicular Joint Abnormality', *Am. J. Sports Med.* 26(5): 610–613, (1998)

Petersen C.M., Hayes K.W., 'Construct Validity of Ciriax's Selective Tension Examination: Association of End-feels with Pain at the Knee and Shoulder', *J. Orthop. Sports Phys. Ther.* 30(9): 512–521, (2000)

Petty N.J. et.al., 'Esame Clinico e Valutazione Neuromuscolo-scheletrica in Terapia Manuale', Edizione Masson, Milan, p.194, (2000)

Platt FW., 'Diagnostic value of the medical history', *Arch. Intern. Med.* 148(4): 984–985, (1988)

Postacchini F., 'Atti del Convegno Internazionale "La Cuffia dei Ruotatori della Spalla"', Rome (2001)

Sandler G., 'The importance of the history in the medical clinic and the cost of unnecessary tests', *Am. Heart J.* 100(6): 928–931, (1980)

Scheibel M., Habermeyer P., 'Current procedures for clinical evaluation of the shoulder', *Orthopade.* 34(3): 267–283, (2005)

Schmitt L., Snyder-Mackler L., 'Role of scapular stabilizers in etiology and treatment of impingement syndrome', *J. Orthop. Sports Phys. Ther.* 29(1): 31–38, (1999)

Schomacher J., *Terapia Manuale: Imparare a Muovere e Percepire*, Edizioni Masson, Milan (2001)

Scott J., Ansell B.M., Huskisson E.C., 'Graphic representation of pain', *Pain* 2: 175–184, (1976)

Smith R., 'What clinical information do doctors need?' *Br. Med. J.* 313: 1062–1068, (1996)

Solem-Bertoft E., Thuomas K.A., Westerberg C.E., 'The influence of scapular retraction and protraction on the width of the subacromial space. An MRI study', *Clin. Orthop. Relat. Res.* 296: 99–103, (1993)

Solomon D.H., Schaffer J.L., Katz J.N., Horsky J., Burdick E., Nadler E., Bates D.W., 'Can History and Physical Examination Be Used as Markers of Quality? An Analysis of the Initial Visit Note in Musculoskeletal Care', *Med. Care.* 38(4): 383–391, (2000)

Tytherleigh-Strong G. et al., 'Rotator Cuff Disease' *Curr. Opin. Rheumatol.* 13: 135–145, (2001)

Valadie A.L. 3RD, Jobe C.M., Pink M.M., Ekman E.F., Jobe F.W., 'Anatomy of Provocative Tests for Impingement syndrome of the Shoulder', *J Shoulder Elbow Surg.* 9(1): 36–46, (2000)

Van Wingerden B.A.M., *Connective Tissue in Rehabilitation*, Scipro Verlag, Vaduz (Liechtenstein) (1995)

Villamira M.A., De Benedittis G., Nobili R., 'Correlazioni tra test psicologici (MMPI e MHQ) nelle sindromi dolorose croniche', *Il dolore* 3: 53–57, (1983)

Wilk K.E., Andrews J.R., Arrigo C.A., 'The physical examination of the glenohumeral joint: emphasis on the stabilizing structures', *J. Orthop. Sports Phys. Ther.* 25(6): 380–389, (1997)

Wolin PM. et.al., 'Rotator Cuff Injury: Addressing Overhead Overuse', *Phys. Sports Med.* 25(6), (1997)

Woodward T.W., Best T.M., 'The Painful Shoulder: Part I, Clinical Evaluation', *Am. Fam. Physician.* 61(10): 3079–3088, (2000)

Woodward T.W., Best T.M., 'The painful shoulder: Part II. Acute and chronic disorders', *Am. Fam. Physician.* 61(11): 3291–3300, (2000)

Box 8.4

Patient – Orthopaedic specialist – Physiotherapist

The team will work better if all its members feel motivated to contribute to the therapeutic project, rather than submitting to it passively.

Collins English Dictionary defines 'motivation' as 'the process that arouses, sustains and regulates human and animal behaviour'.

Accordingly, adopting an attitude towards a patient with a cuff rupture of the type: 'You have a ruptured shoulder tendon, so I advise you to have an operation, then you will have some physiotherapy and everything will be okay', is starting on the wrong foot, because the patient will clearly not have understood the following:

— the nature of the problem;
— if it can be resolved;
— how it can be resolved, what are the chances of success and what are the risks;
— how long can a result be expected to take; and
— what the patient's own role in the process is.

It often happens in clinical practice that after being given an explanation of all five points, the patient nevertheless asks advice on what to do; this happens if I have not communicated the information properly or if the patient has a problem with comprehension or motivation; I then try to summarize it all, then I wait for the patient to ask to be treated. Only after such a request am I convinced of the patient's motivation and willingness to form an active part of the team.

Willingness and ability to communicate are thus of primary importance.

The doctor should try to devote much of the examination time to listening to the patient's account, because this very often gives clues to the diagnosis and also improves the relationship of trust with the patient, who realizes our readiness to listen. It is, therefore, even more important to know how to listen, in the sense of guiding the account, focusing on the most significant information, and also paying attention to emotional reactions (such as body position, hand gestures, tone of voice, look), because these give clues to emotional state and possible reception.

We often dedicate too little time to this phase, at the risk of having incorrectly assessed the problem, inappropriately asking a physiotherapist to resolve the situation or providing the physiotherapist with insufficient information.

The time factor is, however, on the side of the rehabilitation specialist and physiotherapist. As soon as they start seeing the patient regularly, there is decidedly more time available for listening. These specialists thus have a central role in the team, because they should be capable of gathering information on the therapeutic journey and its results, and passing them on to the orthopaedic specialist.

A harmonious team is, then, one in which the orthopaedic specialist succeeds in making a reliable clinical diagnosis and in informing the patient fully about what they can expect (in terms of both treatment and results), obtains the patient's consent and motivation to be treated, and passes all of this on to the rehabilitation specialist who, after making an additional assessment, starts and continues with the therapeutic journey and is always ready to communicate the results obtained. If physiotherapists are asked what they expect, they answer that they want the opportunity and ability to communicate with the orthopaedic specialist.

To achieve this as well as possible, it is first of all necessary to speak the same language: clinical presentations and assessment tools, such as tests, assessment scales, functional tests with or without apparatus, and instrumental examinations, where applicable, should not only be understood by both the physiotherapist and the orthopaedic specialist, but above all be interpreted in the same way.

It should thus be clear that there is not only a disorder-specific objective, but also a patient-specific objective; the same cuff rupture can be approached differently depending on the activity and age of the patient.

A 'vertical' approach should be avoided, since not all patients are suitable for surgery and the best time to discover this is before the procedure, not afterwards; it is also true that an operation can often put an end to long, pointless courses of rehabilitation.

The team should be flexible, in the sense that it should be able to change direction at any time; for example, if an initial approach comprising rehabilitation is correct for painful shoulder due to subacromial impingement, it is also true that the physiotherapist should be prepared to tell the surgeon about any lack of success and to agree to change strategy and adopt a surgical solution.

Since the need to communicate within the team is, therefore, clear, how can we improve the means of doing this? Obviously by means of the complete documentation of cases; this means leaving a trace which allows us to determine precisely, for example, what the ROM of the shoulder was when the patient was first seen (if we wrote it on a form), how extensive was the cuff rupture and what was the outcome of the final suture (if we have taken intra-operative photographs or videos), and what level of functional recovery we obtained after 15 days of treatment (if we recorded the situation at the outset). Trusting everything to memory may be over-optimistic, and may expose therapists to medicolegal problems, an

(Continued)

increasingly common feature of modern clinical practice.

Future means of documentation which should come into current use include CD-ROMs and the Internet.

CD-ROMs can be used for the following:
— to gather a large quantity of data and images;
— to visualize their content easily; and

— to update this content easily on an on-going basis.

The Internet can be used, perhaps by setting up a team website, both to change the availability of time for information from that granted by us to what the patient has available (improved patient approach to the disorder and to the team), and to exchange information and evaluations virtually in real time.

Box 8.5

Patient information – Italian pain questionnaire (IPQ)

(De Benedittis G., Massei R., Nobili R., Pieri A., Corli O.,
'The Italian Pain Questionnaire', *Pain* 35: 53–62, 1988.)

Forename ---------------------------------- Surname ---------------------------------- Age --------------

Test date and centre ---

Instructions

Some of the words or expressions that you find in this form may describe your current pain. Indicate, by putting a cross next to the corresponding sign, which words describe it best. Choose as many words as you want in each group you consider most appropriate to describe your pain. Leave out groups of words which do not seem appropriate to you.

S1	Periodic	❑		E1	Tiresome	❑
	Persistent	❑			Indefinable	❑
					Alarming	❑
S2	Pulsating				Worrying	❑
	Throbbing	❑			Intolerable	❑
S3	Variable	❑		E2	Annoying	❑
	Diffuse	❑			Disturbing	❑
	Fixed	❑			Incapacitating	❑
S4	Piercing	❑		M1	Insistent	❑
	Cutting	❑			Acute	❑
S5	Heavy	❑		M2	Obstinate	❑
	Constrictive	❑			Gnawing	❑
	Biting	❑			Exasperating	❑
S6	Makes the area	❑			Agonizing	❑
	more sensitive to thetouch					
	Sharp	❑				

Present pain intensity (PPI)

0	None	❑
1	Mild	❑
2	Moderate	❑
3	Severe	❑
4	Very severe	❑
5	Excruciating	❑

S7	Aching	❑
	Dull	❑
S8	Burning	❑
	Transfixing	❑
	Lacerating	❑
A1	Debilitating	❑
	Irksome	❑
A2	Nauseating	❑
	Suffocating	❑
A3	Causes agitation	❑
	Distressing	❑
A4	Causes groaning	
	Depressing	❑
	Oppressive	❑

For the examiner's use only

Medical diagnosis:

PRIr   S_ _   A_ _   E_ _   M_ _   T_ _
NWC   _ _
PRIrc   S_ _   A _ _   E _ _   M _ _
PPI   _ _   AV : _ _   VAS: _ _
Self-completion: No ❑   Yes ❑
Selection: free ❑   limited ❑

Box 8.6

Patient information – Subjective shoulder rating scale (SSRS)

(Kohn D., Geyer M., 'The subjective shoulder rating system', *Arch. Orthop Trauma Surg.* 116 [6-7]: 324–328, (1997))

Forename ------------------------------- Surname -------------------------------------
Age --------------------------------- Sport --------------------------------- Occupation ---------------
Date completed

Instructions
Answer every question – put an X in the box ❏ next to the best answer – do not leave blanks for any of the questions below – only one answer is allowed

	Right shoulder	Left shoulder	Score
1. Do you have shoulder pain?			
a) No	❏	❏	35
b) With some movements	❏	❏	30
c) Also at night	❏	❏	20
d) At rest and at night	❏	❏	10
e) Continuous and severe	❏	❏	0
2. How is the shoulder joint function?			
a) Normal	❏	❏	35
b) Slightly limited	❏	❏	30
c) I cannot reach my neck or back	❏	❏	20
d) I cannot reach my forehead or buttocks	❏	❏	10
e) My shoulder is completely stiff	❏	❏	0
3. Are you afraid of dislocation?			
a) No	❏	❏	15
b) It almost dislocates during some movements	❏	❏	10
c) It dislocates but goes back immediately	❏	❏	5
d) It has dislocated several times	❏	❏	0
4. Are you limited in what you do by your shoulder problems?			
a) No	❏	❏	10
b) Sport and work are slightly limited	❏	❏	7
c) I have had to change sport or work	❏	❏	3
d) I have given up sport or work	❏	❏	0
5. Can you work overhead?			
a) Without any problems	❏	❏	5
b) Yes, but with shoulder problems	❏	❏	2
c) Impossible	❏	❏	0

Examiner

Functional examination as part of manual therapy

Box 8.7

Patient Information – The essential points of the functional evaluation

Selection of data for examination

The examiner should decide which aspects should be examined, based on the information provided by the doctor and by the patient.

For example, an athlete with a painful shoulder will have mainly profound physical pain (musculoskeletal pain) originating in the musculofascial, tendon, capsular, ligamentous, osteoperiosteal and joint structures.

Each structure gives rise to different impairments (pain, movement restriction, etc.) and different disabilities.

In order to evaluate the best therapeutic strategy (drawing up the treatment plan), and times and methods of resuming sport, the diagnostic differentiation (the functional and not the medical diagnosis) must be precise as regards the pathogenetic mechanism in operation and the anatomical and functional structure affected.

Gathering selected data

The examiner will then gather the selected data systematically.

For example, dyskinesis of the scapula, capsular retraction, amplitude of movement of a joint, etc.

The data are gathered in various phases and with the patient in various positions (standing upright, sitting, or lying supine) during this practical, systematic approach.

When recording the data, the physiotherapist should avoid using generic terms such as 'limited ROM, dyskinesis of the scapula in active movements'. Such phrasing is not helpful and will cause problems when two successive examinations are compared. It is understood that any parameters or data that are not reported should be considered normal or insignificant.

Analysis and supplementation of data gathered

Because the data are gathered at different times, the physiotherapist should supplement the information obtained, choose the significant information, outline a functional state of the areas examined in accordance with the medical history, and finally draw up a health profile of the patient. Contradictory data may require further investigative procedures (special tests).

Identification of the clinical case

The aim of the physical examination is to obtain a set of appropriate data and to correlate the findings with the history and the data provided by the doctor.

The examiner's ultimate aim is to identify the functional problems of the areas examined.

SECTION III

SURGICAL
TREATMENT

INCLUSION CRITERIA FOR SURGICAL TREATMENT

R. Zini
P. Pirani

Surgery may be indicated in any shoulder disorder, whether traumatic or degenerative, either because of the characteristics of the lesions, which may always require anatomical repair, or because of the failure of previous non-invasive treatment, which may have been medical or for rehabilitation.

Until a few years ago, it was believed that shoulder disorders were divided into categories distinct from one another, and could be classified as relating to instability, i.e. tendon disorders, or to traumatology. The latest classifications of shoulder disorders recognize that the limit between all these fields is blurred; they often overlap, making the diagnosis of disorders and the subsequent inclusion of some of these for surgical treatment more crucial.

Furthermore, procedures have evolved from open surgery (Table 9.II, between pages 398 and 399) to mini-open repair (Table 9.I, between pages 398 and 399), culminating in the development of arthroscopy and all-arthroscopy; arthroscopic techniques are, in any case, used alongside conventional open techniques in cases in which they have not been replaced, offering a wide range of surgical options in any given disorder (Fig. 9.I).

Arthroscopy has increased our knowledge of anatomical variants, joint lesions and above all the biomechanics of the shoulder to a remarkable extent. Owing in particular to a knowledge of the biomechanics of the shoulder girdle, the concept of anatomical repair has been replaced by that of surgical restoration of the balance between the various components; rather than repairing the anatomical damage itself, surgery has begun to aim at restoring the 'functional equilibrium' lost as a result of a trauma or disorder.

Fig. 9.1

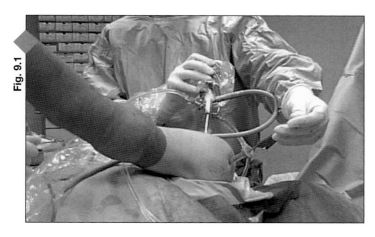

Surgical arthroscopy.

Inclusion criteria for surgical treatment

This has changed how the classification of disorders is viewed, how patients are selected for surgery and how the type of surgical treatment is chosen.

Owing to the mini-invasive nature of the technique, to the ability to reach almost any joint location easily and to developments in technology which guarantee ever better and more stable results, arthroscopy has led not only to a better understanding of disorders, but also to a considerable expansion of the range of surgical indications.

In this chapter we shall address several aspects of selecting surgical treatment, and for specific disorders the reader is referred to the subsequent chapters. There is clearly still a 'no-man's land' in which there is no unanimous agreement, owing to contradictory data in the literature. We have tried to demonstrate aspects of both schools of thought, in the knowledge that these concepts will evolve sooner or later, and probably in the same direction.

The doctor, the athlete and the injury

Patients who participate in sport, particularly at a competitive or at least a serious level, often subject the shoulder girdle to functional overuse, which may develop into inflammation or degeneration of the joint structures. In a smaller number of cases, however, an acute traumatic event occurs which causes an anatomical lesion. It is important to distinguish between the two groups and the patient's history is essential for this. It will be necessary to know when the symptoms started, whether it was after high-energy contact with another player or after a fall, or whether the pain appeared progressively. It is also important to correlate the type of pain and its appearance with the action carried out; the classic example is a volleyball player who feels pain and weakness in the limb in the cocking position for a smash; this strongly suggests posterolateral impingement.

Differentiating between these two main categories of patients is the first step because, in a traumatic event, it is important to stop the athlete or at least to limit athletic movements, until diagnostic tests have ruled out anatomical lesions, whereas in the case of overuse, it is a question of examining the athletic movement or training load, or strengthening muscle structures which are inadequate at that time.

What the athlete requires is to identify the lesion quickly, repair it, recover physical fitness without delay and return to the sport. Often, however, this is at variance with the biology and, in particular, with the clinical course. There are clinical pictures of multidirectional instability which are not easy to identify, particularly when they occur in a patient with laxity who had previously always effectively compensated for this characteristic; in this case the clinical picture may be very indistinct initially and far clearer subsequently, when the lesions have obviously worsened. Rehabilitation treatment often has an excellent chance of resolving the symptoms effectively and identifying the aetiology of the lesion in these cases.

Furthermore, surgical treatment in which the symptoms are unclear is very likely to under- or overestimate the lesions, leading to a poor or incomplete result.

Similarly, a clear clinical picture, treated effectively surgically, will in any case need time for biological repair and recovery; an acute cuff lesion is not firm because four sutures have been applied, but it will become firm when the tendon lesion has healed by the closing of its edges. Other variables are related to the patient's age: the normal process of reduction in calcic tone in athletes over the age of 40 should also be considered, since the anchor inserted holds differently compared to a 20-year-old patient.

If the chances of movement are good, given the motivation of the patient and correct surgical treatment, the implanted surgical material (for example, a reabsorbable or metal anchor or screw, suture material, etc.) is destined to fail during cyclic mobilization if the tendon has not healed or there is no integration between the bone and the synthetic material. It was long believed that the problem could be resolved by creating new materials (reabsorbable sutures made of polylactic acid, the various types of reabsorbable sutures, FiberWire, etc.), failing to take account of the fact that the problem was not simply one of mechanical resistance but also of one of biocompatibility and, though less well known, one of tissue induction. Unfortunately, it is not possible to tell in advance which patients will have osteointegration or healing problems; the only rule is, therefore, to observe biological repair times. The physiotherapist is, therefore, essential, since he or she is in close contact with the patient and can monitor the postoperative course and, above all, check that the structures under repair are not being overused.

Which type of surgery is indicated?

In many cases, the surgeon is able to choose between open surgery and arthroscopy. Neither can be improvised and arthroscopy in particular requires a long learning curve and the availability of substantial technical and instrumental support. Approaching an arthroscopic procedure without the aid of an infusion pump may prove a difficult task, and not having dedicated screws or anchors may mean that the result is inadequate over time. Treating a cuff lesion arthroscopically is currently increasingly suggested even by surgeons specializing in open surgery, since this helps to preserve the integrity of otherwise unaffected muscle and capsule structures. It should be taken into consideration at the same time that reinserting a cuff may be far easier, and above all faster, using a mini-open technique and that surgeons should know how to progress gradually towards more complex techniques, as their arthroscopic dexterity is refined; damage to capsular structures may occur not only by incising the capsule with a bistoury, but also by stressing it by inappropriate manoeuvres to reach components further from the portal or by excessively long hydrodistention times.

A good shoulder surgeon should also give appropriate consideration to and distinguish between techniques that have now become standard and those that are obsolete or borderline. Operating on shoulder instability using transosseus suture during arthroscopy is now obsolete, owing to the high incidence of recurrence and the type of complications compared to open surgery or other arthroscopic techniques. Similarly it is far easier, with the techniques currently available, to reinsert a subscapularis during open surgery than during arthroscopy, and this technique should be left to expert arthroscopists.

The trend is thus towards arthroscopic surgery, but arthroscopy has many potential traps and needs even support staff to be fully trained so that they can contribute to the precise organization of the procedure. Minor aspects which are acquired and valued as time goes on, may prove to be major obstacles during initial experiences, for example, when positioning a patient, having maximum accessibility to arthroscopic manoeuvres, one of the points that should be considered is the distance to be kept between the edge of the bed and the shoulder girdle in the beach-chair position, or the bean bag placed too near the posterior portal. Similarly it is only with time that surgeons can learn to regulate the infusion pump to limit bleeding and excessive distension, or to recognize when turbulence is caused by excessive pumping force or by the presence of a portal in which a cannula has not been positioned.

There are many problems lying in wait for surgeons in arthroscopy. Surgeons should, therefore, approach this technique in the knowledge that it can produce excellent results, if known perfectly and applied rigorously, precisely and with an awareness of one's own resources. Patients cannot know whether surgeons have adequate preparation, but surgeons should know whether what they are preparing to undertake matches their abilities.

What type of patient is eligible?

Major surgery will probably require a period of immobilization, and then of physiotherapy. Will the patient follow our instructions? Will he or she observe biological repair times? Will he or she trust a rehabilitation specialist? A surgical procedure which may itself be perfect might not produce a good result if patient compliance is poor, for example, mobilization too soon after suture of the cuff or lack of mobilization after capsuloplasty may result in the suture giving way or severe joint stiffness. It is particularly important in instability to distinguish between cases of voluntary dislocation of the scapulohumeral joint and cases in which instability is so severe that patients are capable of dislocating it by themselves. The difference may seem subtle but is actually decisive: in the former case the patient will behave in a manner which will lead to instability; in the latter case, it is simply a sign of severe joint laxity.

An acute lesion, particularly in an athlete, is an obvious event that should not escape medical attention or treatment. Degenerative lesions which were initially well compensated or unrecognized because they were underestimated or not reported by the athlete owing to the need to compete may result in a late diagnosis.

It is important to establish, in chronic cases of cuff rupture, the condition of the muscles and tendons before planning intervention. If muscle tissue has already developed into fat, not even the best tendon suture will enable the patient to recover movement. It is more difficult, however, to establish preoperatively with CT and MR images to what extent the retraction of the tendon will allow repair. It is not always appropriate to reinsert the supraspinatus and infraspinatus tendons in their anatomical position because excessive traction may cause pain, loss of function, possible nerve damage to muscles and tendon devascularization.

It is now widely believed that it is useful to perform surgery for cuff rupture after a period of rehabilitation to strengthen the muscles and recover the complete range of movement. The duration of the presurgical rehabilitation period is, however, controversial, ranging from 3 months up to 18 months. A rehabilitation period of 6 months is mostly recommended, but in current practice this period is often shortened in young patients with traumatic cuff rupture, and extended in patients over 50 in whom the mobility of the joint is further limited. This interval between the traumatic event and surgical treatment is seen by patients who are athletes as wasted time. With the exception of fractures, allowing the post-traumatic inflammatory phase to run its course will allow a better evaluation of the integrity of the capsuloligamentous structures and better stability if sutures or other means of synthesis are applied, and will allow an assessment of whether post-traumatic shoulder stiffness has occurred, without this affecting the surgeon's patient.

A further very controversial situation is whether to operate on a patient with a partial tendon rupture or to monitor the clinical course. The type of surgical treatment in this case is also subject to debate, i.e. whether to operate on the damaged region of the tendon or to disinsert the damaged portion and reinsert it with an anchor or screw.

The indication of repairing the cuff and the chances of success in massive cuff lesions are also subject to debate. The advantages of the various techniques are often debated at conferences among arthroscopists and other surgeons. Non-arthroscopists suggest transposition of the tendon when reinsertion is impossible; arthroscopists suggest side-to-side suture or, where tenotomy of the long head is not possible, bursectomy and acromioplasty, pending a reverse prosthesis, without thus weakening the deltoid muscle. It is in any case hoped that such severe cases will never occur in athletes.

When to operate

It will seem obvious, but it should be emphasized that rigorous patient selection is necessary in relation to a precise clinical approach, which will result in surgery being undertaken:
— after a clinical diagnosis of the disorder;
— after confirmation of the disorder with clinical and instrumental examinations;
— when the technique acquired will repair the lesion;
— when it is also possible to deal with associated lesions;
— when the disorder is in the phase in which the maximum result can be obtained; and
— when the patient can have adequate postoperative treatment.

Although any surgical procedure requires the confirmation of the lesion hypothesized on the basis of the history, objective examination and radiographic examinations, purely diagnostic procedures are now performed very rarely, whereas lesions not demonstrated by previous clinical and instrumental examinations are often revealed. A knowledge of the subtypes of disorders in cuff lesions and instability is important for resolving the aetiopathogenesis and to avoid the risk of unnecessary if not harmful surgery. For example, impingement secondary to instability in a young athlete will not benefit from acromioplasty; anterior plication in a patient with multidirectional instability will shift the instability from being predominantly anterior to predominantly inferior or posterior.

Similarly, the mistake should not be made of disregarding radiographic examinations, since arthroscopic or open inspection will focus on certain areas rather than others. For example, the axillary projection of the scapulohumeral joint will reveal the possibility of a mesoacromion in a patient with subacromial impingement not otherwise visualized in anteroposterior projection or in outlet view projection; a patient with cuff rupture and a type III acromion as per Bigliani, not assessed correctly radiographically in outlet view projection, might have an excellent tendon repair but the cause will not have been removed and the tendon disorder will probably recur.

The desire to operate as soon as possible is not always a wise choice. Calcific tendinopathy may often benefit from non-invasive treatments, such as laser therapy or shock waves, or even cold therapy of the calcification; the occurrence of adhesive capsulitis is far more subtle; if this is not recognized preoperatively, it can not only render treatment very difficult, if not impossible, but actually aggravate the capsular inflammation.

If the traumatic event causes the fracture of one of the bone components, surgery is indicated when it is not possible to achieve reduction of the bone components. Particular attention should be paid to the trochanter, dislocation of which can result in impingement, and to the glenoid, reduction of the joint surface in which can lead to instability.

Fractures of the middle third of the clavicle may progress well even in the event of poor consolidation of the fragments. Fracture of the lateral third is, however, more critical since this may develop into a fracture-dislocation if the conoid and trapezoid ligaments give way.

We shall now briefly summarize the indications for surgery in the main shoulder disorders.

Scapulohumeral disorders

Instability

In scapulohumeral instability, it is first of all necessary to diagnose the type.

A traumatic and, therefore, monodirectional origin, occurring acutely after a significant traumatic event in a young patient, needs surgical treatment in our opinion; this may be arthroscopic to reinsert or reconstruct the labrum, or open surgery to reinsert the capsule when the detachment or tear affect the humerus.

A bony glenoid lesion associated with detachment of the labrum (bony Bankart lesion) requires evaluation of the extent of the joint rupture by CT (Burkhart, 2000; Itoi, 2000). The bone component should not be underestimated in instability, since the glenoid surface, which is already smaller than the humeral head, may become the destabilizing factor of the joint.

If the damaged portion of bone is small, the fragment may be removed without subsequently altering the joint kinetics. For lesions amounting to less than 25%, arthroscopy may be performed acutely and the detached bone and labrum reinserted with anchors (Porcellini, 2002). This technique is difficult, however, and requires tested athroscopic skill. If the lesions amount to more than 25% of the glenoid area, open surgery is indicated to synthesize the fragments and reconstruct the glenoid surface anatomically.

Open surgery was once considered preferable to arthroscopy, and was indicated in patients participating in contact sports. This was due to poorer long-term results of arthroscopy with transosseous sutures than with open surgery (Gartsman, 2000). The difference between the two techniques is currently smaller, in particular owing to the use of synthesis material. Surgery is performed increasingly often, however, on young patients who have reported a traumatic dislocation (Arciero, 1994). There is no difference in the result, as regards the time elapsed, between the traumatic event and surgery, consequently the aim is to operate early so as not to increase the time the patient is unable to compete. A significant factor is the number of dislocation events a patient has had (Habermeyer, 1999). The overall damage to the capsuloligamentous structures increases with the number of episodes, and in particular tissue quality is substantially reduced.

A source of great controversy is the indication of arthroscopy after the first scapulohumeral dislocation. Studies of conservative treatment have shown that immobilization does not actually influence the chances of recurrence (Hovelius, 1987), whereas age and type of sport are significant risk factors. Arciero and the West Point team consequently reported their experience with cadets at the Military Academy, noting a substantial reduction in the incidence of recurrences after arthroscopic treatment, compared to conservative treatment. Although the sample of indi-

viduals studied cannot be regarded as a normal group, owing to their physical characteristics and functional requirements, it is nevertheless worth emphasizing that the need for surgery should be considered seriously for lesions reported after a dislocation.

It is unclear why age is such a decisive factor in the recurrence of dislocation; one hypothesis is the greater physical activity or participation in sport that predisposes the patient to recurrence. Sport is, in fact, a further major risk factor. We have no literature data on healing characteristics in different age groups.

Supporters of conservative treatment criticize the need to intervene early, since no parameters exist as yet, in individuals under 30-years-old, which can identify who is actually at risk of recurrence; they consequently suggest operating on individuals who have had two or more episodes, since there are fewer of these, thus avoiding treating patients who might benefit, after the initial dislocation, from conservative treatment (Barber, 2003).

A further criticism directed at those who support intervention is that arthroscopy is not without a risk of recurrence. The long-term results of initial arthroscopy on instability are not encouraging, but it should be noted that the arthroscopy technique and instruments now available are not comparable with those in the past.

A crucial sticking point in this discussion would be resolved if the consequences of treatment after a second dislocation, compared to a single episode, were known as regards the severity of the lesions reported and their ability to be repaired.

In instability of multidirectional and atraumatic origin, treatment should be conservative, restoring the balance of the internal and external rotation muscle forces. In cases in which physiotherapy does not resolve the problem completely, plication treatment of the capsule components involved in the instability is carried out.

SLAP lesions and microinstability

SLAP lesions are of particular interest among labral lesions. Their diagnosis is often neither simple nor immediate. It should be suspected in patients who have reported a trauma and in whom the clinical signs of rotator cuff rupture and instability are indistinct, with pain and significant loss of functional power when performing an athletic movement. Examinations in such cases should include arthro-MR, although it should be kept in mind that they may be negative. Although grade I SLAP can almost be regarded as an accessory finding, the other grades require surgical treatment.

Inclusion criteria for surgical treatment

One of the principal pathological conditions in which SLAP lesions can occur in an athlete is postero-superior microinstability, i.e. a congenital form of laxity which is aggravated during athletic or work movements and in which the humeral head is shifted off-centre in relation to the glenoid surface, resulting in the functional overloading of the posterosuperior anatomical components. There are two different theories in this respect: Jobe (1995) blames the excessive anteroinferior laxity for the labrum and supraspinatus lesion; according to Burkhart (1998), however, the cause is the retraction of the posterior portion of the capsule. This is not a purely theoretical issue from the point of view of treatment, since in the former case plication of the anteroinferior portion of the capsule is required to solve the problem (as well as repairing the labrum and cuff lesion), while in the latter case posterior capsule stretching must be carried out. It is possible for both lesions to be present, i.e. for some patients to have excessive anteroinferior laxity and a further subset to have excessive restriction of the posterior portion of the capsule.

Disorders of the subacromial space

Subacromial impingement

Subacromial impingement occurs in particular in young athletes involved in throwing sports. The shape of the acromion may have an important role, but it should be kept in mind that the incidence of type 3 acromion is fairly low and must not be confused with the possible ossification of the coracoacromial ligament, which occurs with ageing; possible causes of impingement should consequently be sought in patients under 30.

Specific conditions such as os acromiale or scapulo-humeral instability may be latent in athletes; it is important to exclude these causes, since conventional acromioplasty will not be successful. In the case of os acromiale (Hutchinson, 1993), the options, depending on the size of the fragment, are surgery to remove the fragment or osteosynthesis. In instability, acromioplasty and in particular section of the coracohumeral ligament will accentuate the symptoms, since they further reduce the extent to which the humeral head is contained in the glenoid.

It is not possible to make a clinical distinction between the various stages of impingement according to Neer (Bigliani, 1986). Although the first stage benefits from conservative treatment, repair of the tendon lesion is essential in the third stage. Unfortunately,

athletes do not tolerate long periods of inactivity well, and the tendency is to give in to pressure from the patient; this does not detract from the fact that it is a good rule of thumb to carry out conservative treatment and to perform arthroscopic treatment only in cases in which symptoms persist after at least six months.

Rotator cuff rupture

Surgery is indicated as soon as possible in traumatic rotator cuff rupture, in order to repair the lesion anatomically. It should, therefore, be performed before the stumps of the tendon become retracted and before muscle atrophy occurs. It is in any case necessary to identify any anatomical configurations which may have caused impingement and influenced the traumatic event (for example a type 3 acromion as per Bigliani, or a mesoacromion). If any are present, it is important to assess the trophism of the tendon.

In cases where the subscapularis has ruptured, it is important to establish the extent of the lesion. If the rupture is located in the upper part of the tendon, surgery may be performed arthroscopically, by expert hands. If the rupture is complete or the surgeon has less arthroscopic competence, open surgery yields better results, since the tendon can be reinserted and the time required for surgery is short.

In supraspinatus and infraspinatus rupture, the surgical approach is increasingly often arthroscopic, regardless of the number of tendons affected (Gartsman, 2002). The better visualization of the anatomical structures and above all the reduced damage to the periarticular tissues are particularly useful in athletes. Where possible, it is useful to attempt anatomical reinsertion of the tendon, but this will depend on the time that has elapsed since the traumatic event. In situations in which the tendon is severely retracted, a side-to-side technique will be required, given that excessive tension on the tendon heads will in any case result in failure; however, the lesion should not be so severe in athletes.

Disorders of the long head of the humeral biceps

The traumatic rupture of the humeral biceps, particularly of its long head, always involves underlying tendon degeneration when it occurs in the proximal tendon; this is due to the unique anatomical route taken by the tendon from the scapulohumeral joint to the bicipital groove. Muscle ruptures or ruptures at the proximal musculotendon junction occur, but with a far lower incidence; in these cases there is usually serious direct or indirect trauma. Surgery is not indicated in such muscle ruptures, nor is immobilization of the limb. It is important to inform the patient of the possible (but rare) heterotopic ossification formation, which can be very painful in the acute phase and be a source of diagnostic doubt (although surgery to remove it is virtually never necessary) or a cause of functional limitation after the acute phase. When the rupture affects the intra-articular portion, reinsertion of the tendon in its anatomical position is not indicated. Tenodesis is recommended, considering that the majority of athletes are young; tenodesis does not, in fact, restore the bicep's function as a stabilizer of the humeral head in the craniocaudal direction, but besides limiting the retraction of the muscle, it should reduce the occurrence of cramp-like symptoms (Barber, 2001). In any case, arthroscopy may be employed to exclude a SLAP lesion which, if present, should be repaired.

The treatment in cases of tendinosis of the long head of the humeral biceps (LHHB) is controversial. Supporters of the stabilizer role of the LHHB advocate the long-term preservation of the tendon; however, those who do not see this tendon as having a biomechanical role suggest tenodesis. Except in cases of intermittent pain that is controlled well by physiotherapy and pharmacological means, the pain may be very severe and limit the athlete's performance; in patients who undergo tenodesis or in whom tendon rupture was spontaneous, the pain diminishes, allowing activity to be resumed. It is impossible to stabilize the tendon by conservative treatment or surgery in dislocation or subluxation of the LHHB. Bearing in mind the traction exerted on the subscapularis in biceps instability, tenodesis is indicated with repair of the subscapularis, if necessary.

Conclusions

It is clear from the above that it is not easy to lay down precise inclusion criteria for surgery for athletes with shoulder problems.

A surgical indication should be supported by a precise clinical as well as radiographic diagnosis, and the choice between open and arthroscopic surgery should depend on the disorder in question and the latest techniques currently in use.

The individual anatomical lesions must absolutely be evaluated and considered, when choosing the procedure to be performed, in relation to the characteristics of the joint they affect, but the two key figures in the surgical procedure, i.e. the surgeon and the patient,

cannot be underestimated as fundamental factors in the decision. The choice of procedure should ultimately also depend on the characteristics of the surgeon, and their experience and ability, and on the characteristics of the patient, whose physical and psychological support is obviously key to the rehabilitation phase, in order to achieve a full return to athletic activity.

Bibliography

Arciero R.A., Wheeler J.H. Ryan J.B. et al., 'Arthroscopic Bankart repair versus non operative treatment for acute initial anterior shoulder dislocation', *Am. J. Sport. Med.* 22(5): 589–594, (1994)

Barber F.A., Byrd J.W.T., Wolf E.M., Burkhart S.S., 'How would you treat the partially torn biceps tendon?', *Arthroscopy* 17: 636–639, (2001)

Barber F.A., Ryu R.K.N., Tauro J.C., 'Should first time anterior shoulder dislocation be surgically stabilized?', *Arthroscopy* 19: 305–309, (2003)

Bigliani L.U., Morrison D.S., April E.W., 'The morphology of the acromion and its relationship to rotator cuff tear', *Orthop. Trans.* 10: 228–232, (1986)

Burkhart S.S., Morgan C.D., 'The peel back mechanism: Its role in producing and extending posterior type II SLAP-lesion and its effect on SLAP repair rehabilitation', *Arthroscopy* 6: 637–640, (1998)

Burkhart S.S., De Beer J.F., 'Related articles: Traumatic glenohumeral bone defects and their relationship to failure of arthroscopic Bankart repairs: significance of the inverted pear glenoid and the humeral engaging Hill-Sachs lesion', *Arthroscopy* 16(7): 677–694, (2000)

Gartsman G.M., Roddey T.S., Hammerman S.M., 'Arthroscopic treatment of anterior-inferior gleno-humeral instability: Two-to-Five-year follow-up', *J. Bone Joint Surg.* Am. 82-A(7): 991–1003, (2000)

Gartsman G.M., 'Arthroscopic rotator cuff repair', *Artroscopia* 3: 18–25, (2002)

Habermeyer P., Gleyze P., Rickert M., 'Evolution of lesions of the labrum-ligament complex in post-traumatic anterior shoulder instability: a prospective study', *J. Shoulder Elbow Surg.* 8(1): 6–74, (1999)

Hovelius L., 'Anterior dislocation of the shoulder in teenagers and young adults: five-year prognosis', *J. Bone Joint Surg.* 69A: 393–399, (1987)

Hutchinson M.R., Veenstra M.A., 'Arthroscopic decompression of shoulder impingement secondary to Os Acromiale', *Arthroscopy* 9: 28–32, (1993)

Itoi E., Lee S.B., Berglund L.J., Berge L.L., An K.N., 'The effect of a glenoid defect on anterio-inferior stability of the shoulder after Bankart repair: a cadaveric study', *J. Bone Joint Surg. Am.* 82(1): 35–46, (2000)

Jobe C.M., 'Posterior-superior glenoid impingement: expanded spectrum', *Arthroscopy* 11: 530–537, (1995)

Porcellini G., Campi F., Paladini P., 'Arthroscopic approach to acute bony Bankart lesion', *Arthroscopy* 18(7): 764–769, (2002)

SURGICAL SOLUTIONS IN JOINT DISORDERS

G. Porcellini
F. Campi
P. Paladini
M. Paganelli

Knowledge of the pathophysiology of the shoulder has substantially improved the surgical treatment of trauma in athletes over the last 10 years. The aim for these patients is both to heal the disorder and for them to return to the same level of athletic performance as before the traumatic event. Athletes characteristically repeat a movement, often beyond normal physiological limits, resulting in gross pathological pictures typical of a given athletic movement. These disorders due to overuse, as well as contact injuries, should, therefore, be interpreted dynamically, i.e. during the movement performed by the athlete during the sport, so that the gross pathological damage can be evaluated correctly to determine the appropriate surgical, arthroscopic and arthrotomic indications which may not necessarily result in recovery of shoulder function, particularly as regards the athletic movement. The constitution of the athlete needs to be evaluated in this respect, such as in the case

of ligament laxity or the posture and muscle use specific to the sport in question, for example multidirectional laxity in swimming.

A diagram of the various disorders, using the glenoid plane, is shown below for a better understanding of the disorders which may affect the glenohumeral joint (Fig. 10.1).

SLAP lesion

Lesions of the superior glenoid labrum, which extend in an anterior and a posterior direction, were described by Andrews (1985) as a result of the transmission of forces along the long head of the biceps. Andrews attributed the symptoms due to instability in throwing athletes to the inability of the biceps to lower the humeral head and to centre it on the glenoid during

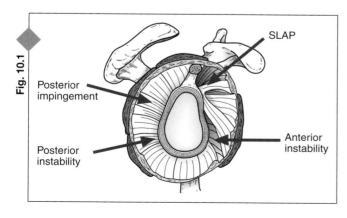

Fig. 10.1

SLAP

Posterior impingement

Posterior instability

Anterior instability

Glenoid plane with disorders.

movements in abduction. The acronym SLAP (superior labral lesion from anterior to posterior) was coined by Snyder (1990) for the same category of lesions of the upper portion of the glenoid labrum. Snyder divided these lesions into four types:

— *Type I:* marked fibrillar degeneration of the superior glenoid labrum, which remains firmly adhered to the sides of the lesion and anchors the biceps attached to the superior labrum;

— *Type II:* fibrillar degeneration of the superior glenoid labrum similar to type I, with avulsion of the glenoid labrum and the biceps tendon from the underlying glenoid (Table 10.I, between pages 398 and 399);

— *Type III:* bucket handle lesion of the superior labrum with the central portion of the lesion in articulation and the peripheral portion firmly adhering to the glenoid and to the intact long head of the biceps; and

— *Type IV:* similar to type III, with extension of the rupture inside the long head of the biceps.

Maffet (1995) described further SLAP lesions associated with type II:

— *Type V:* which extends in a superior direction until the long head of the biceps becomes separated;

— *Type VI:* with an unstable flap of the labrum associated with the separation of the long head of the biceps; and

— *Type VII:* in which the separation of the labrum and the biceps extends to the middle GHL.

Ryu (1997) finally added the type VIII SLAP lesion, with a posterior Bankart lesion associated with SLAP II, and type IX with anterior and posterior Bankart lesions combined with SLAP II. The most frequent mechanism of injury is a fall on the upper limb extended forwards (Snyder 1990) or a low distraction trauma, traumas in abduction and external rotation, in anterior traction and in upwards traction (Maffet 1995). The most useful diagnostic tests for identifying SLAP lesions are those involving traction on the long head of the biceps (LHB), i.e. flexion of the shoulder against resistance to the supinated forearm, a joint rotation and compression test and a SLAP apprehension test (Berg, 1998). None of the tests is, however, capable of predicting a SLAP lesion accurately and precisely. Diagnosis thus needs to be supplemented by an imaging technique, although CT, MR and arthrography alone are not sufficiently sensitive and accurate to predict this disorder (Cartland 1992; Hunter, 1992; Smith, 1993) (Fig. 10.2). The treatment of SLAP lesions depends on the type: debridement for type I, debridement and fixing the labrum and LHB for type II (Table 10.II, between page 398 and page 399), removal

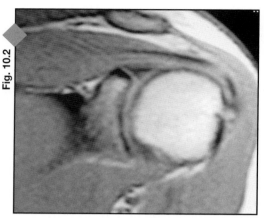

Fig. 10.2

MR image of a SLAP lesion.

of the bucket handle for type III, fixing the LHB if the lesion is smaller than 50% and tenotomy and tenodesis of the LHB if the lesion is greater than 50% for type IV (Rames, 1993; Mileski, 1998). It is important to determine whether disorders which may be associated with SLAP lesions are present, since they may adversely affect the outcome of the treatment, for example rotator cuff lesions, distal clavicular osteolysis and entrapment of the suprascapular nerve by a glenoid cyst (Berg, 1997; Chochole, 1997; Snyder, 1990).

SLAC lesion

Anterosuperior shoulder instability caused by a SLAP lesion may be associated with a rotator cuff lesion in its anterosuperior portion, known as a superior labrum, anterior cuff lesion (SLAC) (Savoie, 2001) (Fig. 10.3). This lesion occurs in particular in patients involved in overhead sports and is manifested clinically by positive instability and rotator cuff tests. Arthroscopic surgery has proved to be very useful in this case too, and is virtually indispensable for treating these lesions, which are not accessible to open surgery, through 360°.

Ganglion cyst associated with SLAP

SLAP lesions may be associated with sublabral cysts which develop along the neck of the glenoid with a valve mechanism, and may even compress the suprascapular nerve, ultimately causing symptoms which may actually mimic a rotator cuff lesion. Such cysts are clearly demonstrated by MR (Fig. 10.4) and may be treated non-invasively (Leitschuh, 1999) or invasively,

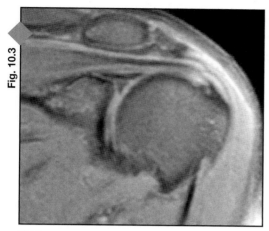

SLAC

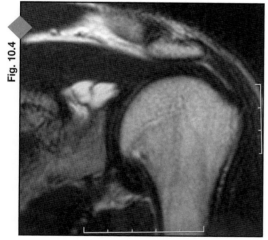

Sublabral cysts along the neck of the glenoid.

by suture or debridement of the SLAP lesion, which contributes to the formation of the valve mechanism which prevents the fluid that has penetrated the cyst escaping further into the joint space. Arthroscopy also appears to be the most accurate and conclusive diagnostic and therapeutic instrument in SLAP lesions associated with glenoid cysts.

Anterior instability

The treatment of anterior, post-traumatic and constitutional instability has altered vastly over the last few years as regards both the steep increase in technological resources available, and the change in prospects for the treatment outcome. Although, until a few years ago, a shoulder without recurrences would have been classified as a good result of surgery to stabilize the glenohumeral joint, a good outcome can now only be defined as such if, as well as avoiding recurrent shoulder dislocations, complete joint function is restored and the patient is, therefore, able to return to the same level of participation as before the traumatic episode. Arthroscopy in the last 10 years has undoubtedly given us a better understanding of the biomechanics and gross pathology of the unstable shoulder (Table 10.III, between page 398 and page 399) and, after the initial attempts and their failures due to inadequate materials (staples) and inexperience on the part of the surgeon, it now appears to be more selective and effective.

The typical advantages of arthroscopy have been clearly described in the literature:
— evaluation of the joint through 360°;
— minimal aesthetic damage with less postoperative pain;
— a smaller deficit in the postoperative ROM;
— no disinsertion of the subscapularis;
— faster return to competition for the athlete; and
— less likelihood of secondary glenohumeral osteoarthritis.

Not all unstable shoulders have the same gross pathological damage, and they should therefore not all be treated arthroscopically; open surgery is still indicated for lesions such as large glenoid and humeral bone detachments. Small bone detachments, up to 25% of the whole surface of the glenoid (bony Bankart lesion), in relatively acute traumas, can be treated selectively by arthroscopy (Porcellini, 2002). A severe capsule disorder (excessive thinning or hyperlaxity) requires open surgical techniques, such as capsular shifts as per Neer, or transpositions of the coracoid as per Latarjet. One of the limits and at the same time the advantages of arthroscopy is the need for the surgical phases to be performed perfectly and the patient and athlete selected correctly. Alterations of scapulohumeral rhythm and voluntary dislocations should be evaluated and treated by an alternative method, with the aid of the physiotherapist, sport therapist and sport injury doctor; sports involving a high risk of injury should also be evaluated carefully, since a higher percentage of recurrences is reported in the literature if treated arthroscopically. Postoperative recovery times for athletes should be evaluated on an individual basis and special attention paid to any joint stiffness which may impede athletic movements and increase the rehabilitation period.

The ideal criteria for selecting arthroscopy are the following:
— a history of trauma;
— Bankart lesion on MR;
— small Hill-Sachs lesion (posterior indentation fracture of the humeral head);
— anterior capsule (IGHL) of good consistency without severe laxity; and
— any associated secondary lesions which lend themselves well to arthroscopic treatment (rotator cuff lesions, SLAP, or mobile bodies).

This technique should obviously be performed by an expert surgeon, since the learning curve is very long and needs special skill in both diagnosis and treatment; mini-anchors or microscrews should, in fact, be introduced into the anterior glenoid rim to suture the labrum and capsule at the most appropriate tension, so as to recreate the stabilizing mechanism of concavity compression. Surgical treatment should also be followed by careful, specific rehabilitation, with a programme for the recovery of passive joint function (joint manipulations) and active joint function (strengthening of the internal and external rotator muscles in water and with elastic bands) monitored periodically by isometric and isokinetic tests. It is, therefore, vital that the surgeon, physiotherapist and sport injury doctor work well as a team when treating an athlete, each contributing their own knowledge, to achieve a faster and safer return for the patient to previous athletic levels.

Bony Bankart lesion

Scapular fractures account for 3–5% of all fractures of the shoulder girdle and approximately 1% of all fractures in general. They are usually caused by a high-speed trauma in motorcycle accidents or falls from a height, often associated with acromioclavicular or sternoclavicular dislocation, clavicular fracture (floating shoulder) or the very rare scapulothoracic dissociation. In the early 1990s, Goss introduced the concept of the superior shoulder suspensory complex as a ring formed by soft tissue and bone, comprising the glenoid, the coracoid, the coracoclavicular ligaments, the distal portion of the clavicle, the AC joint and the acromion. It follows that damage to a single component of this complex will not affect the whole system, but considering that fragments of possible fractures of the glenoid neck are directly connected to the clavicle by the coracoclavicular ligaments, damage to two components of the superior suspensory complex may cause a problem with stability and require surgical treatment. An anatomical classification is, therefore, useful for determining the

most appropriate treatment for these lesions. Numerous classifications have been proposed for scapular fractures, but the fractures associated with instability are fundamentally the intra-articular fractures of the glenoid which Ideberg (1995) divided into five types:
— *Type I:* avulsion of the glenoid rim (anterior: IA; posterior: IB), usually due to traumatic glenohumeral dislocation;
— *Type II:* transverse fractures of the glenoid cavity with upper triangular decomposition;
— *Type III:* oblique glenoid fractures affecting the upper region (they may be associated with an acromioclavicular joint lesion);
— *Type IV:* horizontal fractures affecting the entire scapular body; and
— *Type V:* combination of type II and IV fractures.

Lesions of the glenoid rim (Table 10.IV, between page 398 and page 399), defined as acute fractures or bone erosion associated with recurrent instability, often go unrecognized on a standard X-ray. Although some authors (Hovelius, 1983) do not regard such lesions as capable of significantly influencing glenohumeral stability, others (Rowe, 1981) report a fairly high incidence of recurrent dislocations associated with them. The incidence of anterior glenoid rim fracture associated with anterior glenohumeral dislocation varies from 5.4 to 32% (Rowe, 1981) and the reason for this disparity may be incorrect initial radiographic interpretation. The importance of the size of the fragment removed or loss of bone substance in maintaining instability has been reported in the literature (De Palma, 1983), and Bigliani produced a further classification of this type of lesion in 1998, determining the type of treatment according to his experience:
— *Type I:* bone fragment detached with the labrum inserted (Fig. 10.5);
— *Type II:* bone fragment consolidated in an incorrect position with the labrum detached (Fig. 10.6);
— *Type IIIA:* anterior glenoid erosion of less than 25% of the total surface area (Fig. 10.7); and
— *Type IIIB:* anterior glenoid erosion of more than 25% of the total surface area.

In type III the glenoid generally assumes an 'inverted pear' shape (Burkhart, 2000) (Fig. 10.8), which causes serious problems as regards containment of the humeral head. Containment depends essentially on the result of two geometric variables:
— the 'depth effect' due to glenoid concavity; and
— the length of the glenoid arc which resists dislocation of the humeral head, due to axial loads.

These biomechanical and gross pathological findings and classifications have led, over the years, to

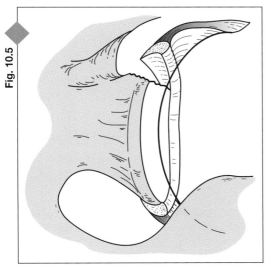

Fig. 10.5

Type I lesion of the glenoid rim.

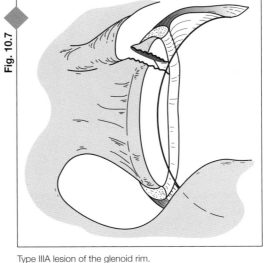

Fig. 10.7

Type IIIA lesion of the glenoid rim.

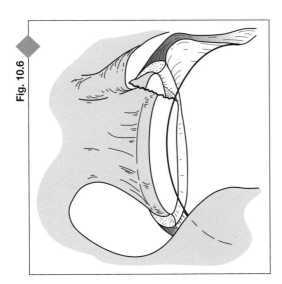

Fig. 10.6

Type II lesion of the glenoid rim.

changes in the type of treatment, from conservative to exclusively arthrotomic-surgery, and finally arthroscopy in selected cases. Bigliani's work is a key part of this trend. In 1998 Bigliani stated that 'open' surgery was the treatment of choice at that time for this type of lesion, and in a description of arthroscopic techniques for the stabilization of unstable shoulder, Warner (1996) listed bony Bankart lesion as one of the strict contraindications to this technique. De Palma had already recommended in 1983 open reduction with internal fixation for open glenoid fractures with glenohumeral instability, while in 1991 Gazielly and Godeneche proposed surgery involving coracoid transposition for cases of glenohumeral instability in which a bony lesion of the glenoid had been demonstrated. It was nevertheless not until 1997 that, thanks to studies by Heggland and Parker, the first attempts at arthroscopic stabilization were observed, although the authors reported their failure to complete the procedure as closed surgery. The following year Cameron (1998) proposed a further arthroscopic method, i.e. the reduction and synthesis of a glenoid fracture with a malleolar screw inserted through the fibres of the subscapularis. Our technique (Porcellini 2002) for arthroscopic stabilization of bony Bankart lesions involves blended anaesthesia (supraclavicular block and general anaesthesia) and placing the patient in a lateral supine position. After diagnosis and evaluation of the lesion performed via the classic posterior and anterosuperior portals, we begin stabilization by creating a further anteroinferior (mid-glenoid) portal. In this phase, visualization is achieved through the anterosuperior portal and the scapular neck is abraded through the mid-glenoid portal, removing clots and fibrous tissue between the glenoid and the bone fragment with the labrum inserted. The same portal is used to insert three mini-anchors along the fracture rim: the first in the lower portion of the fracture, the second in the centre and the third in the upper portion (Fig. 10.9). The function of the

Surgical solutions in joint disorders

Fig. 10.8

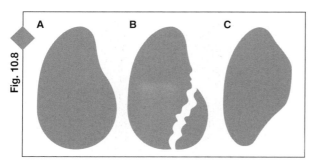

Type III lesion of the glenoid rim with characteristic 'inverted pear' glenoid.

Fig. 10.9

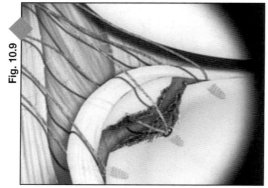

Arthroscopic stabilization of bony Bankart lesions through the anterosuperior portal with Mini-Revo sutures.

first and third screws is to bring the capsule and labrum in contact with the fracture rim, while the central screw will raise the bone fragment to the level of the glenoid cartilage.

To conclude, on the basis of our experience and the results of our studies, the indications for the arthroscopic treatment of bony Bankart lesions remain valid for isolated acute lesions in which the bone fragment accounts for less than 25% of the entire glenoid surface. According to Bigliani, Gazielly and Godeneche, the open procedure remains valid for chronic lesions, when the fragment accounts for more than 25% of the glenoid and where capsule lesions are also present.

Posterior instability

Posterior instability is defined as the result of symptoms reported by the patient owing to excessive posterior glenohumeral translation.

The classification of posterior dislocation has been summarized clearly by Romsey (1999) as follows:
— acute; and
— chronic (fixed long-term).

Whereas for recurrent subluxation it is as follows:
— psychogenic;
— dysplasic; and
— acquired.

Acute posterior dislocation is rare (5%) and half of all cases unfortunately go unrecognized on initial examination. The failure to recognize acute posterior dislocation, and the resulting absence of treatment, leads to chronic posterior dislocation. The indications for the treatment of this lesion depend on the time that has elapsed since the trauma, the proportion of the humeral head involved, the patient's age and the damage to the humeral head and glenoid cartilage. The techniques we currently use are the following: McLaughlin procedure, reduction with a humeral bone graft, and arthroplasty or hemiarthroplasty. Surgical treatment in recurrent subluxation is aimed at patients with painful, involuntary instability, which hinders daily activities and sports. The surgeon should be extremely careful to exclude patients who have a tendency towards voluntary posterior subluxation of the shoulder, to release emotional tension or as a psychogenic tic. Such forms should be treated with the help of a psychologist and with physiotherapy. Dysplasic forms should be examined carefully before deciding on surgery, since they result in an increase in glenoid retroversion and humeral retrotorsion; these bone deformities should be carefully evaluated by CT with a view to possible glenoid osteotomy or the use of a posterior bone graft. A further important requirement, before attempting surgery, is a careful study of scapulothoracic rhythm dysfunction. Warner (1992) clearly outlined this problem, noting that the anterior serratus has a fundamental role in scapulothoracic dysfunction, resulting in impaired glenohumeral stability. The largest group of patients consists, however, of those suffering from acquired recurrent posterior subluxation, posterior Bankart lesion, elongation of the posterior band of the IGHL and an increase in the rotator interval; the anterosuperior part of the capsule has an important role in posteroinferior stability (importance of the coracohumeral ligament). Posterior bony Bankart lesions are, unlike the anterior form, extremely rare in our experience. We have moved from open surgery with posterior access to the use of arthroscopy in all cases to make a differential diagnosis between unidirectional and multidirectional forms. Owing to the versatility of this procedure, in contrast with open surgery, access can be gained to the posterior structures (labrum, posterior capsule) (Table 10.V, between page 398 and page 399) and anterior structures (rotator interval) for effective stabilization of this lesion. We tend to prefer, when stabilizing these lesions, to use miniscrews and non-reabsorbable thread for posterior Bankart lesions and suture of the rotator interval with endoarticular PDS stitches and retensioning of the IGHL, whereas we do not use techniques involving shrinkage of the capsule. The literature results for this technique have been very poor in the past (Hawkins, 1996); things are now changing thanks to better gross pathological classification and the treatment of soft tissue. Pollock and Bigliani (1993) report 80% of good results with careful retensioning of the posteroinferior pouch of the IGHL and our experience tends to support this, with excellent results being achieved, particularly in patients with reverse Bankart lesion due to a unidirectional posterior traumatic dislocation, whereas patients with multidirectional laxity may, in some cases, be left with slight instability, which should be kept under control by correct balancing of the internal and external rotators.

Posterosuperior impingement

Internal impingement between the inferior surface of the rotator cuff and the posterosuperior portion of the glenoid and the glenoid labrum is entirely normal and physiological. The supraspinatus tendon is pinched between the greater tuberosity and the posterosuperior surface of the glenoid, when the arm is abducted at 90° in maximum external rotation. In this position, the humeral head is translated 4 mm in a posterior direction. The glenohumeral ligaments and the static and dynamic stabilizer muscles in the normal shoulder allow this posterior translation and prevent anterior

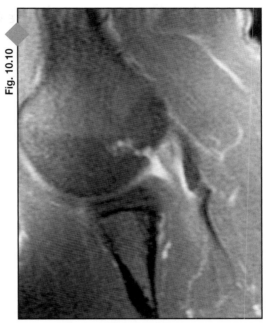

Fig. 10.10

MR arthrography in the ABER position to evaluation cuff lesion and impingement on the upper rim of the glenoid.

instability. In athletes, repeated throwing, fatigue and repetitive movement, for example, the smash in volleyball, can weaken the stabilizer muscles, causing pathological impingement between the posterosuperior surface of the glenoid and the rotator cuff which is damaged as a result. Damage to the lower trapezius and the anterior serratus can cause a loss of scapular synchrony and lead, as a result, to hyperangulation and a relative increase in glenoid anteversion. The impaired balance of the weakened internal rotators, in contrast with the external rotators, can be evaluated clinically using Zaslav's test (2001). MR and in particular MR arthrography in the abduction and external rotation position (ABER) (Fig. 10.10), can be used for a correct evaluation of the cuff lesion and impingement on the upper rim of the glenoid. Usually we additionally conduct an isometric study of these muscle groups using a machine developed for this purpose, which can identify the difference in the force exerted by these muscle groups. Clinically, patients with internal impingement syndrome complain of posterior pain, usually alleviated by the relocation test; the ROM is complete and there is no increase in external rotation; the tests for impingement (Neer, Hawkins and Yocum) are all positive. A very interesting study by Crockett (2002) found osseous adaptation in young baseball pitchers.

An increase in humeral retroversion (40°) in the dominant limb is a positive factor for a good level of play and for lower susceptibility to rotator cuff injury; there is no posterior capsule contracture in these players and the posterior soft tissue is not strained. Internal impingement may represent the evolution of various conditions, such as anterior capsule laxity or posterior capsule contracture with an associated SLAP lesion (peel back mechanism). Dynamic evaluation, conducted arthroscopically, is the best way of confirming a diagnosis of internal impingement, both in primary and secondary cases. As regards treatment, the surgical solutions we use, once physiotherapy has been unsuccessful, are debridement performed arthroscopically or in some cases tendon suture for primary cases, while in secondary cases we treat the associated lesion by stabilizing the Bankart or SLAP lesion if present, or by carrying out plication of the IGHL and suture of the cuff where damaged.

Cartilage erosion

Cameron (2002) demonstrated and drew up guidelines for an increasingly frequent problem in glenohumeral joint disease, i.e. osteoarthritis in young patients. Sport, which involves exceeding and repeating technical movements, can lead to arthropathy of the shoulder with the early onset of osteoarthrosis (Cameron, 2003). For the treatment of such cases (Table 10.VI, between page 398 and page 399), we tend to use surgical arthroscopy, which allows us to remove the inflamed synovial membrane and cartilage debris. Cartilage lesions, after careful cleaning of debris, are pierced using appropriate instruments to allow revascularization followed by the formation of a fibrocartilaginous membrane (Frisbie, 2003); this can limit further damage in a joint which will nevertheless subsequently undergo rapid deterioration in terms of both gross pathology and results.

Bibliography

Andrews J.R., Carson W.J., MCleod W.D., 'Glenoid labrum tears related to the long head of the biceps', *Am. J. Sport Med.* 13: 337–341, (1985)

Berg E.E., Ciullo J.V., 'A clinical test for superior glenoid labral or 'SLAP' lesions', *Clin. J. Sports Med.* 8: 121–123, 1998.

Berg E.E., Ciullo J.V., 'The SLAP-lesion: A cause of failure after distal clavicle resection', *Arthroscopy* 13: 85–89, (1997)

Bigliani L.U., Newton P.M., Steinmann S.P., Connor P.M., McLiveen S.J., 'Glenoid rim associated with recurrent

anterior dislocation of the shoulder', *Am. J. Sport Med.* 26(1): 41–45, (1998)

Burkhart S.S., De Beer J.F., 'Traumatic glenohumeral bone defects and their relationship to failure of arthroscopic Bankart repairs: significance of the inverted-pear glenoid and the humeral engaging Hill-Sachs lesion', *Arthroscopy* 16(7): 677–694, (2000)

Cameron B.D., Galatz L.M., Ramsey M.L., Williams G.R., Iannotti J.P., 'Non-prosthetic management of grade IV osteochondral lesions of the glenohumeral joint', *J. Shoulder Elbow Surg.* 11(1): 25–32, (2002)

Cameron M.L., Kocher M.S., Briggs K.K., Horan M.P., Hawkins R.J., 'The prevalence of glenohumeral osteoarthrosis in unstable shoulders', *Am. J. Sports Med.* 31(1): 53–55, (2003)

Cameron S.E., 'Arthroscopic reduction and internal fixation of an anterior glenoid fracture', Case report, *Arthroscopy* 14(7): 743–746, (1998)

Cartland J.P., Crues J.W., Stauffer A., Nottage W., Ryu R.K.N., 'MR imaging in the evaluation of SLAP injuries of the shoulder: Findings in 10 patients', *AJR Am. J. Roentgenol.* 159: 787–792, (1992)

Chochole M.H., Senker W., Meznik C., Breitenseher M.J., 'Glenoid labral cyst entrapping suprascapular nerve: dissolution after arthroscopic debridement of an extended SLAP-lesion', *Arthroscopy* 13: 753–755, (1997)

Crockett H.C., Gross L.B., Wilk K.E., Schwartz M.L., Reed J., O'Mara J., Reilly M.T., Dugas J.R., Meister K., Lyman S., Andrews J.R., 'Osseous adaptation and range of motion at the glenohumeral joint in professional baseball pitchers', *Am. J. Sports Med.* 30(1): 20–26, (2002)

De Palma A.F., 'Fractures and fracture-dislocations of the shoulder girdle', In: De Palma A.F. (eds.) *Surgery of the Shoulder*, 3rd ed. JB Lippincott, Philadelphia, pp. 367–369, (1983)

Frisbie D.D., Oxford J.T., Southwood L., Trotter G.W., Rodkey W.G., Steadman J.R., Goodnight J.L., McIlwraith C.W., 'Early events in cartilage repair after subchondral bone microfracture', *Clin. Orthop.* 407: 215–227, (2003)

Gazielly D.F., Godeneche J.L., 'The use of coracoid transfer for recurrent anterior glenohumeral instability', In: Watson M.S. (eds.), 'Surgical disorders of the shoulder', Churchill Livingstone, London, pp. 355–362, (1991)

Goss T.P., 'Double disruptions of the superior shoulder suspensory complex', *J. Orthop. Trauma* 7(2): 99–106, (1993)

Hawkins R.J., Janda D.H., 'Posterior instability of the glenohumeral joint. A technique of repair', *Am. J. Sports Med.* 24(3): 275–278, (1996)

Heggland E.J.H., Parker R.D., 'Simultaneous bilateral glenoid fractures associated with glenohumeral subluxation/dislocation in a weightlifter', *Orthopaedics* 20: 1180–1183, (1997)

Hovelius L., Eriksson K., Fredin H., Hagber G., Hussenius A., Lind B., Thorling J., Weckstrom J., 'Recurrences after initial dislocation of the shoulder. Results of a prospective study of treatment', *J. Bone Joint Surg. Am.* 65(3): 343–349, (1983)

Hunter J.C., Blatz D.J., Escobedo E.M., 'SLAP-lesions of the glenoid labrum: CT arthrographic and arthroscopic correlation', *Radiology* 184: 513–518, (1992)

Ideberg R., Grevsten S., Larsson S., 'Epidemiology of scapular fractures. Incidence and classification of 338 fractures', *Acta Orthop. Scand.* 66(5): 395–397, (1995)

Leitschuh P.H., Bone C.M., Bouska W.M., 'Magnetic resonance imaging diagnosis, sonographically directed percutaneous aspiration, and arthroscopic treatment of a painful shoulder ganglion cyst associated with a SLAP-lesion', *Arthroscopy* 15(1): 85–87, (1999)

Maffet M.W., Gartsman G.M., Moseley B., 'Superior labrum biceps tendon complex lesions of the shoulder', *Am. J. Sports Med.* 23: 93–98, (1995)

Mileski R.A., Snyder S.J., 'Superior labral lesions in the shoulder: pathoanatomy and surgical management', *J. Am. Acad. Orthop. Surg.* 6: 121–131, (1993)

Pollock R.G., Bigliani L.U., 'Recurrent posterior shoulder instability. Diagnosis and treatment', *Clin. Orthop.* 291: 85–96, (1993)

Porcellini G., Campi F., Paladini P., 'Arthroscopic approach to acute bony Bankart lesion', *Arthroscopy* 18(7): 764–769, (2002)

Rames R.D., Karzel R.P., 'Injuries to the glenoid labrum, including SLAP-lesions', *Orthop. Clin. North Am.* 24: 45–53, (1993)

Romsey M.C., 'Disorders of the shoulder: Diagnosis and Management', Williams Iannotti Lippincott, London, (1999)

Rowe C.R., Zarins B., 'Recurrent transient subluxation of the shoulder', *J. Bone Joint Surg. Am.* 63(6): 863–872, (1981)

Ryu R.K.N., 'Classification and treatment of SLAP injuries', 14th Annual Meeting, *Arthroscopic Surgery of Shoulder*, San Diego, pp. 255–260, (1997)

Savoie F.H. 3rd, Field L.D., Atchinson S., 'Anterior superior instability with rotator cuff tearing: SLAC-lesion', *Orthop. Clin. North Am.* 32(3): 457–61, ix, (2001)

Smith A.M., McCauley T.R., Jokl P., 'SLAP-lesions of the glenoid labrum diagnosed with MR imaging', *Skeletal Radiol.* 22: 507–510, (1993)

Snyder S.J., Karzel R.P., Del Pizzo W., Ferkel R.D., Friedman M.J., 'SLAP-lesions of the shoulder', *Arthroscopy* 6: 274–279, (1990)

Wang D.H., Koehler S.M., 'Isolated infraspinatus atrophy in a collegiate volleyball player', *Clin. J. Sport Med.* 6(4): 255–258, (1996)

Warner J.J., Lephart S., Fu F.H., 'Role of proprioception in pathoetiology of shoulder instability', *Clin. Orthop.* 330: 35–39, (1996)

Warner J.J., Micheli L.J., Arslanian L.E., Kennedy J., Kennedy R., 'Scapulothoracic motion in normal shoulders and shoulders with glenohumeral instability and impingement syndrome, A study using Moire topographic analysis', *Clin. Orthop.* 285: 191–199, (1992)

Zaslav K.R., 'Internal rotation resistance strength test: a new diagnostic test to differentiate intra-articular pathology from outlet (Neer) impingement syndrome in the shoulder', *J. Shoulder Elbow Surg.* 10(1): 23–27, (2001)

CHAPTER 11

SURGICAL SOLUTIONS IN MUSCLE AND TENDON DISORDERS

R. MINOLA
L. CASTELLANI
P. SUMMA
M.C. GIORDANO

The method is the means of achieving the result: accuracy and a systematic approach to analysing the patient and the reliability of the surgical procedure will determine the reproducibility and consistency of the results.

The diagnosis of rotator cuff disorder in an athlete thus requires a detailed history and a rigorous object-ive examination, the examination being based on a knowledge of anatomy and on an interpretation of the movement responsible for the injury as a function of shoulder biomechanics.

The treatment is chosen according to the injury:
— reparable anatomical lesion = reparative surgery = optimal choice;
— functional lesion = rehabilitation of the movement = optimal choice;
— non-reparable anatomical lesion = reconstructive and replacement surgery of the damaged part and/or functional rehabilitation = optimal choice;
— non-reparable anatomical lesion = palliative surgery = non-optimal choice.

The ability to obtain consistent, reproducible results for the patient thus depends on the clinician's ability to analyse the traumatic event (microtrauma or macrotrauma), to interpret it with the aid of the objective examination and radiological images, and finally to use surgery, where necessary, according to the technique most appropriate to the injury.

An adequate classification is, therefore, necessary in order to make a therapeutic choice. The classification is based on the time elapsed since the trauma, on the site and type of anatomical damage, whether the lesion can be repaired, and finally whether associated anatomical lesions are present.

Classification of rotator cuff lesions

Duration of the symptoms

A knowledge of the chronology of the injury is essen-tial for a correct therapeutic choice.

A severe acute lesion is, in fact, operable once the initial post-traumatic inflammation has subsided to reduce the risks of stiffness and pain, while an acute lesion in a previously damaged area can be tackled promptly to avoid causing chronic lesions, and so on.

We divide lesions as follows, based on the symp-toms reported:
— *acute lesion:* symptoms reported within a month, generally of traumatic origin;
— *subacute lesion:* disorder occurring one to six months previously, generally on a microtraumatic or macrotraumatic basis; and
— *chronic lesion:* disorder occurring more than six months previously, generally on a degenerative and microtraumatic or macrotraumatic basis.

Site of the lesion

The topographical site of the lesion provides import-ant information on the nature of the lesion and may indicate the need for additional surgical procedures, such as subacromial or coracoid decompression, or tenodesis of the long head of the biceps.

Knowing or suspecting the topography of the lesion preoperatively may be important for planning the position of arthroscopic portals, as we shall see below.

We divide lesions as follows:

- **simple,** which can in turn be divided into the following:
  — *anterior:* isolated lesions of the subscapularis which may be accompanied by medial subluxations or frank dislocations of the long head of the biceps;
  — *anterosuperior:* lesions of the upper part of the subscapularis and the anterior part of the supraspinatus;
  — *superior:* lesions of the supraspinatus only, with no involvement of the long head of the biceps or the subscapularis;
  — *posterosuperior:* lesions of the supraspinatus and the infraspinatus;
  — *posterior:* lesions of the infraspinatus tendon only;
- **complex:**
  — *anterosuperior and posterosuperior:* extensive lesions involving all the rotator cuff tendons to a varied extent.

Degree of reparability

Classifying lesions on the basis of their extent and the involution of the muscle tissue is important for planning the type of repair, for quantifying the difficulty of the procedure and for predicting the patient's chances of recovery as far as possible.

The classification we use identifies the damage simply and realistically, defining the degree of repair that is possible:

— *early:* in which the tendon(s) is (are) substantially disinserted from the bone but not retracted, and valid muscle tissue is present. These are the lesions with the most favourable prognosis and they require firm reinsertion of the tendon in the bone (Table 11.I, between page 398 and page 399, Fig. 11.1);

— *late:* in which the tendon(s) is (are) not only disinserted from the bone but are also retracted (but not beyond the glenoid), and the muscle tissue is still valid or hypotrophic (up to 50% of its normal volume, evaluated by preoperative MR) (Table 11.II, between page 398 and page 399, Fig. 11.2). These lesions still have a favourable prognosis, they need a detailed analysis of the geometric shape of the lesion to be able to reattach the tendon correctly to the bone, they require adequate mobilization of the tendon from its fibrotic adhesions, and the reinsertion of the tendon in the bone requires one or more

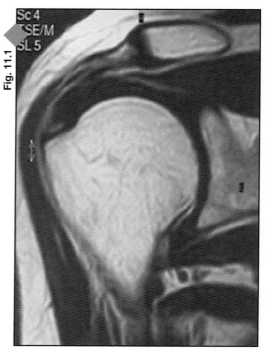

Fig. 11.1

MR image of an early lesion.

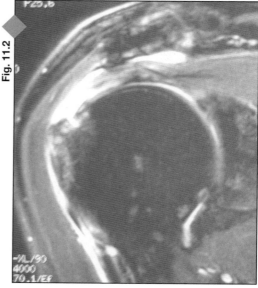

Fig. 11.2

MR image of a late lesion.

anchors, in some cases to improve the hold of the repair to the bone. Reduction in the extent of the lesion with side to side sutures is useful;

— *too late:* in these cases the tendons have become disinserted (as far as the glenoid or more medially), and the muscle tissue is not valid (more than 50% of its normal volume, evaluated by preoperative MR) (Table 11.III, between page 398 and page 399, Fig. 11.3). These lesions have a poor prognosis, but they may benefit from balancing the lesion by tendon reinsertion with subscapularis or infraspinatus anchors, with selective suture according to which side is most involved.

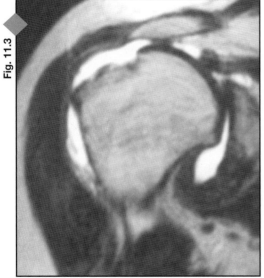

Fig. 11.3

MR image of a lesion that is too late, with the tendon rim at the glenoid.

The aims of this partial suture are restoring the balance of the muscle pair, increasing the stability of the margins of the lesion, and stabilizing the lesion or slowing its progress.

Decision-making strategy for repairing the rotator cuff

Acute lesion (within one month of the trauma or the onset of the symptoms).

The aim of surgery is to reinsert the tendon anatomically in the bone:

— the natural footprint of the tendon in the bone, i.e. the physiological area of contact between

bone and tendon (Table 11.IV, between page 398 and page 399) is recreated by implanting a sufficient number of medial and lateral anchors (Dugas, 2002);

— the surgical technique may be performed entirely arthroscopically or, when required, by transdeltoid access (mini-open surgery);

— surgery performed in an acute patient with firm sutures, with no tendon or muscle hypotrophy observed (early repair), ensures faster rehabilitation;

— biotechnologies can be used postoperatively to improve healing quality and reduce the time required for repair.

Subacute lesion (within one to six months of the trauma or the onset of the symptoms).

There are, in fact, two scenarios:

— *early:* the patient has suffered a trauma which has damaged the rotator cuff. Patients tend to go to an Accident and Emergency Department where rest and treatment for the pain are recommended. Owing to the persistence of the symptoms, the patient then turns to a specialist;

— *late:* the patient already had damage, tolerated to a varying extent, which worsened after further trauma or sport-related stress.

The strategy is thus defined as follows:

• *early:* the procedure is the same as for a patient with an acute lesion; and

• *late:* the objective is to restore mobility to the tendons so that they can be reinserted in the bone:

  — in order to reattach the tendons in a physiological position, the type of lesion, generally an anterior or posterior L-based lesion, must be understood;

  — to reduce the suture tension and the apparent extent of the damage, side to side sutures (from medial to lateral) can be used;

  — the anatomical footprint must be recreated as in early lesions;

  — the procedure can be performed entirely arthroscopically or by transdeltoid access, used only for fixing tendons to bone;

  — surgery performed on a patient with more fragile tendon tissue or with muscle hypotrophy (late repair) requires prolonged and closely monitored rehabilitation in order for the result to be valid;

  — biotechnologies can be used postoperatively to improve healing quality and to reduce the time required for repair.

Chronic lesion (When the patient is evaluated more than six months after the trauma or the onset of the symptoms).

There are, in fact, two scenarios:
— *late:* the patient already had damage, tolerated to a varying extent, which worsened after further trauma or sport-related stress; and
— *too late:* in these cases the tendons have become disinserted (as far as the glenoid or more medially), and the muscle tissue is not valid (more than 50% of its normal volume, evaluated by preoperative MR).

The strategy is defined as follows:
• *late:* the procedure is the same as for a patient with a reparable chronic lesion;
• *too late:* the aim is to stabilize the lesion overall and to reinsert the tendon in the bone where possible:
　— the anterior (subscapularis) and posterior (infraspinatus) muscle and tendon pairs are recreated and balanced;
　— side to side sutures are used to reduce tension and the extent of the damage without limiting joint volume and to reduce the risk of stiffness;
　— the surgical technique can be performed entirely arthroscopically or, for the final phase of fixation to the bone, by transdeltoid access;
　— balanced repair requires controlled mobilization;
　— surgery performed on a patient with more fragile tendon tissue and with muscle hypotrophy (late repair) requires prolonged and closely monitored rehabilitation in order for the result to be valid;
　— biotechnologies can be used postoperatively in selected cases to improve healing quality and to reduce the time required for repair; and
　— in selected cases (individuals under 50–55-years-old), muscle-tendon transfer from the pectoralis major to an anterior subscapularis defect, or from the latissimus dorsi to a posterior infraspinatus defect, may be considered.

Surgical technique

Surgery of the rotator cuff is and will be largely arthroscopic, or mini-invasive.

The advantages of arthroscopic suture over open surgery are: the preservation of the deltoid and its periosteal insertion, reduced postoperative pain, simplified rehabilitation, in particular passive joint recovery, detailed evaluation of associated disorders and their treatment (such as SLAP lesion, instability, etc.) and a better cosmetic result (Gartsman, 1998; Stollteimer, 1998; Tauro, 1998).

Positioning the patient

When planning the procedure, the surgeon has until now had two choices of position: lying on the side or the beach-chair position.

These positions both have their advantages and drawbacks, but the value of defining a single standard for shoulder surgery justifies the choice of the beach-chair position. This position has been chosen for the following reasons:
— reproducibility and a systematic approach to the surgical procedure;
— greater reliability with locoregional anaesthesia which can be combined with sedation or general anaesthesia;
— the evaluation of the intra-articular anatomy is not affected by excessive static traction which minimizes associated disorders, such as instability;
— the ability to perform a dynamic evaluation of the shoulder in all the physiological planes in order to understand better the effect of the injury; and
— the tissue can be repaired with adjustable tension and in a physiological position.

Furthermore, a final dynamic test can be performed to assess the quality and stability of the repair carried out.

Beach-chair position The patient is placed on the operating couch in a seated position with supports and with the chest flexed at between 60° and 80° in relation to the floor. The half of the chest on the affected side should be free in a posterior direction to allow the arthroscope to be manoeuvred freely. The head and neck are supported by a headrest with the head slightly flexed.

The legs should be flexed with a cushion underneath and held in place with Velcro straps.

It is important that the patient's lumbosacral region is completely supported at the back.

Finally, the beach-chair position allows traction to be applied with the arm in slight abduction and in 80° anterior flexion: a traction apparatus will provide movement that is readily adjustable in both the lateral plane and in rotation.

Portals

The first portal is the standard posterior portal, located 2 cm below and 1 cm medially in relation to the posterolateral angle of the acromion, in the 'soft spot'.

The second standard portal is anterior and is performed out-in with the spinal needle, lateral in

relation to the coracoacromial ligament. It is placed according to the location of the lesion:
— for repairing the subscapularis tendon, the portal is created at the tendon insertion in order to position the anchor;
— for a SLAP or Bankart lesion, two portals are generally used, i.e. the anterosuperior portal and the anteroinferior portal; and
— for lesions of the superior or posterosuperior rotator cuff, the anterior portal located in the rotator interval is sufficient.

Initial phase of arthroscopy and evaluation of damage

The procedure starts with a static and dynamic evaluation in the air of the glenohumeral joint.

The insertion of the long head of the biceps is examined and it is moved from its groove to determine whether there is any extra-articular damage.

Joint stability is evaluated and any capsule or labral lesions are repaired during the same surgical procedure.

The cuff insertion area is evaluated, along with the mobility of the tendon, whether it is damaged, and the extent of any partial tears.

Lesions of the subscapularis

Damage to the subscapularis muscle tendon is easier to evaluate with the arm in internal rotation, and it is important that it is repaired before other tendon lesions (Wright, 2001). When repairing the subscapularis tendon, it is first of all necessary to remove scar tissue from the humerus, using the motorized system, to create a bleeding bone bed to help the healing process.

The mobility of the bone in the tendon and its reduction is then evaluated (Table 11.V, between page 398 and page 399). If the supraspinatus is damaged, a second superior portal through it is useful, as an accessory portal, otherwise one will be created above the head of the biceps.

The anchor is positioned with a double suture through the anterior portal and the two threads are taken into the accessory portal. At this point:
— the double thread of a suture is frozen using Klemmer forceps;
— one end of the other suture is frozen; and
— a pusher is positioned at the other end of the same thread.

An instrument, called a penetrator, is introduced through the anterior portal, piercing the tendon. The keyhole incision is then opened, the thread picked up using the pusher and the penetrator led out with the thread. This will be the post for tying the knot.

If a U suture is preferred, the same procedure is repeated with the other end. Otherwise the other end is recovered through the superior portal to make a sliding or non-sliding knot, depending on whether the thread slides in the anchor.

The same steps are performed with the other suture. For lesions measuring more than 1.0–1.5 cm, two anchors are used to reattach the tendon to the bone.

Portal placement for the subacromial space

As a rule, all the portals for access to the subacromial space should be made 1–2 cm below the inferior profile of the acromial bone, except MIP for minimal invasive portals, which are made in a superior location for the positioning of the anchor.

A posterolateral portal (PL) is always created in the subacromial space (1–2 cm below the posterior acromial angle). The aim is to achieve better visualization of the space and to make it easier to manage the instruments, particularly in the lateral region of the cuff tendons.

Preparation and evaluation of the lesion

With the optical device in the PL portal, bursectomy is carried out through the anterior portal using the shaver and the vaporizer, in order to visualize the entire cuff lesion. The phase involving the vaporizer is important for obtaining acceptable haemostasis in order to visualize the procedure.

Once bursectomy has been performed, lateral access must be created by means of the out-in technique with a spinal needle. This access must be centred on the lesion, since it will allow visualization of the whole suture procedure.

Once the optical device has been placed in a lateral position, the lesion can be evaluated in three dimensions, providing an accurate assessment of both the extent of the lesion on the trochanter (in the antero-posterior direction), and the degree of retraction of the tendons (in the lateromedial direction).

Using the grasper through either the anterior or the posterolateral portal, the degree of retraction of the lesion must be evaluated along with the possibility of reduction of the tendon. One of the factors determining the success of the cuff suture is, therefore, the degree to which the damaged tendon can be reinserted in the bone and how easy this is. If mobility is inadequate, the adhesions will be freed and the coracohumeral ligament released. This is carried out by visualizing the ligament through the lateral portal and releasing it through the anterior portal by means of radiofrequencies in order to reduce the risk of bleeding from the fat covering the muscle belly of the supraspinatus or, anteromedially, clotting the branch of the thoracoacromial artery.

To obtain greater tendon excursion, if subacromial cleaning is insufficient, superior capsule release can be carried out from 1 o'clock to 10 o'clock, to section the capsule expansions above the superior glenoid labrum, without going too far owing to the presence of the suprascapularis nerve approximately 1.5–2 cm from the glenoid rim.

Once the lesion has been analysed, suturing is planned. The bone bed is cleaned and traces of the damaged tendon insertion removed. The bone must be pared down to bleeding tissue to provide essential support for the repair substances, but not too much to weaken the bone which will receive the anchors. The tendon margins can also be pared to remove degenerative tissue.

If a side to side suture is planned, the lesion will be visualized through the lateral portal. The procedure begins by placing the first suture medially 1 cm from the apex of the lesion. The suture can be passed through the tendon directly, using either a suture leader or a penetrating grasper.

In the former case, a 20° up suture leader preloaded with a reabsorbable thread of adequate size (at least No. 2), will be used through the anterior or posterolateral portal, depending on whether there is less of the tendon present in an anterior or posterior position. The suture leader will initially pass through the first margin of the lesion in a surface-deep direction, and then the second margin in the opposite direction.

The thread is recovered from the eyelet of the suture leader using a crochet hook through the opposite portal and the other end of the thread is recovered through the principal portal, through which a sliding knot will be made. The same procedure is repeated at a distance of a centimetre as necessary.

The same procedure can be performed with two penetrating graspers. One of the instruments is loaded with a non-reabsorbable thread of appropriate size. Always starting from the margin where the least amount of the tendon is present, the penetrating grasper is passed through straight in a surface-deep

direction. The penetrating grasper is passed through the opposite portal so as to pierce the tendon lesion from the other margin, again in a surface-deep direction. The thread is taken from the first instrument and pulled through the tendon, and then led out. The other end of the thread is recovered through the principal portal and a sliding knot is made.

Positioning of the anchors

A percutaneous superior accessory portal (MIP) is prepared at an angle of 45° to the bone plane, through which an anchor is positioned with a double thread of a different colour.

Fixing in the bone is performed according to the two deadman angles described by Burkhart: the first is the angle which is obtained perpendicular to the anchor and the suture: the smaller this angle, the smaller the risk of the anchor being pulled out of the bone. The second is obtained in the direction of the force vector of the repaired tendon (i.e. parallel to the bone) and the suture: the smaller this angle, the smaller the tension on the suture and the risk of rupture. Ideally these two angles should be less than 45°. In practical terms, this is obtained by positioning the anchor in the direction of the tendon to be reattached and positioning the knot medially in relation to the anchor eyelet.

In order to reproduce the anatomical insertion of the tendon in the bone (footprint), we position the first anchor medially and subsequent anchors laterally to the tendon (Table 11.VI, between page 398 and page 399).

The suture is prepared once the first anchor has been positioned medially, adjacent to the joint cartilage of the head. The thread leading towards the tip of the anchor is initially frozen with Klemmer forceps and the other thread is prepared for the suture.

The more lateral end is held in the anchor with Klemmer forceps and the other end is prepared with a pusher, always making sure that it is held in place.

The penetrating grasper is introduced through the posterolateral or posterior portal and passed in a surface-deep direction through the tendon lesion; the thread is then picked up with the aid of the pusher. This thread is then released from the pusher and the penetrating grasper is withdrawn through the posterolateral portal with the thread. The same procedure is repeated with the other end and a sliding knot is made, if the thread slides adequately in the tissue. The second thread is released and the same procedure repeated.

In accordance with the principle of positioning the anchors according to the footprint, the second and subsequent anchors are placed in a lateral position in order to reproduce the anatomical insertion of the tendon (Fig. 11.4).

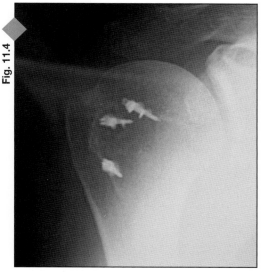

Fig. 11.4

X-ray image following arthroscopic suture of the supraspinatus and subscapularis (anterosuperior lesion). Note the position on the trochanter of the two medial and lateral anchors to recreate the footprint.

The tendon can also be sutured with the suture leader. For a right shoulder, a suture leader inclined to the left is chosen, if it passes through the posterior part of the tendon through the posterior or posterolateral portal; if, however, it passes through the anterior portal, a suture leader inclined to the right is chosen.

After the anchor has been positioned through the MIP, the thread of the more medial anchor is led through the desired portal which becomes the working portal. The suture leader is loaded with the thread and passed through the tendon into the position we have chosen, in a deep-surface direction.

The thread on the suture leader is led through the opposite portal (accessory portal) using a crochet hook and both instruments are removed at the same time; the thread is then led through the accessory portal to the principal portal. A sliding or a non-sliding knot is made.

Acromioplasty

Arthroscopic acromioplasty must be performed correctly to prevent possible complications associated with the failure of the surgery. Approximately 5 mm of the thickness of the anterior acromion is removed, using the diameter of the shaver blade or acromizer as a measuring guide. After identifying the anterolateral angle, the bone tissue is removed from the outer rim of the acromion using the posterior optical device and the instrument through the mediolateral access, extending in an anteroposterior direction and then in a lateromedial direction. The bone resection is carried out in the anterior portion of the acromion to avoid future instability.

Postoperative management

For lesions defined as early, the patient is permitted to use the limb actively with 50% of joint function and therefore does not need a brace during the day. The limb should, however, should be braced at night for four weeks.

A randomized prospective study is under way in which 50% of the patients undergo postoperative cell stimulation therapy for three weeks and 50% have simulated therapy.

During the first four weeks, patients are asked to perform passive mobilization (in water or dry) equivalent to 80% of their joint function. Active use of the limb, equivalent to 80% of joint function, is permitted from the 30–35th day after surgery.

For lesions defined as late, the patient is permitted to use the limb actively with 50% of joint function, and therefore does not need a brace during the day. The limb is braced at night for four weeks.

During the first four weeks, patients are asked to perform passive mobilization (in water or dry) equivalent to 80% of their joint function. Active use of the limb, equivalent to 80% of joint function, is permitted from the 40–50th day after surgery.

For lesions defined as too late, the patient is permitted to use the limb actively with 50% of joint function, and therefore does not need a brace during the day and the limb is braced at night for four weeks.

During the first four weeks, patients are asked to perform passive mobilization (in water or dry) equivalent to 80% of their joint function.

Active use of the limb, equivalent to 80% of joint function, is permitted from the 40–50th day after surgery.

Bibliography

Dugas J.R., Campbell D.A., Warren R.F., Robie B.H., Millett P.J., 'Anatomy and dimensions of rotator cuff insertions', *J. Shoulder Elbow Surg.* 11(5): 498–503, (2002)

Surgical solutions in muscle and tendon disorders

Gartsman G.M., Khan M., Hammerman S.M., 'Arthroscopic repair of full-thickness tears of the rotator cuff', *J. Bone Joint Surg.* 80-A(6): 832–840, (1998)

Stollteimer G.T., Savoie F.H., 'Arthroscopic rotator cuff repair: Current indications, Limitations, Techniques and Results', AAOS Instructional Course Lectures Vol. 47: 59–65, (1998)

Tauro J.C., 'Arthroscopic rotator cuff repair: Analysis of technique and results at 2- and 3-year follow-up', *Arthroscopy* 14: 45–51, (1998)

Wright J.M., Heavrin B., Hawkins R.J., Noonan T., 'Arthroscopic visualization of the subscapularis tendon', *Arthroscopy* 17(7): 677–684, (2001)

SECTION IV

REHABILITATION, TRAINING AND PREVENTION

REHABILITATION: CULTURAL MODELS, WORKING MODELS AND SCOPE

M. Testa

Rehabilitation today is still commonly based on a biomedical view of health with the disease at the centre.

This view is represented in the international classification of diseases (ICD) (www.who.int/classifications/icd/en/). This system does not, however, provide sufficient information about rehabilitation and is not exhaustive as regards a series of disorders characterized by an often unclear multifactorial aetiology, where the pain and disability aspects take precedence over clearly identifiable gross pathological components that can be attributed to the clinical picture.

The biomedical model is applied mostly to infectious diseases and applies less well to disorders with a chronic degenerative course, where psychoaffective and social components tend to have an important role, and also because of their influence on pain which is often perceived out of proportion to the nociceptive stimulus.

Rehabilitation has the person, not the disease, as the object of its action, and thus necessarily has to refer to a model that is different from but complementary to the biomedical model, capable of describing the person's health more extensively and including social and environmental aspects in this view.

Rehabilitative physiotherapy, by its nature, requires far greater active involvement by the patient than a pharmacological treatment or a surgical procedure. The physiotherapist cannot proceed without a knowledge of the state of health of the individual to be rehabilitated, not only as regards the presence of disorders, but also as regards an awareness of the different domains of health, disability and problems of participation caused by the disorder.

The use of a model to interpret the state of health, such as that proposed by WHO (world health organization), first in the form of the international classification of impairments, disabilities and handicaps (ICIDH-2) and currently in the form of the international classification of functioning (ICF) (www.who.int/classifications/icf/en/), becomes necessary for physiotherapists and rehabilitation specialists in general. It allows a truly 'holistic' approach to the individual, who becomes the focus of the work of various health professionals, and this also allows professional boundaries to be bridged and good interdisciplinary relations to be developed between the various specialists, based on the patient's requirements.

The use of this model which, as we emphasize, is not in opposition but complementary to the biomedical model (www.who.int/classifications/icd/en) is supplemented by the use of a further cultural model, strongly characterizing the actions of the physiotherapist, i.e. the multidimensional load/carriability/adaptability model (Hagenaars, 2002).

This tool for interpreting state of health provides a dynamic view of the organism that is continually added to and adapted in each area of health as a function of the internal or external requests that reach the individual.

The ICF and the multidimensional load/carriability/adaptability model form a cultural framework for the rehabilitation specialist's evaluation, aimed at constructing a prognostic health profile (PHP) (Testa, 2004); this is a real working tool which also provides a basis for the choice of outcome, all the information for defining objectives, and the strategies and therapeutic techniques for obtaining the best quality procedure and the best way of meeting the patient's expectations.

Fig. 12.1

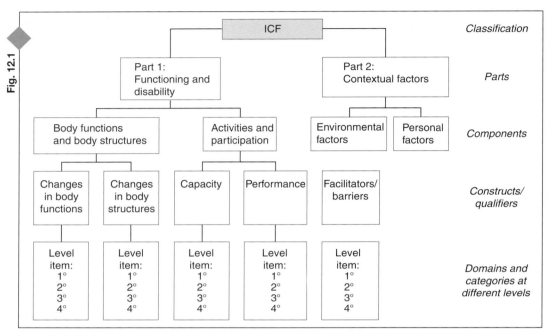

The structure of the ICF.

We shall, in this chapter, examine these various aspects and try to explain their applicability to clinical practice, with a few examples.

Use of the ICF in rehabilitation practice

The health needs of the patient/individual cannot be assessed solely on the basis of the medical diagnosis; the consequences of the disease also need to be considered.

The ICD is not, therefore, a sufficient tool to meet this need. Historically, a change in perspective was brought about by the growing incidence of chronic disorders which, unlike acute infections in which diagnosis leads via appropriate therapy to the resolution of the health problem, need greater attention to be paid to their repercussions on the individual's quality of life.

WHO replied to this challenge in 2000 with a review of the ICIDH, producing first the ICIDH-2 and then the ICF, which is no longer a classification of the consequences of disease; it has made a further cultural leap to become a classification of the components of health (www.who.int/classifications/icd/en).

The ICF provides a scientific model for the study of forms of disability and function in daily activities which allows a common language to be developed to gather data for use in research and in health management, in terms of planning social well-being. Although, at first sight, this model seems to be remote from clinical practice and useful only for managing health at the level of government political strategy, combination with other models for interpreting the actual experience of individual patients provides specialists with a common arena for interdisciplinary cooperation at its highest level, with the person and their needs, rather than the disorder, at its centre. Health is thus understood as a dynamic equilibrium which can be continually adjusted, on the basis of not only health and medical conditions, but also biological-genetic and psychosocial-behavioural factors. The therapeutic strategy should, therefore, also include ways of reinforcing the individual's behaviour aimed at developing health (Fig. 12.1) (Table 12.1).

Multidimensional load/carriability/ adaptability model and the PHP

The cultural foundations of the biopsychosocial approach provided by the ICF are applied in our clinical rehabilitation practice, although incorporated in an interpretational model of the patient's functional state

Table 12.1

Why it is important to know the ICF

- Allows universal communication
- Facilitates studies of health and disability
- Facilitates and necessitates an evaluation of outcome
- Allows a comparison of different measures
- Supports care policies
- Provides a cultural framework in which other models relevant to individual professional figures can be incorporated

which considers the local and general carriability (Hagenaars, 2002) of the individual in the various areas of health, i.e. biological, psychological and social. This consideration will inform and guide our history taking and will enable us to construct appropriate diagnostic and therapeutic strategies to meet the needs and expectations of our patient. The key tool in this model is the PHP. It is constructed on the basis of the belief that the health of the individual is the result of dynamic relations between the domains of biology, psychology and social interaction or participation. Consequently, the specialist will aim to identify the disorders present and to classify them in the separate areas as impairment, disabilities or participation problems, and to recognize the relations existing between these in a specific area and between disorders present in different areas. The evaluation must additionally take into account personal and external factors affecting the individual which intensify the specific clinical conditions in a positive or negative sense.

The history taking is a vital part of this process, constituting an opportunity for both gathering information and establishing a relationship with the patient who can explain the expectations of which he or she is both aware and unaware, the latter often being predominant.

We can describe two phases: an initial phase involving the critical collection of information, and a second phase of analysis and interpretation, which precedes and determines a targeted physical examination.

The first phase involves the collection of demographic data, reference data (such as the medical diagnosis), whether other disorders are present, which drugs are being taken, and the patient's expectations as regards our therapy. The patient's complaints are listed, classifying them according to the categories of impairment, disability and participation. These categories are situated

temporally and any changes in them over time are identified, the result of diagnostic tests or previous therapeutic measures are analysed, and coping strategies determined. An attempt is made to identify any links between individual impairments, between the impairments and the disability, and between the disability and participation.

Once the temporal dynamic picture of the disturbances and the patient's current state have been defined, we enter a second, more interpretational, phase in which we try to determine whether there is a balance between environmental requirements and the individual's ability to respond to them, evaluating patient capacity for both local and general adaptation, and the compensatory strategies implemented, whether positive or negative.

The link between load and carriability and coping strategies should be analysed not only in the present, but also historically, based on data obtained previously.

All the information gathered, analysed and interpreted is used to identify a procedure for evaluation, aimed at demonstrating the impairments, disabilities and participation problems exhibited by the patient as objectively as possible. To achieve this, the traditional tools of physical examination will be used to assess impairments and disabilities, along with questionnaires for the objective evaluation of disabilities and participation problems.

At the end of the evaluation, we shall have sufficient information to be able to establish a link between the patient's complaints and the corresponding impairments and disabilities, or to determine a lack of coherence typical of chronic conditions, in which there is often no longer a proportional link between nociception and pain behaviour. We shall also have identified the elements which will form the basis of our planned manual therapy and targeted therapeutic practice, and outlined opportunities for interdisciplinary cooperation. It will also be possible to agree the conditions of treatment with the patient to obtain not only informed consent, but also full cooperation in order to achieve the objectives set, if these were not made clear at the outset.

Choice of outcome

The choice of outcome is crucial to constructing the therapeutic plan. Since the result of the treatment must be measured, the choice of what to measure and how to measure it becomes critical to the validity of the measurement made. This choice will be determined by considering how well the measurement matches the patient's requirements and the therapist's objectives. For example, if the patient's expectations include reduction of pain and not an increase in the range of motion of the shoulder, it will be advisable to choose a VAS rather than a measurement of angle. If the objective is to recover a particular ability without pain, the use of compensatory strategies, if this does not constitute a risk factor for the subsequent progression of the disorder, is valid; consequently it is not the individual components of the movement which will be assessed, but the effectiveness of the movement itself.

If the patient's problems relate specifically to participation, a clinimetric scale such as SF-36 (McHorney, 1993; Ware, 1992) or the sickness impact profile (SIP) (Jensen, 1992) for quality of life, is preferable to a questionnaire for measuring disability or impairment, such as the shoulder pain and disability index (SPADI) (Bot, 2004; Heald, 1997; Roach, 1991) or the simple shoulder test (Roddey, 2000).

The structure of the ICF is again helpful for choosing the outcome measurement that will be used based on the health domain most affected by the disorder and by the individual patient's needs and expectations.

Clearly these are only the general motivations for the choice of outcome and the method of measuring it. The tool will also be chosen on the basis of its scientific validity.

The tests most commonly used for the shoulder are the SPADI, the SST and the shoulder severity index (SSI) (Beaton, 1998).

It may sometimes be useful to combine these specific tools for the shoulder with a VAS (Banos, 1989; Carlsson, 1983) and with the McGill pain questionnaire (MPQ) (Burckhardt, 1984) (translated into Italian and validated as the IPQ (De Benedittis, 1988)). The IPQ is used to identify and determine the emotional component of pain, distinguishing it from the physical component. It provides useful information on the patient, on his or her experience of the disorder, and on how the experience of pain changes according to the various treatment phases.

Physiotherapist's skills in the various areas of impairment, disability and problems of participation

The following is not intended as a detailed description of the operational limits of the physiotherapist, but to provide points for consideration regarding the opportunities for taking action in the various areas of health.

- As regards participation, the role of the therapist as we see it is limited to providing support via

counselling and the use, if necessary, of cognitive and behavioural strategies with the patient and his or her family and friends.

- If, however, the case treated falls within the skills of the physiotherapist, this area will be strongly influenced by the success of measures in the areas of disability and impairment. If this does not happen, it will be necessary to review the clinical rationale, to reconsider the links between the areas of impairment, disability and participation, and to reorganize the therapeutic approach, if necessary by including interdisciplinary cooperation in the rehabilitation plan.

- An approach aimed specifically at disability involves the use of targeted therapeutic exercises closely adapted to the movement in question. Ability can be regarded as the application of physiology to the situation and therapeutic exercise will be designed as 'situational', i.e. it will have as its principal objectives not the recovery of a range of motion or the expression of strength or speed, but the ability to use this capacity in a more effective and qualitatively better manner to achieve the objective of the movement itself.

- As we know, there are numerous clinical states in impingement syndromes which seem to recognize instability (Jobe, 1991) or impaired timing of muscle activation in movements by the upper limb (Toyoshima, 1974) as predisposing factors for shoulder impingement. These alterations concern the timing of scapular movement and the ability to stabilize the scapular segment and the shoulder girdle in preparation for movement. Upper arm movements cannot take place without the involvement of axial structures (spinal column) (Comerford, 2001), in which the muscle groups are inserted which are responsible for the stabilization and coordination of the movement of the shoulder girdle as a function of the movement of the upper limb. Similarly, the contribution of the lower limbs to the preparation and optimization of upper limb movements (think of throwing) cannot be disregarded (Young, 1996). When designing therapeutic exercises, the physiotherapist should give due consideration to such factors, and should abandon as soon as possible exercises focused on the glenohumeral joint alone which have fairly limited neuromotor and biomechanical significance. Occupational therapy or training is a borderline area. It is also an area that provides great opportunities for interdisciplinary cooperation between the various professionals concerned with movement as a means of recovering or promoting health; in the case of an athlete we can talk about therapeutic training.

- Impairment is tackled by the physiotherapist principally by manual therapy, i.e. by means of mobilization and manipulation of the joints and muscle structures involved or responsible for the patient's dysfunctional clinical state.

Impairment can be divided into anatomical and functional. These two categories are closely linked: anatomical damage can often alter a function which is, in turn, responsible for the patient's symptoms (for example, a capsuloligamentous lesion following glenohumeral dislocation with instability and pain). The anatomical impairment is important only if this link seems clear. In these cases, if compensation strategies are not an option (in the previous example, strengthening of shortened internal rotators, modifying movements used at work or in sports), surgery is required and rehabilitation will have a support function for optimal healing and functional recovery.

The functional impairments we encounter on a daily basis include pain, instability and hypomobility.

- Pain is a condition that is defined by the international association for the study of pain (IASP) (www.iasp-pain.org/defsopen.html) as an unpleasant sensory and emotional experience, associated with actual or potential tissue damage, or described as such.

This definition emphasizes not only that the experience of pain is not always the response to anatomical damage, but also that previous experiences significantly influence the personal experience of pain (Fig. 12.2). These psychosocial aspects must be taken into consideration when designing therapeutic strategies for rehabilitation, since they alone are capable of influencing the improvement perceived by the patient. The use of cognitive and behavioural techniques, or at least a careful meta-analysis of the relationship with the individual patient, is of particular relevance, so as to

Fig. 12.2

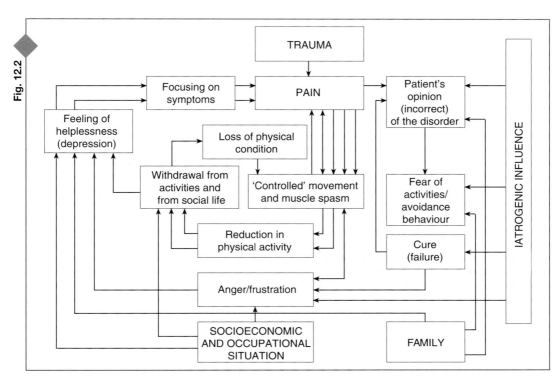

Influence of biomedical, physiological, psychological, socioeconomic and iatrogenic factors on the development of disability (modified from MAIN, 2000).

Rehabilitation: Cultural models, working models and scope

monitor relational conditions, avoiding generating false beliefs and expectations for the patient which can activate a nocebo response (Benedetti, 2003).

Apart from these aspects, our aim will be to reduce the pain, partly by therapeutic action with this objective, when pharmacological therapy is not possible or in cases of myofascial pain caused by trigger points (Testa, 2003), but largely as a result of improving the joint
and muscular dysfunction responsible for the clinical symptoms.

- The category of instability referred to above relates not to macroscopic instability phenomena which result in dislocation of the joint, but to microinstability, often caused by difficulty maintaining the humeral head in the angle of inclusion of the glenoid, rather than by anatomical lesions (Lazarus, 1996; Lippit, 1993), during movements of the upper limb. These forms of instability can be associated with either hypermobility or hypomobility of the joint, or with changes in muscle function, understood as incorrect timing of activation or insufficient ability to stabilize the components of the shoulder girdle.

Constitutional hypermobility is believed to be a predisposing factor to the development of instability (Hakim, 2003), whereas in the case of hypomobility, capsule 'tightness' may cause arthrokinematic changes, principally affecting the components of translation of joint head movement (Tyler, 2000).

As regards inadequate muscle activation, which is undoubtedly responsible for arthrokinematic changes, it is not yet clear whether it is a consequence of inhibition due to joint disorders (inflammation and pain) (D'Ambrosio 2003; Smiderle, 2003; Young, 1987, 1993), or is due to the development and use by the patient of incorrect motor strategies.

There are few studies in this area concerning the shoulder, however there are some relating to the lumbar spine (Hodges, 2000) and cervical spine (Falla, 2004). In any case, the principles on which the working hypotheses for the lumbar and cervical spine are based are applicable to all the joints.

The therapeutic measures recommended by the physiotherapist in this case will be based largely on therapeutic exercise, aiming to progress from recovery of recruitment capacity and control of muscles with the primary function of stabilization, to the incorporation of this recovered ability into the usual work- and sport-related movements.

Table 12.2

Effects of immobilization on joint structures

- Proliferation of fibroadipose tissue in the synovial space
- Proliferation of fibroadipose tissue on the cartilage surface
- Proliferation of synovial cells with resulting hypertrophy of the synovial membrane
- Whole-thickness ulceration of the cartilage at pressure points
- Synovial, capsule and cartilage adhesions with fissuring at the insertion sites
- Changes in the rotation centres of the joint with a resulting change in joint kinematics
- Increase in joint temperature (usually lower than body temperature) and activation of collagenase with enzymatic degradation of collagen and proteoglycans
- Increased synthesis of collagen in ligaments
- Loss of parallel arrangement of collagen fibres
- Random arrangement of collagen fibres
- Defects of continuity in collagen fibres
- Osteoclastic reabsorption at the muscle-tendon insertion sites
- After eight weeks of immobilization, the muscle-tendon insertions reach only the periosteal level

- Hypomobility is a problem that confronts the physiotherapist on a daily basis, both when it causes pain and resulting disability in relation to the development of a form of joint instability, and when it is the single cause of disability as in frozen shoulder.

We shall not look in detail at the possible causes of joint hypomobility due to a capsuloligamentous disorder, which forms part of the pathophysiology of individual pathological events; we do, however, consider it important to note the consequences of immobilization for the physiology of the joint and the connective tissues of which it is composed (van Wingerden, 1995), in order to provide useful references for determining the dosage of any therapeutic measure (Table 12.2).

The clinical result of immobilization and, by analogy, of acquired hypomobility (although of different severity) is that lesions appear very rapidly, but resolve fairly slowly: it takes a year for hypertrophy of a tendon to resolve and for ligaments the time is even longer. Furthermore, joint immobilization maintained for more than four weeks is believed to cause irreversible loss of elasticity of the capsuloligamentous tissues.

A synovial joint is an anatomical structure whose function is manifested in particular through movement, and even the partial restriction of this has fairly important functional consequences and clinical repercussions.

When immobilized, the shoulder tends to lose its full range of motion rapidly and the intra-particular temperature tends to rise to 37°, at which temperature the collagenase produced by the synovial cells attacks the joint tissues, as occurs in rheumatoid arthritis and osteoarthritis (Bland, 1994).

Besides affecting connective tissues, immobilization alters the physiology of the joint receptors, and this has consequences for tone and the recruitability of muscle structures functionally connected to the joint and the consequent development of clinical conditions similar to the instability described above (Schaible, 1991).

Furthermore, the development of an altered articular environment, associated with a reduction in inhibitory modulation of the primary afferent fibres, encourages the sensitization of type IV receptors which have a typically nociceptive function (Heppelmann, 1997; Schaible, 2002).

Physical exercise and manual therapy can help repair the damage caused by immobilization to connective tissue, allowing reintegration of proprioceptive afferences with the modulation activity of nociceptive afference and the development of correct patterns of muscle activation.

Case report

The aim of this section is to demonstrate the concepts described above, implemented in daily practice. In the case described, the biopsychosocial model and the multidimensional load/carriability model form the background to the clinical rationale. These constitute the PHP through which the patient's clinical picture will be described and the building blocks positioned for constructing the therapy, and for choosing the outcome and the method of measuring it.

We do not intend to propose particularly innovative rehabilitation techniques here, but we do aim to emphasize, using a practical example, the value of incorporating a biopsychosocial view in the evaluation and to show to what extent this view influences the technical

aspects and the way they are proposed and included in a recovery process.

This process focuses on the health of the individual rather than solely on the dysfunctional regions. It will also become apparent how it provides added value in rehabilitation practice and determines the choice of appropriate therapeutic techniques and dosages, which can only benefit the quality of interaction with the patient.

Prognostic health profile

T.G., a 50-year-old man, married with children, who is left-handed, takes part in sport and gardening, and works as a businessman, carrying out administrative tasks for the company which he owns.

He has had insulin-dependent diabetes since the age of 30. He has had three back operations for recurrent slipped disc.

In January 2001 he began to experience persistent pain in his left shoulder which was diagnosed as tendinopathy of the supraspinatus with primary acromiohumeral impingement, treated arthroscopically (three months later) by bursectomy and acromioplasty, and finding substantial degeneration of the insertion point of the supraspinatus. The postoperative course was abnormal with very intense pain, and rehabilitation was impossible. Despite the pharmacological therapy managed by the internal specialist and a cautious approach to rehabilitation, the patient had a further capsulotomy procedure through 360° and debridement of the acromioplasty following a diagnosis of frozen shoulder (10 months later).

On admission he presented with elevation of 100°, abduction of 80°, external rotation of 10°, internal rotation to the homolateral side, a Jobe test positive for pain, and a negative palm up test. Arthroscopy showed the following: the long head of the biceps in position, a reduced joint space, a closed rotator cuff interval and a subacromial space with significant tissue adhesion. The patient was discharged with instructions to keep a brace on for 10 days to relieve pain, to take analgesics as required and to carry out passive mobilization exercises for the first few days.

The patient's current postoperative state shows virtually complete inability as regards the shoulder joint and a very high level of joint pain and reactivity; the preoperative functional values are therefore regarded as reference and baseline values. The shoulder surgery perception (SSP) scale which measures pain and disability, the patient's principal problem, was adopted as a measure of outcome (baseline SSP 51/60).

Carriability was greatly reduced on both a general physical level and locally in the shoulder region. A reduction in psychological carriability was also observed.

The patient was particularly worried and tired. He was discouraged and did not believe that his problem could be solved. He wanted to recover his lost abilities and to improve his level of participation in sport and work which, already substantially reduced after his back operations, were further reduced after the first shoulder operation. Nevertheless, his call for help 'to get rid of the pain, to recover at least some joint function ... the minimum for good quality of life' contained elements that suggested the activation of positive coping mechanisms in response to the disorder and the correct rationalization of his current state of health; this was confirmed by a VAS score of 5, consistent with the musculoskeletal type of the disorder, while the VAS score was 9 following the first operation.

Therapy

Therapy of the impairment will be aimed at reducing pain and joint reactivity, increasing joint amplitude, improving joint stability and reinforcing coping strategies and rationalization of the situation (objectives).

This will be done by using joint mobilization manoeuvres which preserve the arthrokinematics, combined with analgesic techniques and informing the patient about his general health, and the need for and type of rehabilitation; the rehabilitation specialist will seek to control verbal and non-verbal anxiogenic messages so as not to disturb the rationalization and coping process which is activated independently by the patient (strategies).

The specialist will use his or her skill and participation to develop movement strategies with the patient to allow him to resume daily activities and work as soon as possible, strengthening his active coping ability, and preference will be given in parallel to therapeutic exercises aimed at recovering the ability to perform the movements involved in both daily and work activities and, where possible, leisure activities or sports. Reduced loads will be used to stimulate positive reinforcement mechanisms and to avoid the patient becoming frustrated.

The patient will initially have five sessions a week for four weeks, then three sessions a week for two weeks, and then two sessions a week as necessary.

Bibliography

Banos J.E., Bosch F., Canellas M., Bassols A., Ortega F., Bigorra J., 'Acceptability of visual analogue scales in the clinical setting: a comparison with verbal rating scales in postoperative pain', *Methods Find Exp. Clin. Pharmacol.* 11(2): 123–127, (1989)

Beaton D., Richards R.R., 'Assessing the reliability and responsiveness of five shoulder questionnaires', *J. Shoulder Elbow Surg.* 7(6): 565–572, (1998)

Benedetti F., Pollo A., Lopiano L., Lanotte M., Vighetti S., Rainero I., 'Conscious expectation and unconscious conditioning in analgesic, motor, and hormonal placebo/nocebo responses', *J. Neurosci.* 23(10): 4315–4323, (2003)

Bland J.H. (ed.)., Disorders of the cervical spine. Diagnosis and medical management. WB Saunders, Philadelphia (1994)

Bot S.D., Terwee C.B., Van Der Windt D.A., Bouter L.M., Dekker J., De Vet H.C., 'Clinimetric evaluation of shoulder disability questionnaires: a systematic review of the literature', *Ann. Rheum. Dis.* 63(4): 335–341, (2004)

Burckhardt C.S., 'The use of the McGill Pain Questionnaire in assessing arthritis pain', *Pain* 19(3): 305–314, (1984)

Carlsson A.M., 'Assessment of chronic pain. I. Aspects of the reliability and validity of the visual analogue scale', *Pain* 16(1): 87–101, (1983)

Comerford M.J., Mottram S.L., 'Functional stability retraining: principles and strategies for managing mechanical dysfunction', *Manual Ther* 6: 3–14, (2001)

D'Ambrosio C., Smiderle M., Testa M., 'Alterazioni del reclutamento muscolare all'arto inferiore dopo distorsione di caviglia: ruolo della propriocezione. Scienza della riabilitazione', vol. 4, no. 2, April–June (2003)

De Benedittis G., Massei R., Nobili R., Pieri A., 'The Italian Pain Questionnaire', *Pain* 33(1): 53–62, (1988)

Falla D., Jull G., Hodges P.W., 'Feedforward activity of the cervical flexor muscles during voluntary arm movements is delayed in chronic neck pain', *Exp. Brain Res.* 5, (2004)

Hagenaars L.H.A., Bernards A.T.M., Ostendoorp R., *The Multidimensional Load/Carriability model*, Nederlands Paramedisch Instituut, Amersfoort 2002, 1st English ed.

Hakim A., Grahame R., 'Joint hypermobility. Best Pract. Res.', *Clin. Rheumatol.* 17(6): 989–1004, (2003)

Heald S.L., Riddle D.L., Lamb R.L., 'The shoulder pain and disability index: the construct validity and responsiveness of a region-specific disability measure', *Phys. Ther.* 77(10): 1079–1089, (1997)

Heppelmann B., 'Anatomy and histology of joint innervation', *J. Peripher. Nerv. Syst.* 2(1): 5–16, (1997)

Hodges P.W., 'The role of the motor system in spinal pain: implications for rehabilitation of the athlete following lower back pain', *J. Sci. Med. Sport* 3(3): 243–253, (2000)

Jensen M.P., Strom S.E., Turner J.A., Romano J.M., 'Validity of the Sickness Impact Profile Roland scale as a measure of dysfunction in chronic pain patients', *Pain* 50(2): 157–162, (1992)

Jobe F.W., Pink M., 'Shoulder injuries in the athlete: the instability continuum and treatment', *J. Hand Ther.* 4: 69–73, (1991)

Lazarus M.D., Sidles J.A., Harryman D.T. II, Matsen F.A. III., 'Effect of a chondral-labral defect on glenoid concavity and glenohumeral stability. A cadaveric model', *J. Bone Joint Surg. Am.* 78(1): 94–102, (1996)

Lippit S., Matsen F., 'Mechanisms of glenohumeral joint stability', *Clin. Orth. Rel. Res.* 291: 20–28, (1993)

Main C.J. et al., *Pain management: an interdisciplinary approach*, Churchill Livingstone, Edinburgh (2000)

McHorney C.A., Ware J.E. JR, Raczek A.E., 'The MOS 36-Item Short-Form Health Survey (SF-36): II. Psychometric and clinical tests of validity in measuring physical and mental health constructs', *Med. Care.* 31(3): 247–263, (1993)

Roach K.E., Budiman-Mak E., Songsiridej N., Lertratanakul Y., 'Development of a shoulder pain and disability index', *Arthritis Care Res.* 4(4): 143–149, (1991)

Roddey T.S., Olson S.L., Cook K.F., Gartsman G.M., Hanten W., 'Comparison of the University of California-Los Angeles Shoulder Scale and the Simple Shoulder Test with the shoulder pain and disability index: single-administration reliability and validity', *Phys. Ther.* 80(8): 759–768, (2000)

Schaible H.G., Neugebauer V., Cervero F., Schmidt R.F., 'Changes in tonic descending inhibition of spinal neurons with articular input during the development of acute arthritis in the cat', *J. Neurophysiol.* 66(3): 1021–1032, (1991)

Schaible H.G., Ebersberge A., Von Banchet G.S., 'Mechanism of pain in arthritis', *Ann. N.Y. Acad. Sci.* 966: 343–354, (2002)

Smiderle M., Spairani L., Testa M., 'L'inibizione riflessa del quadricipite dopo trauma al ginocchio: aspetti fisiopatologici e indicazioni terapeutiche. Scienza della Riabilitazione', vol. 4, no. 2 Apr–Jun (2003)

Sulli., *Fisiopatologia dell'artrosi*

Sulli., *Variazione milieu articolare con sensibilizzazione dei recettori*

Testa M., 'Lezioni di teoria, metodologia e pratica clinica della terapia manuale. Master in Riabilitazione dei disordini muscolo-scheletrici', University of Genoa, School of Medicine and Surgery, Academic year 2003/4

Testa M., Barbero M., Gherlone E., 'Trigger Point: Update for the Clinical Aspects', *Europa Medico Physica* 39: 20–27, (2003)

Toyoshima S., Hosikikawa T., Miyashita M. et al., 'Contribution of the body parts to throwing performance', In: Nelson R.C., Morehouse C.A. (eds.) *Biomechanics* IV, University Park Press, Baltimore, p. 169, (1974)

Tyler T.F., Roy T., Nicholas S.J., Gleim G.W., 'Quantification of posterior capsule tightness and motion loss in patients with shoulder impingement', *Am. J. Sport. Med.* 28: 668–673, (2000)

Van Wingerden B.A.M. (eds), 'Ligaments and capsule', In: *Connective Tissue in Rehabilitation*, Scipro Verlag, Valduz (Liechtenstein) (1995)

Ware J.E. JR, Sherbourne C.D., 'The MOS 36-item short-form health survey (SF-36). I. Conceptual framework and item selection', *Med. Care.* 30(6): 473–483, (1992)

Young A., 'Current issues in arthrogenous inhibition', *Ann. Rheum. Dis.* 52(11): 829–834, (1993)

Young A., Stokes M., Iles J.F., 'Effects of joint pathology on muscle', *Clin. Orthop.* 219: 21–27, (1987)

Young J.L., Herring S.A., Press J.M., Casazza B.A., 'The Influence of the Spine on the Shoulder in the Throwing Athlete', *AJST* 7(1): 5–17, (1996)

www.iasp-pain.org/defsopen.html

www.who.int/classifications/icf/en/

www.who.int/classifications/icd/en

CHAPTER 13

POSTOPERATIVE REHABILITATION

M.L. VOIGHT
T.A. BLACKBURN JR.
B.J. HOOGENBOOM

A substantial amount of information on the diagnosis and treatment of shoulder girdle lesions has appeared in recent years. The frequency of shoulder injuries has increased since the population has generally become more active. The shoulder is particularly prone to injury, since it involves a delicate balance between mobility and stability (Kibler, 1998; Paine, 1993; Peat, 1986).

The safe and effective rehabilitation of the shoulder requires a knowledge of the anatomical and biomechanical characteristics of the shoulder complex. When working on a patient who has recently undergone surgery, the therapist must be familiar with the surgical technique, the potential and associated complications of the surgery and the tissue healing times. As with all therapeutic protocols, it is essential to perform a full examination comprising static, dynamic and functional tests to determine the level of involvement/healing of tissues throughout the postoperative recovery period. Based on the result of the tests, a rehabilitation programme can be designed which will preserve the degree of healing of the tissues and the patient's response to surgery.

The principal objective of any rehabilitation programme is to return the athlete to a pain-free condition with a high level of functionality as quickly and as safely as possible. Patients in whom conservative treatment has been unsuccessful often need to undergo surgery. These patients need a cautious, reasonable postoperative approach to rehabilitation, based on state of the art knowledge. Whether the patient is in the post-traumatic or postoperative phase, there are basic principles that will determine the choice of strategy and clinical approach to the rehabilitation of the shoulder (Table 13.1).

Principles of rehabilitation

There are many other specific principles in addition to the six basic guidelines for rehabilitation which must be taken into account before undertaking a rehabilitation programme for a shoulder injury or surgical procedure.

— The first principle of rehabilitation of the shoulder is to emphasize the treatment of the shoulder girdle as a whole, rather than the

Table 13.1

The six basic guidelines for rehabilitation

Rehabilitation standards

1   The effects of immobilization must be minimized as far as possible, by following guidelines for the surgical repair of tissues

2   A surgical stabilization or tissue scar should never be placed under excessive strain

3   The patient should meet specific criteria before going on to the next stage in the rehabilitation protocol

4   The rehabilitation protocol should be based on the latest clinical and functional studies

5   The rehabilitation protocol should be personalized and adapted to each patient, based on his or her expectations

6   Rehabilitation should be a process in which the doctor, physiotherapist, trainer, patient and his or her family work together to achieve common goals

Postoperative rehabilitation

glenohumeral joint alone. The shoulder girdle is a complicated system formed by the glenohumeral, acromioclavicular, sternoclavicular and scapulothoracic joints, and an intricate network of muscles, tendons, ligaments and other connective tissue structures (Peat, 1986). An optimally functioning shoulder girdle needs normal arthrokinematics of all the joints involved, adequate muscle resistance and strength and correct neuromuscular and proprioceptive control. A therapist who tries to treat 'the shoulder' by considering the glenohumeral joint in isolation rather than the shoulder girdle, may create problems for the patient. This is particularly true in postoperative rehabilitation, even if the surgical technique used involved only a single joint (e.g. treatment of a Bankart lesion) or structure (e.g. treatment of a SLAP lesion) of the shoulder girdle. To obtain complete functional recovery, attention must be paid to all aspects of the shoulder girdle during rehabilitation.

— The second principle of shoulder rehabilitation involves obtaining a stable scapular base on which the humerus can act. This is the concept of proximal stability for distal mobility (Kibler, 1998; Paine, 1993). The scapula acts as a stable support base for anchoring the 17 muscles that take origin from or are inserted in it (Peat, 1986). The scapula is closely associated with the position of the humeral head during movement and helps to maintain a complicated balance between the glenohumeral joint and the scapulothoracic joint. This association enables the precise movement of the humeral head and maintains the correct recruitment of the muscles of the glenohumeral joint (Kibler, 1998). The scapula also has the ability to stabilize itself at any point in the movement arc of the upper limb during a large range of functional activities. Exercises that focus on scapular control can be started early in postoperative rehabilitation following surgery on the glenohumeral joint.

— The third principle of rehabilitation is a therapeutic approach which acknowledges the shoulder girdle as an integral part of the upper limb and kinetic chain of the trunk. This principle derives from the first two. The voluntary movement schemes used in daily life and in sport are exceedingly complex. Both involve the action of the muscles of the joints of the upper limb, the trunk and the lower limbs, to perform movements synergically. The optimal

treatment should, therefore, emphasize the upper limbs, but should also concern the trunk and lower limbs (Kibler, 1995a, 1995b; Kibler, 1993). It is, therefore, possible, by treating the shoulder girdle, to rehabilitate other areas of the kinetic chain or to prevent their functional decay.

— The fourth principle of rehabilitation of the shoulder girdle involves determining the functional planes of movement. Most of the exercises are performed in the scapular plane (Fig. 13.1) or anterior to the scapular plane, which is generally the safest and most convenient.

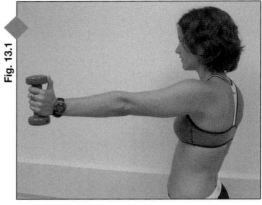

Fig. 13.1

Abduction in the scapular plane.

Exercises performed in this plane ensure correct biomechanical alignment for the function of the rotator cuff muscles and avoid straining the soft tissues in the perioperative period (Moseley, 1992; Townsend, 1991). Exercises performed in the coronal plane may, on the other hand, cause impingement and strain of the rotator cuff tendons, while exercises performed in the frontal plane may strain anterior structures repaired surgically, such as the capsule, the glenohumeral ligaments and the labrum.

— The fifth principle involves using short levers to strengthen the shoulder muscles, particularly at the start of the rehabilitation programme. During the 'protected' phase of rehabilitation, the loads should be applied with the arms close to the body and the elbows flexed, increasing the levers as the rehabilitation progresses.

— The sixth principle of rehabilitation concerns the adoption of postures in which the neuromuscular recruitment is most likely to strengthen the muscles of the shoulder girdle. Recent EMG studies have identified specific positions and optimal activities to achieve this (Blackburn, 1990; Moseley, 1992; Townsend, 1991). This principle arises from the following concept: isolated movement schemes strengthen weak muscles, while combined movement schemes restore functional activity. The specific exercises and positions which demonstrate this principle will be discussed below.

— The seventh principle involves designing an exercise programme ranging from the simplest to the most complex, gradually reproducing the forces and loads to which the athlete will be subjected on returning to the sport. In accordance with the concept of always respecting pain, this principle also involves a progression from non-stressful (non-painful) positions to positions which may potentially cause pain, but which are necessary for a complete functional recovery. This rehabilitation principle helps the athlete to restore correct kinaesthetic sensitivity and proprioception of the upper limb in relation to functional performance. The muscle and the joint need to be re-educated to allow the athlete to discriminate between joint movement and position, and direction, amplitude and speed of movement (Kibler, 1995a, 1995b; Voight, 1996). In order that the muscles and soft tissues (both normal and after surgery) can adapt and respond appropriately to increasing loads, they must be subjected to a progressive, controlled load, in increasingly demanding positions and manoeuvres.

— The eighth and final principle postulates that functional stability will ensure a good functional outcome. A shoulder is functionally stable when there is a normal arc of movement, adequate strength and proprioception and normal neuromuscular control. Achieving functional stability through surgery and the correct rehabilitation of the shoulder girdle will ensure a return to the desired level of functionality or that preceding the injury.

The rehabilitation protocol

There are detailed rehabilitation protocols in the literature for the various types of surgical reconstruction, but they are often based on clinical observation and personal experience. No randomized prospective studies have ever been conducted into the results of these protocols. There are many reasons why in vivo studies

on this subject are limited. It is extremely difficult to plan studies which include a multitude of variables, such as the techniques adopted by various surgeons, types of patients, individual variability in the elasticity of connective tissue and the patient's return to work or sport. It is also difficult to extrapolate the functional result of one surgeon and one rehabilitation group to those of others. It is consequently essential to base any guideline for the treatment of the shoulder on the healing times required by the surgical technique and on the biomechanics of the movement which may strain and damage the suture. The suture, in this case, refers to the point of insertion of tissues manipulated to allow a reduction in the translation of the glenohumeral joint. A knowledge of the resistance of scar tissue at various times will make it possible to design progressive exercises for a complete and safe return to work or sport.

It is difficult, bearing these concepts in mind, to design a rehabilitation protocol which incorporates all the variables mentioned. Numerous demands must be met before therapists can plan complete rehabilitation protocols which will meet the needs of the majority of patients undergoing surgery for anterior shoulder instability. Which movement may strain the suture line? When will the suture bear more intense exercises? Finally, when will the suture be able to bear the workload of a return to work or sport?

Limits of healing

The rate of healing of collagen tissue must be studied and understood in order to answer these questions and to provide adequate guidelines for rehabilitation. The injury, or in this case the surgery, of a vascularized tissue starts with a series of events, known overall as inflammation and healing (Reed, 1996). The inflammation and healing processes of tissues have been extensively studied. These processes generally last for 60 days and lead to the final maturation of collagen tissue, which may last for up to 360 days. The rehabilitation specialist must be capable of gaining the maximum benefit from the body's natural capacity for repair, to be sure that the capsule of the glenohumeral joint is completely healed in the direction of application of the loads.

The tissue healing or proliferative phase (3rd–20th day) begins after the initial inflammatory phase immediately following surgery (1st–3rd day). Fibroblasts start to synthesize collagen scar tissue around the suture (Reed, 1996). This scar tissue strengthens the fold in the capsule, made by the surgeon to reduce the inadequacy of the tissue. Intramolecular and intermolecular bonds develop between the new collagen filaments, and these bonds may be damaged by excessive strain on the suture. The scar tissue matures and is remodelled by subtle strains which allow the shoulder to recover its complete function gradually. For three weeks following surgery, the suture can bear only minimal strain owing to the weakness of these bonds. The rehabilitation programme in this early phase of healing must be designed to reduce pain and to minimize inflammation, to support the other parts of the kinetic chain, to increase muscle resistance and strength, and to prevent postoperative complications.

From the 21st to the 60th day, the scar tissue becomes progressively stronger and susceptible to remodelling. The load on the suture in the late phase of healing should, therefore, be increased moderately, in order to have better control over the outcome of tissue healing. Remodelling reaches its culmination between the first and the eighth week (Reed, 1996).

A knowledge of the surgical procedures for anterior shoulder instability will also help the rehabilitation specialist understand the healing process. The majority of the many surgical techniques for restoring anterior shoulder stability fall into five categories. These are: open capsulorrhaphy, arthroscopic capsulorrhaphy and thermal capsulorrhaphy (thickening of the capsule), the Bristow procedure and subscapular techniques (e.g. Magnuson-Stack and Putti-Platt). The Bankart procedure involves repairing the capsulolabral complex; it is rarely used alone but is combined with one of the other capsulorrhaphy techniques.

Before the surgical and rehabilitation guidelines were reviewed, there were few points to be noted. There were no scientific data which confirmed that a capsulorrhaphy performed according to a given technique would heal in a given time in patients of a certain type. The theories about collagen healing were based on a generic knowledge of inflammation and the processes of repair. These theories can be associated with various protocols suggested by and based on the experience of various surgeons and physiotherapists. Unfortunately, these guidelines were not supported by any type of clinical study.

The progressive nature of the rehabilitation protocol is the art concealed by the science of rehabilitation. There are many reasons for increasing the workload on the suture line gradually. The aspects which deserve most attention are the patient's possible generalized ligament laxity, the type of stabilizing method adopted and the possibility that the procedure will involve re-doing a previous repair. Repeated traumas or a lesion which occurred a long time ago may adversely affect tissue quality. The surgeon must

be consulted frequently in the initial phases of rehabilitation, to adapt the rehabilitation programme and assess the results. This interaction will provide much information which will help to maintain the movement arc within a safe range. For example, an anterior capsulorrhaphy procedure on the shoulder of a throwing athlete is usually performed using a surgical technique which requires the positioning of the arm during the postoperative period in the plane of the body with a few degrees of external rotation and abduction. This ensures that the athlete will have an adequate range of motion for throwing correctly, if the shoulder recovers adequately. By contrast, the stabilization of the shoulder of an American football player requires postoperative positioning in the scapular plane with 45° external rotation. A good result in this type of patient does not depend on the maximum degree of joint function. There must be an exchange of information between the surgeon and the physiotherapist to clarify which type of movement and which range is being permitted postoperatively, so that early progressive mobilization does not adversely affect the outcome of the surgical repair.

Surgical techniques and rehabilitation

Open capsulorrhaphy

Open capsulorrhaphy is considered the gold standard for anterior shoulder stabilization, owing to a success rate of 91–96% and the assurance of no subsequent episodes of subluxation or dislocation (Satterwhite, 1997). Generally, a patient without hyperlaxity who undergoes capsulorrhaphy, with or without a Bankart procedure, will achieve 45° of external rotation and 90° of elevation in the scapular plane in the immediate postoperative period (Jobe, 1991). These movements do not stress the suture and allow rehabilitation to begin in this range. After three weeks, the soft tissues will be sufficiently healed to be able to resume gentle active or passive work at the suture. At this point in the rehabilitation programme, a small amount of strain must be applied to allow the tissues to heal with adequate length and strength. At six weeks, passive stretching of the suture may begin in order to obtain the joint function required for the type of activity performed. At 12–16 weeks, the scar should be sufficiently mature to allow most movements to be performed and at 24 weeks, the patient may return to sport-related activities.

Patients with hyperelastic connective tissue must wait until the 8th–10th week following surgery, depending on the joint function achieved, before starting stretching. It is essential in this type of patient to obtain most of the joint function without onerous stretching exercises, giving preference to active mobilization exercises. Nevertheless, some patients fail to achieve sufficient joint function and need to start stretching early. The progress in both active and passive joint function needs to be monitored closely in all patients. The rehabilitation approach to a capsulorrhaphy with or without a Bankart procedure is similar. A Bankart lesion is rarely present in the absence of capsule laxity.

Bristow procedure

The Bristow procedure involves the transposition of the apex of the coracoid process to the glenoid labrum, fixing it on the anterior glenoid. Consolidation will be complete within six weeks (Phillips, 1998). Care must be taken to rotate the elbow, since the short head of the biceps and the coracobrachial are moved together with the bone section. Since the soft tissues are unaffected, active or assisted active mobilization can be started within a week of surgery. Stretching may be started as soon as it is tolerated. At six weeks, once the bone has consolidated, these patients may begin a more aggressive programme of stretching and muscle strengthening (in other words, at this point the patient may perform stretching as permitted by pain and inflammation). A return to sport-related activities may be expected as early as the 12th week, but in general it is better to wait until the 16th–24th week.

Transposition of the subscapularis

In the technique introduced by Magnuson and Stack, the anterior capsulomuscular wall is strengthened by transposing the capsule and the tendon of the subscapularis muscle lateral to the humerus (Phillips, 1998). The Putti-Platt procedure is a variant of the subscapularis transposition; the rehabilitation guidelines are similar to those for capsulorrhaphy, but with the additional drawback that it does not correct any capsular or labral defect that may be present (Phillips, 1998). The recovery of joint function necessary for sport-related activities may be limited by this surgical technique, depending on the tension of the subscapularis.

Arthroscopic capsulorrhaphy

Arthroscopic capsulorrhaphy has been used by surgeons because it results in the formation of less reactive fibrous tissue than open capsulorrhaphy (Christensen, 1993). The open technique involves arthrotomy which requires operation on most of the tissues to reach the capsule. It is, however, possible with arthroscopy to subject the suture to strain too quickly during early mobilization of the shoulder. Patients should be able to elevate the arm actively in the scapular plane to 90° in the early postoperative period, but should avoid increasing the joint range before six weeks. Active mobilization is possible in the first six weeks within the safe range (which is pointed out by the surgeon with the aim of not straining the suture). In our experience, these limitations are similar to those applying to the open technique, but we stress once again that the shoulder should not be mobilized beyond its limit before the tissues have healed sufficiently. If the patient needs to return to very heavy work, the soft tissues should be given time to heal adequately, and this generally occurs within six months of the surgical procedure.

Guanche (1996) conducted a comparative study of open and arthroscopic reconstructions performed on the shoulders of patients with isolated Bankart lesions. Only pendulum exercises and those using an elastic band were prescribed in the first four weeks after surgery. This period was then followed by progressive rehabilitation with work or sport being resumed at four months. Despite this conservative attitude, 5 of the 15 patients in the arthroscopy group reported a subluxation or dislocation on follow-up at 17 to 42 months, whereas only a single patient out of 12 in the open group reported a similar event (Guanche, 1996). The authors concluded that the impossibility of arthroscopically mobilizing the glenohumeral ligaments may cause recurrent instability (Peat, 1986). The arthroscopic procedure is operator-dependent and the absence of a large incision conceals the fact that extensive work has been performed within the shoulder. This may be a further reason for proceeding with slightly more conservative rehabilitation in these patients, compared to those who have undergone open surgery.

Thermal capsulorrhaphy

Thermal capsulorrhaphy is a relatively new technique, with few studies to support rehabilitation guidelines. It involves heating the capsule by laser or with a radiofrequency generator (RF). As a result of the temperature to which the tissue is exposed, the collagen is denatured and shortens accordingly. The resistance of the denatured tissue and its healing capacity are still under investigation. Hayashi noted that the collagen and cell morphology in vivo returns to normal histologically 7 to 38 months after surgery (laser) (Hayashi, 1999). There are no studies in humans evaluating capsule resistance after thermal treatment, or the fate of the shoulder capsule during the remodelling process (Naseef, 1997). Selecky (1999) has performed studies on cadavers, comparing resistance in capsules subjected to laser treatment and untreated capsules, and found that tissue which has undergone thermal treatment is less prone to laceration in the treated area. Schaefer (1997) has however suggested, on the basis of animal models, that the biological response of connective tissue to laser causes further impairment of tissue integrity, besides that attributable to the immediate effect of the laser. Even when sufficient capsule shrinkage is obtained, this tissue may lengthen over time, becoming longer than before surgery (Imhoff, 1995; Schaefer, 1997).

The authors recommend waiting six weeks before forcing mobilization, since only a few patients seem to have a reduction in joint function. The glenohumeral joint should be evaluated frequently, to prevent the development of contractures. Strengthening exercises can be started early, provided they are performed within a safe range. Suture lines can never be overstrained, but denatured collagen must also be protected for a period.

Ellenbecker and Mattalino recently published the short-term follow-up of a group of 20 patients who underwent thermal capsulorrhaphy (Ellenbecker, 1999). At 12 weeks, 4 of the 20 patients regained complete external rotation (mean 86.6°) and 12 patients completely regained external rotation strength. A review of the surgical technique showed that these patients had all undergone Bankart arthroscopic repair and capsule retensioning using the Suretac system (Ellenbecker, 1999). The thermal component had been used to strengthen the fixing. It is, however, difficult to evaluate the result of this technique without a comparable control group in which thermal capsulorrhaphy was performed without the Suretac system. These results appear to be promising and it will be interesting to see whether these patients recover complete external rotation, maintain stability and can resume participation in overhead sports.

Surgery of the glenoid labrum

Lesions of the glenoid labrum have been associated with shoulder instability. Bankart lesion is a disorder that affects the inferior anterior labrum. It must be treated to ensure the stability of the capsulolabral complex and to restabilize the glenohumeral joint.

Lesions of the superior labrum (SLAP lesions) have been described by Snyder as a wide variety of lesions of the labrum and the insertion point of the long head of the biceps in the supraglenoid tubercle (Snyder, 1990), ranging from degeneration of the superior labrum to bucket handle ruptures and avulsion of the long head of the biceps (Snyder, 1990).

SLAP lesions characterized by degeneration or minor lacerations can be treated arthroscopically and simply need time for the symptoms to resolve. Patients can start mobilization, strengthening and proprioceptive exercises as soon as they feel ready.

Lesions that require the fixing of the labrum and biceps tendon generally need three weeks of protected mobilization, generally consisting of 90° of maximum elevation in the scapular plane and 45° of external rotation. Between the 3rd and 6th week, mobilization may be increased cautiously, and after the 6th week, the workload may be increased. These patients should, in fact, be treated as if they had shoulder instability, concentrating on strengthening the biceps in patients who also have tendinitis of the long head of the biceps. Care should be taken not to overstrain the long head of the biceps, as after a Bristow procedure, since it is inserted in the superior labrum.

Biomechanical limits

When the shoulder is in a neutral position, the capsule is not particularly stressed. The principal limits on anterior translation, when the arm is by the side, are the superior and middle GHLs (Bowen, 1991). At 45° of abduction, the middle GHL acts by limiting anterior translation (Bowen, 1991). When the upper limb is elevated to 90° with the humerus in the scapular plane, the capsule is placed under slight tension. It is when the arm increases the elevation to more than 90°, as far as complete elevation, that the tension on the anterior bundle of the inferior capsule or the glenohumeral ligament complex gradually increases (O'Brien, 1988).

When the arm is held in a posterior direction in the scapular plane, the tension on the anterior capsule increases in accordance with the degree of horizontal abduction of the arm. If external rotation is added to this movement, the tension on the anterior capsule is increased further (O'Brien, 1990; Turkel, 1981).

Following surgery to prevent anterior translation, exercises in the scapular plane cause only slight tension on the suture line, unless they are performed overhead.

When the tissue has healed, the work can be increased with exercises in internal rotation and posterior to the scapular plane. The exercises should be performed in the scapular plane, until adequate tissue repair has occurred (generally around the 6th week following surgery).

Exercises

Rehabilitation is necessary, after static stability has been restored surgically, to recover the complete joint function and dynamic stability of the glenohumeral joint. The example of a patient with a loose shoulder caused by a cerebrovascular accident is sufficient to illustrate how much of a fundamental role the muscles have not only in movement, but also in glenohumeral joint stability. The position and stabilization of the scapula provide a solid base for humeral movements (Kibler, 1998; Paine, 1993). This base also allows the rotator cuff muscles (supraspinatus, infraspinatus, teres minor and subscapularis), the deltoid and the long head of the biceps brachii to maintain the dynamic stability of the glenohumeral joint (Wilk, 1993).

An exercise programme can be started immediately after surgery within a movement arc which does not place the suture under severe tension. Passive or active anterior elevation can be achieved early between 90° and 135°. External rotation and horizontal abduction movements stress the suture greatly and should be regulated according to the progress of healing, and the surgical technique used. The risk of adhesions or shoulder stiffness can be kept to a minimum by early mobilization. Grade III and IV joint mobilization exercises should be started no earlier than after six weeks and only if it is essential to increase joint mobility. Mobilization exercises should be performed in series of 5–10 repetitions, 3–5 times daily and maintained for 30 seconds.

Exercises to strengthen the shoulder muscles can already be planned during the protected rehabilitation period, with emphasis on exercises for the muscles of the scapula.

Moseley (1992) has studied which are the best exercises for positioning and stabilizing the scapula (Figs. 13.2–13.4, see Fig. 13.1). Townsend (1991) maintains that the exercises described in Figures 13.4 and 13.5 should be strictly included in any shoulder rehabilitation protocol aimed at overhead athletes. Blackburn (1990) believes that the exercises shown in Figures 13.5 and 13.6 are better for the rotator cuff. In contrast with Blackburn, Townsend (1991) has

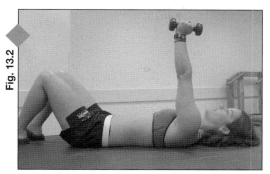
Fig. 13.2

Pushup without load – OKC – with weight (scapular protraction).

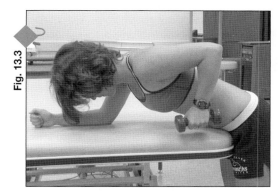
Fig. 13.3

Bent row.

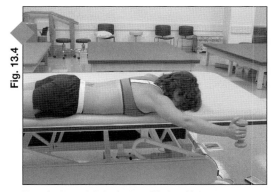
Fig. 13.4

Prone horizontal abduction, modified position.

documented a better EMG response by the shoulder muscles during elevation in the scapular plane in internal rotation in a seated or upright position. The authors maintain that horizontal abduction exercises in external rotation, performed in a prone position, are

Postoperative rehabilitation

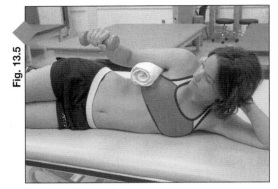

Fig. 13.5

External rotation on the side.

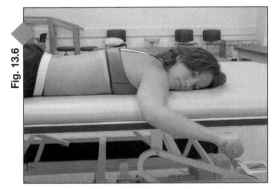

Fig. 13.6

External rotation 90°/90° in a prone position.

excessive in the early rehabilitation period (Fig. 13.5). Strengthening a weak rotator cuff with the arm elevated in the scapular plane in internal rotation may allow the humeral head to move in a superior direction, thus causing impingement with the majority of the muscles at which this exercise is aimed. In the final analysis, the key to using these exercises is the ability to alter position, to keep the movement at all times within the safe range for early mobilization in the postoperative period. The humerus must be kept in the scapular plane (Fig. 13.1), or slightly further forwards and the glenohumeral joint must not be externally rotated before the surgeon declares the tissue healing process to be complete. Strengthening exercises should be performed in 3–5 series of 10 repetitions, once or twice daily; progressively higher weights may be used starting from 2 kg, and increasing the load as tolerated. Dumb-bells (Fig. 13.2), wrist weights, elastic bands or other suitable aids can be used. Isometric exercises for the shoulder girdle can be done at home, with 2–3 daily sessions consisting of

2–3 series of 10 repetitions, maintaining the position for six seconds in each direction. They should be performed in flexion, abduction, adduction, extension, and internal and external rotation, with submaximal force and with the limb in the frontal plane.

When the patient's joint mobility allows and the rotator cuff is strong enough to stabilize the glenohumeral joint, the patient may start to use machines. The patient's position on the machine should not involve him or her exceeding the safe range of motion or placing the repaired tissues under excessive strain. For example, the majority of less recent machines for strengthening the pectorals place the patient's shoulder in extreme horizontal abduction. This may result in instability at any time, but particularly in the first 3–4 months after surgery. The latest machines provide adjustment for the lever arms and for increasing the weight by small amounts, making them suitable for patients who have recently undergone surgery. Patients may start strengthening exercises with machines after they have achieved adequate mobility and have passed four out of five muscle tests without other symptoms. If possible, it is useful to increase the weights by one kilogram every 3–5 series of 10 repetitions. This should, in any case, be done cautiously.

Attention should be paid to the position of the hands and the amplitude of the movement when using the bench press and shoulder press. The hands should be closer than normal, to prevent stress on the anterior capsule when lowering the weight, and care should be taken to avoid the elbow going below the plane of the body. These recommendations also apply to flexion movements. These guidelines should be followed for at least four weeks after surgery.

Lephart (1994) has described a loss of proprioception in the shoulder related to instability. Proprioceptive exercises allow the coordination of inputs received by all the muscles of the shoulder. These exercises consist of small movements (leaning against the wall or table), rhythmic stabilization (Voss, 1985) (Figs. 13.7 and 13.8) and proprioceptive neuromuscular facilitation (PNF) of the scapula (Voss, 1985), and may be performed from the second week following surgery. Wilk and Arrigo maintain that weight lifting should be started early in the conservative treatment of unstable shoulder, to develop dynamic shoulder stability (Wilk, 1993). These techniques can be used safely in the protected rehabilitation phase, without jeopardizing the surgical outcome. The patient can regulate the load by using the healthy upper limb and the lower limbs (Fig. 13.9). Rhythmic stabilization is performed at 90° flexion against submaximal resistance to the upper limb in all the movement planes (Fig. 13.7).

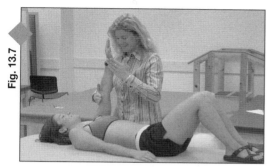

Manual rhythmic stabilization.

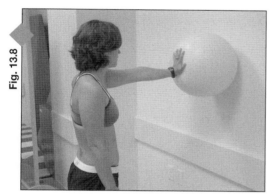

Transfer of load, minimum load, ball against the wall.

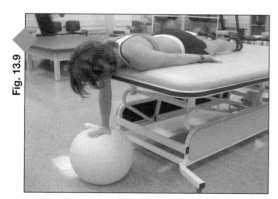

Transfer of load, minimum load, alternative position.

be performed after six weeks. During the restrictive, active and functional phases of rehabilitation, the patient may additionally use various oscillating machines, throw a medicine ball, use neuromuscular training apparatus and exercise with heavy weights (Figs. 13.10–13.15, see Fig. 13.4). Proprioceptive training can be carried out in the form of OKC or CKC activities. Various aids are useful for this type of exercise, such as inflatable balls and unstable surfaces (Figs. 13.8, 13.9, 13.12, 13.13). The progression of

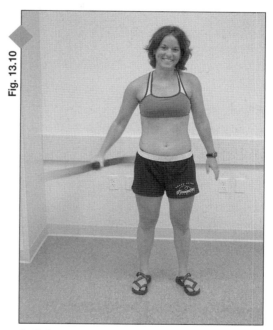

Oscillations with an oscillating rod, safe ROM.

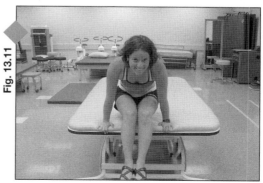

Pushup with load – CKC – seated.

This technique can also be performed in internal and external rotation at 45° of abduction in the scapular plane. To increase the proprioceptive stimuli and the level of difficulty, patients are asked to close their eyes during the exercise. PNF can be implemented at the first postoperative session and diagonal movements can

Postoperative rehabilitation

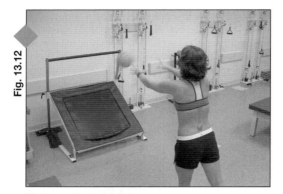

Fig. 13.12

Mini-trampoline, two-hand pass.

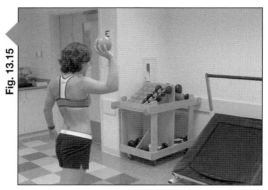

Fig. 13.15

Mini-trampoline, one-handed in the functional range.

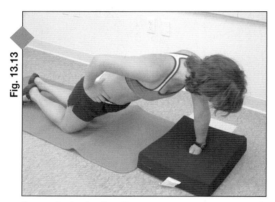

Fig. 13.13

Progressive load, soft surface.

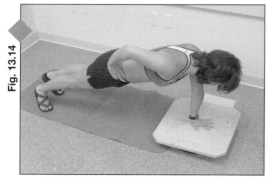

Fig. 13.14

Full load on an unstable surface.

When the athlete enters the active phase of rehabilitation, isokinetic exercises can be used to continue strengthening work and stamina training on the dynamic stabilizers of the shoulder. It can start at the higher velocities (240–300°/second), then progress to programmes with greater amplitude, for example, from 180 to 300°/second. At the end of the active phase, an isokinetic test can be performed on the internal and external rotators at 180 and 300°/second. If the result shows a deficit in strength and resistance of less than 15%, specific training for a return to sport-related activity can be started. This moment indicates the start of phase IV. Functional exercises, depending on the previous surgical stabilization, for American footballers and wrestlers, include traditional flexion movements with monolateral and bilateral support (Tippett, 1995). Tippett and Voight

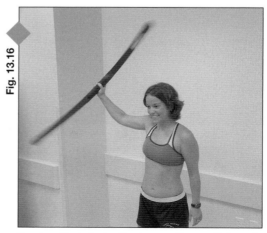

Fig. 13.16

Proprioception in the functional range with an oscillating rod.

proprioceptive exercises should be based on the symptoms and on the rate of healing. Proprioceptive exercises can be performed daily in 3 series of 15 repetitions at 15–30 seconds.

recommend that the training programme should additionally include spinning (axial rotation) on a single arm, which can be used as both an exercise and a functional test (Tippett, 1995). This exercise allows the injured limb only to be subjected to a load, in such a way that the arm and the feet are the only points in contact with the ground. The athlete rotates around the arm which remains fixed, clockwise and anticlockwise, for a given time or number of turns. Overhead athletes can use, as part of their functional rehabilitation,

plyometric exercises with elastic bands, a medicine ball or oscillating rods (Fig. 13.16). Some of these are plyometric exercises for internal and external rotation at 90° abduction, the two-hand pass, throwing a ball diagonally and in elevation, and throwing a baseball one-handed (Wilk, 1993). For overhead athletes, a functional improvement should lead to a training programme for throwing and to a return to sport-related activity within six months of surgery (Mellion, 1995). For athletes from other sports, a careful specific

Table 13.2

General guidelines for shoulder repair for anterior instability or glenoid labrum injury: phase I

Phase	Objectives	Therapy
0–3 weeks 'Protective'	*Control of pain/oedema*	• Cryotherapy, electrostimulation
		• Grade I, II mobilization
	Mobilization (protected ROM) (10–25 repetitions 2–3 times daily)	• Brace for three weeks
		• Passive anterior elevation (PAE) in the scapular plane (SP) from the second day according to medical limitations
		• Passive external rotation (ER) in the SP and abduction (ABD) and ER according to medical limitations
		• Pendulum exercises
		• Active mobilization for all movements
	Strengthening (protected ROM) (3–5 series × 10 repetitions twice daily) (0–2.5 kg)	• Start of isometric exercise by flexion, adduction (ADD), ABD, extension (EXT), internal rotation (IR) and ER
		• Strengthening
		• Flexion/extension wrist
		• Flexion/extension elbow
		• Raising shoulders with scapular ADD (retraction)
		• Abduction in the scapular plane (Fig. 13.1)
		• Pushups (Fig. 13.2)
		• Bent row (Fig. 13.3)
		• Modified prone horizontal abduction (Fig. 13.4)
		• ER on the side (Fig. 13.5)
		• ER 90°/90° prone (Fig. 13.6)
		• IR with limb adducted
	Proprioception (protected ROM) (10–25 repetitions once daily)	• Rhythmic stabilization (Fig. 13.7)
		• Transfer of load (Figs. 13.8 and 13.9)
		• Oscillations (oscillating rods) in a limited range (Fig. 13.10)
	Cardiovascular fitness (30–60 min (3–5 times/week))	• Bicycle
		• Step
		• Walking

Postoperative rehabilitation

Table 13.3

General guidelines for shoulder repair for anterior instability or glenoid labrum injury: phase II

Phase	Objectives	Therapy
3–6 weeks 'Restrictive'	*Mobilization* • PROM/AROM • 60°–90° ER • 45°–60° IR • 135°–155° ABD • 135°–165° elevation	• Active mobilization against the suture in all directions
	Strengthening 3 to 4/5 manually	• Increase the exercises in Table 13.2 for the whole joint function available • Increase weights as tolerated • Pushups from a seated position (Fig. 13.11)
	Proprioception Difference of 30% or less between the injured side and the healthy side	• Increase the intensity and load according to the exercises in Table 13.2 for the whole joint function available • Plyotoss, two-hand pass (Fig. 13.12)
	SDA All daily sedentary activities	No restrictions Proceed as tolerated

Table 13.4

General guidelines for shoulder repair for anterior instability or glenoid labrum injury: phase III

Phase	Objectives	Therapy
6–12 weeks 'Active'	*Mobilization* • PROM/AROM • 90° + ER • Complete IR • 60°–180° ABD	• Gradual increase in passive stretching • Grade III and IV mobilization techniques • Bar • Overhead pulley

	Strengthening
	• 4-4+/5 manually
	• Isokinetic difference of 15% or less
		• Gradually increase the weights up to 2.5 kg
		• Use machines
		  — Bench press
		  — Military press
		  — Seated row
		  — Lat pull down
		  — Biceps
		  — Triceps

	Proprioception Difference of 15% or less	• Proprioceptive exercises with full load in a CKC (Fig. 13.14) • Progress to proprioceptive exercises in an OKC and CKC close to the maximum limit of the joint range
	Activity • Light, non-repetitive overhead • Lift light weights	• SDA as tolerated • Do not perform sport-related activities

Table 13.5

General guidelines for shoulder repair for anterior instability or glenoid labrum injury: phase IV

Phase	Objectives	Therapy
12–24 weeks 'Functional'	*Mobilization* • AROM/PROM • Obtain full or sufficient joint function to participate in a sport	• Progressive AROM and passive range of motion (PROM)
	Strengthening • 5/5 MMT • <10% isokinetic difference	• Continue exercises with machines • Continue with free loads • Military press • Bench press • Shoulder press • Row • Lateral raise
	Proprioception • <10% proprioceptive difference	• Load on unstable surfaces • Throwing one-handed (Fig. 13.15) • In elevated functional positions (Fig. 13.16)
	Activity • Gradual progression to all activities	• Return to sport-related activity (from partial to complete, from simple to complex) • Return to overhead disciplines, such as throwing, tennis or golf

training programme needs to be designed, which will ensure a safe, full return to sport-related activity.

Postoperative treatment

Given that the patient's state of tissue healing and progress in relation to specific functional criteria will determine their rehabilitation, we have designed a rehabilitation programmed divided into phases each lasting three weeks. These guidelines are not, however, intended as a protocol based on time since surgery and the times are simply given as a guide. Personalized modifications and variations of the requirements for each individual patient are, therefore, possible. The surgeon should be able to insert specific dates in the patient's programme depending on the type of procedure performed and should at all times be available for consultation. Tables 13.2–13.5 give general guidelines for a shoulder which has undergone repair for anterior instability or glenoid labrum injury. These guidelines may not suit patients with significant instability or hyperlaxity, or those who have undergone thermal capsulorrhaphy or repeated repair procedures. The time limits in these cases should be longer and based principally on the doctor's assessments.

Conclusions

The constant, high-level use of the shoulder complex places it at risk, both of overuse and soft tissue damage. Huge loads and angular velocities are generated in the shoulder complex at many points and these can cause tissue to give way with the consequent need for surgery. The rehabilitation therapist should understand the wide range of stresses and strains that can damage a shoulder, in order to recognize and prevent them and to be able to treat them adequately in a shoulder that has been damaged or operated on. Although no recognized studies have been published in the literature on the results obtained in patients who have undergone shoulder stabilization or glenoid labrum repair, some knowledge will help to plan the correct rehabilitation programme for the recovery of joint function and muscle tone. Therapists should know how to combine their knowledge of how tissues heal with the biomechanics for each type of surgical procedure, in order to plan a rehabilitation programme which does not overstrain the suture. They must design effective exercises for the recovery of the muscles of the shoulder girdle, including proprioceptive and functional exercises. No single generic protocol will suit every patient, but a programme based on a number of basic points, aided by any suggestions by the surgeon, will help patients to achieve their maximum functional level.

This chapter has discussed the basic principles of shoulder rehabilitation, applying them following various types of surgical procedures.

The rehabilitative process should follow a well-organized route, based on the latest clinical concepts and on scientifically proven evaluations, in order to achieve the best functional outcome for the athlete.

Bibliography

Blackburn T.A., McLeod W.D., White B., WOFFORD L., 'EMG analysis of posterior rotator cuff exercises', *J. Athletic Training* 25: 40–45, (1990)

Bowen M.K., Warren R.F., 'Ligamentous control of shoulder stability based on selective cutting and static translation experiments', *Clin. Sports Med.* 10: 757–782, (1991)

Christensen K.P., 'Arthroscopic vs. open Bankart procedures: A comparison of early morbidity and complications', *Arthroscopy* 9: 371–374, (1993)

Ellenbecker T.S., Mattalino A.J., 'Glenohumeral joint range of motion and rotator cuff strength following arthroscopic anterior stabilization with thermal capsulorrhaphy', *J. Orthop. Sports Phys. Ther.* 29(3): 160–167, (1999)

Guanche C.A., Quick D.C., Sodergren K.M., Buss D.D., 'Arthroscopic vs. open reconstruction of the shoulder in patients with isolated Bankart lesions', *Am. J. Sports Med.* 24(2): 144–148, (1996)

Hayashi K., Massa K.L., Thabit G., Fanton G.S., Dillingham M.F., Gilchrist G.W., Markel M.D., 'Histological evaluation of the glenohumeral joint capsule after laser assisted capsular shift procedure for glenohumeral instability', *Am. J. Sports Med.* 27(2): 162–167, (1999)

Imhoff A.B., 'The use of lasers in orthopedic surgery', *Oper. Tech. Orthop.* 5: 192–203, (1995)

Jobe F.W , Giangarra C.E., Kvitne R.S., Glousman R.E., 'Anterior capsulolabral reconstruction of the shoulder in athletes in overhand sports', *Am. J. Sports Med.* 19(5): 428–434, (1991)

Kibler W.B., 'Evaluation of sports demands as a diagnostic tool in shoulder disorders', In: Matsen F.A., Fu F., Hawkins R.J. (eds.), *The Shoulder: A balance of mobility and stability*, AAOS, Rosemont, pp. 379–395, (1993)

Kibler W.B., 'Biomechanical analysis of the shoulder during tennis activities', *Clin. Sports Med.* 14: 79–85, (1995a)

Kibler W.B., Livingston B., Bruce R., 'Current concepts in shoulder rehabilitation', *Adv. Oper. Orthop.* 3: 249–300, (1995b)

Kibler W.B., Perry J., 'The role of the scapula in athletic shoulder function', *Sports Med.* 26: 325–337, (1998)

Lephart S.M., Warner J.J.P., Borsa P.A., Fu F.H., 'Proprioception of the shoulder joint in healthy, unstable, and surgically repaired shoulders', *J. Shoulder Elbow Surg.* 3(6): 371–380, (1994)

Mellion M.B., Walsh W.M., Shelton G.L., 'Baseball and Softball', In: *The Team Physician's Handbook*, 3rd ed. Hanley and Belfus, Philadelphia, pp. 570–584, (1995)

Moseley J.B., Jobe F.W., Pink M., Perry J., Tibone J., 'EMG analysis of the scapular muscles during a shoulder rehabilitation program', *Am. J. Sports Med.* 20(2): 128–134, (1992)

Naseef G.S., Foster T.E., Trauner K., Solhpour S., Anderson R.R., Zarins B., 'The thermal properties of bovine joint capsule: The basic science of laser- and radiofrequency-induced capsular shrinkage', *Am. J. Sports Med.* 25(5): 670–674, (1997)

O'Brien S.J., Neves M.C., Arnoczky S.P. et al., 'The anatomy and histology of the inferior glenohumeral ligament complex of the shoulder', *Am. J. Sports Med.* 18(5): 449–456, (1990)

O'Brien S.J., Schwartz R.E., Warren R.F., Torzilli P.A., 'Capsular restraints to anterior/posterior motion of the shoulder', *Orthop. Trans.* 12:143, (1988)

Paine R.M., Voight M.L., 'The role of the scapula', *J. Orthop. and Sports Phys. Ther.* 18: 386–391, (1993)

Peat M., 'Functional anatomy of the shoulder complex', *Phys. Ther.* 66: 1855–1865, (1986)

Phillips B.B. 'Recurrent dislocations.' In: Campell's *Operative Orthopedics*, 9th ed. Mosby-Year Book, St. Louis (1998)

Reed B.V., 'Wound healing and the use of thermal agents', In: Michlovitz S.L. (ed.), *Thermal Agents in Rehabilitation*, 3rd ed. F.A. Davis Co., Philadelphia, pp. 3–29, (1996)

Satter White Y.E., 'Shoulder Instability', In: *Diagnostic and Operative Arthroscopy*, 1st ed. W.B. Saunders Co., Philadelphia, pp. 105–113, (1997)

Schaefer S.L., Ciarelli M.J., Arnoczky S.P., Ross H.E., 'Tissue shrinkage with the Holmium: Yttrium aluminum garnet laser: A postoperative assessment of tissue length, stiffness, and structure', *Am. J. Sports Med.* 25(6): 841–848, (1997)

Selecky M.T., Vangsness T., Liao W., Sadaat V., Hedman T.P., 'The effects of laser induced collagen shortening on the biomechanical properties of the inferior glenohumeral complex', *Am. J. Sports Med.* 27(2): 168–172, (1999)

Snyder S.J., Karazel R.P., Del Pizzo W., Ferkel J.F., Friedman M., 'SLAP-lesions of the shoulder', *Arthroscopy* 6: 274–279, (1990)

Tippett S.R., Voight M.L., 'Functional Progressions for Sport Rehabilitation', 1st ed. *Human Kinetics*, Champaign (1995)

Townsend H., Jobe F.W., Pink M., Perry J., 'Electromyographic analysis of the glenohumeral muscles during a baseball rehabilitation program', *Am. J. Sports Med.* 19(3): 264–272, (1991)

Turkel S.J., Panio M.W., Marshall J.L., Girgis F.G., 'Stabilizing mechanisms preventing anterior dislocation of the glenohumeral joint', *J. Bone Joint Surg.* 63 A(8): 1208–1217, (1981)

Voight M.L., Hardin J.A., Blackburn T.A., Tippett S.R., Canner G.C., 'The effects of muscle fatigue on and the relationship of arm dominance to shoulder proprioception', *J. Orthop. and Sports Phys. Ther.* 23: 348–352, (1996)

Voss D.E., Ionta M.K., Myers B.J., *Proprioceptive Neuromuscular Facilitation*, 3rd ed. Harper and Row, Philadelphia (1985)

Wilk K.E., Arrigo C.A., 'Current concepts in the rehabilitation of the athletic shoulder', *J. Orthop. Sports Phys. Ther.* 187(1): 365–378, (1993)

MANUAL THERAPY IN REHABILITATION

A. Foglia

The management of disorders of the shoulder complex is clearly multidimensional. Passive manual movement is only one of the possible options. The choice of therapy is based on an interpretation of both the subjective and physical examinations and on the priority accorded these. The review of manual therapy techniques given is rather artificial, since therapeutic planning needs to take into account all the possible techniques available. This chapter will consider only the joint mobilization techniques we consider most useful in daily clinical practice.

The principles underlying the choice of passive mobilization techniques have been described in detail by other authors, such as Austin, Jones, Magarey and Maitland. Akeson, Woo and Frank have helped to clarify phenomena such as joint stiffness, and the mechanical properties of biological tissue and the structural and functional changes in connective tissue due to immobilization are now better understood.

This chapter will not address the physiological and biomechanical mechanisms which make passive mobilization effective (van Wingerden, 1995).

The author of this chapter sets great store by management based on an examination of damage (both organic and functional), which takes into account an increased knowledge of the pathomechanics and pathophysiology of the structures within the shoulder complex (von Eisenhart-Rothe 2002, 2005) and the influences of the nociceptor components (Barden 2004; Myers 2003, 2004; Warner 1990, 1996).

Passive manual mobilization as a training stimulus: general principles

Mobilization in rehabilitation and training: this is the two-fold subject that will be addressed.

For a better understanding of the factors which have led to the terms mobilization and training being addressed, it is useful to look at some definitions in greater detail.

First of all, sport injury rehabilitation refers to all the measures (treatments and specialized rehabilitation procedures) which aim to minimize the sequelae of an injury and to maximize the residual post-traumatic functional and physical abilities of an athlete.

Rehabilitation training is, however, a systematic process which aims to modify the performance capacity of a given musculoskeletal region, by the application of appropriate physical workloads.

The use of the expression physical workloads arises owing to the need to make the stimuli applied to the patient/athlete in the course of a therapeutic process quantifiable in some way and consequently measurable.

We have tried, in our proposal, to apply the principles of athletic training to manual therapy, because the passive mobilization of biological tissue is also a physical stimulus and a stress to which the organism responds by adaptation.

Any physical stimulus applied as part of athletic training is comparable with that applied in manual therapy.

Manual therapy in rehabilitation

Adaptation as a phenomenon of development is expressed by a global, aspecific reaction by the body, codified by Selye in his general adaptation syndrome (GAS) theory, according to which any external stimulus is regarded as a form of stress (Calligaris, 1997).

The body has the innate ability to respond to any external action which may disturb its internal equilibrium (homeostasis) with a reaction (specific to the external stimulus and proportional to its magnitude) which aims to restore the fundamental and essential equilibrium (Bellotti, 1999).

To restore homeostasis, the organism makes a provisional adjustment of its functions, which ceases when its external cause is withdrawn.

These are, therefore, temporary changes. If, however, the body is subjected to a series of homogeneous stimuli close together and of increasing magnitude, its response would be to make increasingly stable and established changes (Fig. 14.1).

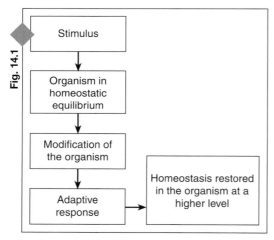

Fig. 14.1

Stimulus-adaptation sequence in athletic training (modified from Bellotti, 1999).

But that is not all: the body responds to any external stimulus which may upset its equilibrium with a reaction which exceeds the 'destabilizing' action and raises the initial normal level, giving rise to the phenomenon of overcompensation.

Physical workload is one of the external stimuli which interfere with the body's internal state of equilibrium, as is manual therapy (mobilization, manipulation, capsular stretching, etc.) in the field of rehabilitation.

Hence the need to understand the size of an external load, in order to carry out the essential task of monitoring in the therapeutic process.

Parameters specific to the physical stimulus are, therefore, necessary to ensure that the external load (C) is appropriate (for example, manipulation rather than mobilization) and to allow its planned administration (for example, one therapeutic session per week rather than three).

Intensity of the stimulus

This refers to the intensity of the individual stimulus in relation to maximum individual capacity.

A physical stimulus for training should be greater than the individual's load capacity, in order for the morphological and functional changes of adaptation to take place.

Stimuli below the load capacity threshold will not result in adaptation and the overall effect of excessive stimuli may lead to overload (Fig. 14.2).

Since the functional properties (load capacity) of a damaged tissue are subjected during rehabilitation to continual change, the functional limits of the structure to be rehabilitated should be examined closely (functional evaluation), so that rehabilitation training is effective.

Duration of the stimulus

This refers to the duration of a single stimulus.

The higher the intensity of a stimulus, the shorter its duration should be (manipulation) and vice versa, the longer the duration of the stimulus, the lower its intensity should be (grade I mobilization: see the section Grades of mobilization).

Frequency of the stimulus

This refers to the number of individual stimuli in relation to one unit of time.

It is common practice in rehabilitation to work serially, i.e. according to a given mobilization technique carried out several times.

Volume of the stimulus

This is the total of all the individual stimuli in one session of treatment.

The volume of the stimulus can be regarded as the product of the intensity of the stimulus, its duration and frequency (Fig. 14.3).

Fig. 14.2

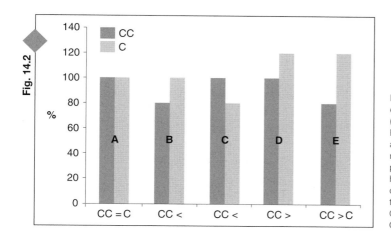

Diagram of the relationship between external load and load capacity. In A load (C) is appropriate to load capacity (CC). In B CC is reduced, whatever the reason, and a normal load will result in a reduction. In C load is reduced in the presence of normal CC, and this will not have an optimal training effect, i.e. CC will diminish. In D CC is normal, C is of a training level and CC will increase. In E CC is reduced and the load is excessive: CC will diminish further.

Fig. 14.3

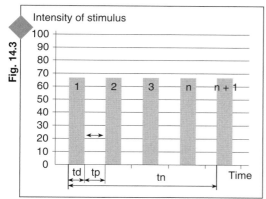

Volume of the stimulus (modified from Einsingbach T., Klumper A., Biedermann L., *Fisioterapia e Riabilitazione sportive*, Edizioni Marrapese, Rome 1991).
td: duration of stimulus; tp: stimulus interval; tn: duration of load; n: duration of stimulus.
Intensity of stimulus × duration of stimulus × frequency of stimulus = volume of stimulus.

Because adequate and logical adaptive responses correspond to the total external loads 'administered' over time to a biological tissue (the raising of the load capacity threshold (CC)), it is vital that the following principles are observed:
— principle of specificity;
— principle of progression; and
— principle of individualization.
Clinical experience in physiotherapy has shown that physical workload alone is insufficient to explain the resulting practical results.

Simply identifying a load for a patient to work with (one cycle of manual therapy for 10 sessions) does not mean that its effects can be generalized to different patients with the same disorder, or even the same individual at different times.

The concept of physical workload (a defined quantity of specific motor stimuli) must be considered alongside the concept of local load capacity, i.e. the result of immediate reactions at the site of the lesion to the external stresses produced by the external training load.

There are many factors which characterize the local load capacity of a tissue or a musculoskeletal region; one of these is the biological healing process of a tissue.

Figure 14.4 shows the various phases in the healing process, which are important for planning rehabilitation treatment.

The organism's aim, as mentioned above, is to return to homeostasis, although it should be noted that the curve rises to a higher level shortly before this condition is reached, and this is known as overcompensation (Fig. 14.5).

The external stimulus, in this case joint mobilization, is simply a 'causal agent' of a 'particular effect', which is different for each individual, for each clinical condition, and also for the same individual at different times in the course of the disorder, depending on the extent of the organic and functional damage to the shoulder, official age, athletic age, psychological condition, social status, etc.

Generalizing a manual therapy technique or a 'training' workload for the same individual or for several individuals is inconceivable.

A classic principle of the theory of training, i.e. the individualization of stimuli (load), should in our opinion, form one of the cornerstones of joint mobilization.

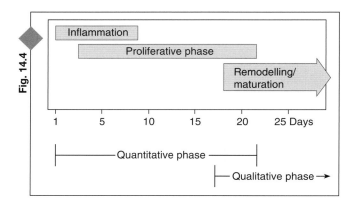

Fig. 14.4

Phases in the healing process (from Van Wingerden, 1995).

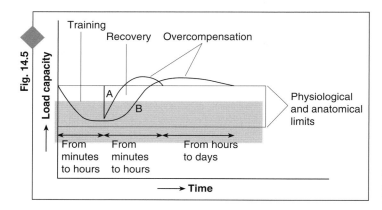

Fig. 14.5

Return of the organism to homeostasis and overcompensation (from Van Wingerden, 1995).

Grades of mobilization

— *Grade 1:* a small amplitude movement performed at the start of the range (this can be used if the tissue is very reactive, or in the warm-up phase of a pain-relief or treatment session);
— *Grade 2:* a larger amplitude movement at a distance from the painful ROM;
— *Grade 3:* a large amplitude movement which reaches the limit of the range: pain limit (this is used with moderately reactive tissue); and
— *Grade 4:* a small amplitude and high velocity movement beyond the limit (restrictive barrier) of the range available remaining within the physiological limit of the joint (this is used in the absence of pain and with the aim of gaining the few degrees still missing from the range of motion to achieve full joint amplitude) (Fig. 14.6).

Grade 1 and 2 techniques are used for their neurophysiological effects (reducing pain), while the aim of

Grade 3 and 4 techniques is to cause mechanical changes in the tissues (Evans, 2002), although there is also a neurophysiological effect.

It is evident from the above that the concept of load or external stimulus should be considered alongside the concept of internal load (Fig. 14.7).

It is necessary, when modulating the intensity and quantity of the manual stimulus, to know how to take advantage of the phenomenon of overcompensation, which is a natural process in every individual, how to support it and how to increase the external load and load capacity of the organism over time (Fig. 14.8).

Pain is also, on the one hand, a factor of 'disturbance' of load capacity (local and general) and, on the other, a guiding symptom during rehabilitation.

Pain is the best guide for modulating the amplitude, intensity, frequency and quantity of physical stimulation. Within certain limits, appropriately measured stimuli will cause stable, lasting morphofunctional modifications in proportion to the rate they are applied.

Fig. 14.6

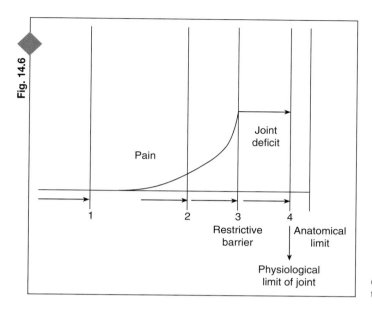

Graph of amplitude of movement in relation to degrees of mobilization.

Fig. 14.7

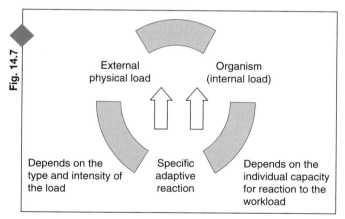

External load and internal load (modified from Bellotti, 1999).

The principle of frequency is closely related to the principle of recovery between the various stimuli, which depends in turn on the intensity of the treatment, the structures involved in the adaptation process and how well the individual tolerates the stimulus (Fig. 14.9).

The cockpit model, a teaching model devised by colleagues at the Vrije Universiteit Brussel (VUB) on the Master's course in 'Manual Therapy' (Fig. 14.10) may be useful when making a coherent choice between parameters in order to plan the therapeutic session (training) (Fig.14.11).

Assuming that each parameter is represented by a scale of values, they should be constantly monitored

to check that the various indicators are in proportion to one another:

— *joint position:* neutral (pain-free or resting position) or in a specific position (in proximity to the restriction);
— *rhythm;* slow, i.e. below the respiratory rate (approximately 18 cycles per minute) or fast, i.e. above this rate;
— *direction of passive manual movement:* direct, i.e. towards the limitation, or indirect (in the opposite direction to that of the limitation);
— *stage:* grade 1 for tissue that is highly reactive, grade 4 (manipulation) for recovery of PROM in the absence of pain;

Fig. 14.8

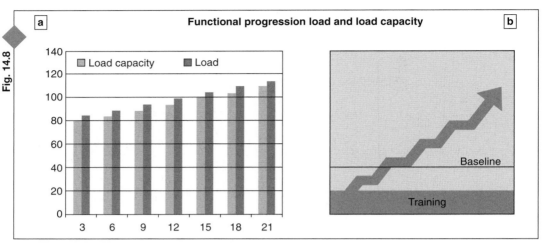

Principle of functional progression.

Fig. 14.9

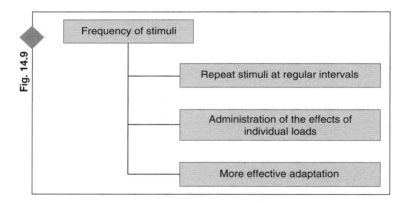

Frequency of stimuli (modified from Bellotti, 1999).

— *amplitude of movement;*
— *components:* i.e. how many components are included in the technique: an 'angular' mobilization technique (abduction) or an 'accessory' mobilization technique (translation) or finally a mixed technique (abduction and translation);
— *types of components:* traction, compression, translation, axial rotation, etc.; and
— *number of repetitions.*

Joint mobilization

Physiological joint movement is characterized by the dynamic combination of a passive component (osteokinematic and arthrokinematic), an active component (property of periarticular structures) and a neural component.

A reduction in joint movement is caused by a loss of or change in one or all of the above components.

Passive manual movement, constituting a specific physical stimulus, helps the physiotherapist to manage the tissue and functional modifications of the damaged structures (Bang, 2000).

Rehabilitation specialists have access, in their daily clinical practice, to various treatment techniques, each of which are useful for obtaining set objectives.

These include, for example, passive (or active) static lengthening techniques used essentially to condition

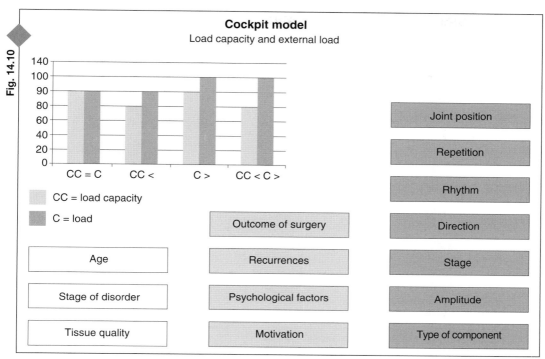

Fig. 14.10

Cockpit model (by kind permission of Dr E.J. Barbaix, VUB, Department of Manual Therapy).

contractile structures. These techniques aim as far as possible to improve the extendibility of the muscle and tendon complex, one of the properties of contractile structures.

Therapeutic exercise also involves the use of techniques aimed at the afferences of the area affected by the disorder (proprioceptive training).

There are many other solutions specific to muscle training which are sometimes necessary to increase the dynamic control of a joint. Besides the therapeutic procedures described above, there is also mobilization in all its forms, i.e. passive, active or assisted active, mechanical or manual.

Passive joint mobilization

Passive joint mobilization, a procedure which will be described in this chapter, is a particular passive manual movement which can be performed at variable amplitudes, directions and speeds.

For this type of therapy, the physiotherapist needs to understand the anatomical, physiological and histological characteristics of the joints forming the

shoulder joint complex. The physiotherapist will also need to be familiar with the various morphofunctional changes related to shoulder disorders and their clinical implications.

The normal physiology of the shoulder joint involves the coexistence, as mentioned above, of arthrokinematic movements (movement between joint surfaces), osteokinematic movements (movement between bones) and neuromuscular movements (dynamic joint stability). Owing to the morphological and functional characteristics of inert capsule tissue, a joint can have a degree of elasticity, which is known in manual therapy as joint play (Fig. 14.12).

Joint play is a basic requirement of normal joint function; this is why passive mobilization techniques are used to try to improve it.

The physiotherapist's primary aim in the rehabilitation of musculoskeletal disorders is to increase as far as possible the patient's residual motor abilities (as a result of the disorder).

The aim of the joint mobilization techniques suggested in this chapter is to restabilize the arthrokinematics and osteokinematics of the joints forming the shoulder.

Manual therapy in rehabilitation

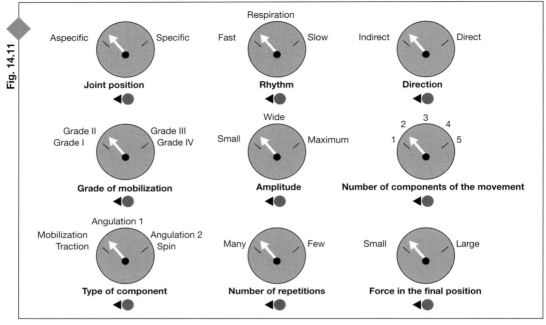

Fig. 14.11

Factors relating to external load and load capacity (local and general).

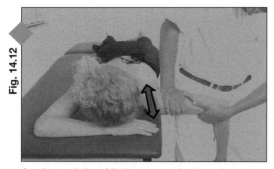

Fig. 14.12

Anterior translation of the humerus: evaluation and treatment.
Joint play: this is a range in which mobilization occurs without any soft tissue resistance.
Beyond this range the tissues are under tension, stretch and begin to offer initial mild resistance.
N.B.: the arrow shows the joint play to be tested or treated.

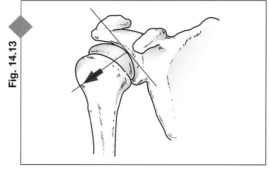

Fig. 14.13

Traction: the dark arrow shows the direction of traction.

Intrinsic joint mechanics can be rehabilitated by traction and translation. Both techniques can be used at the same time for evaluation and treatment.

Traction is the movement carried out along a line perpendicular to the plane of the joint surface, drawn from the centre of the curvature of the concave end of the joint. This direction does not, in the majority of cases, correspond to the longitudinal axis of the diaphysis of the bone on which

traction is being performed (see the orientation of the humeral glenoid in relation to the humeral head) (Fig. 14.13).

In translation movements, the bone to be mobilized is moved in line with the curvature of the joint ends to be mobilized, to avoid contact which in the glenohumeral joint would place the fibrous labrum at risk (Figs. 14.14 and 14.15a). Translation movements are, therefore, possible only if they are performed together with a traction component.

Translation movements can be performed with the joint heads in various positions. In the early phase of rehabilitation or in a warm-up, translation movements should be carried out in a resting (neutral) position and may subsequently be performed in a more specific position (approaching the limit of the range, or barrier). Translation movements are also performed in different directions, particularly those corresponding to osteokinematic limitations.

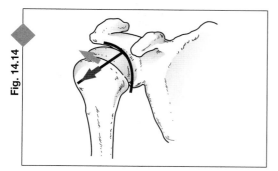

Fig. 14.14

Translation: the dark arrow shows the traction component, while the light arrow shows the direction of translation.

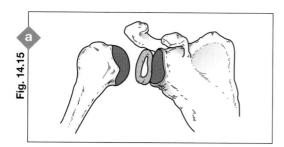

Fig. 14.15

a

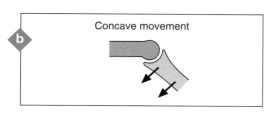

b

Concave movement

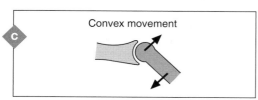

c

Convex movement

(a) The glenoid labrum; **(b)** rotation and translation in concave on convex movement; **(c)** and in convex on concave movement.

The concave-convex rule

In biomechanics movement is described in terms of rotation and translation. Specific conventional terminology has been developed in clinical practice, and this needs to be known in order to be able to understand the concave-convex rule.

'Arthrokinematics' refers to movements of the joint surfaces in relation to one another. An 'arthrokinematic movement' is always associated with the 'movement of one bone in relation to another' (osteokinematics).

A roll movement occurs when the joint surfaces correspond point for point. The term 'roll', referring to the convex bone head on the concave bone head, is used in clinical practice to describe a component of angular movement. Translation occurs when, during movement, one point on a joint surface comes successively into contact with many points on the corresponding joint surface. The translation of the convex surface on the concave surface is conventionally defined as a 'slide' movement. A 'swing' movement is the name conventionally given to the rotation of the concave bone head on the convex bone head.

A 'glide' movement is the clinical name conventionally given to translation of the concave bone head on the convex surface. Consequently, if a joint has to be moved across the concave bone end, for example, the acromion on the clavicle, this is called a swing-glide (a swing along with a glide in the same direction) (Fig 14.15b).

If, however, the joint has to be mobilized across the convex bone end, for example, the humeral head on the glenoid, this is called a roll-slide (a roll movement along with a slide movement in the opposite direction) (Fig. 14.15c). A spin component, i.e. a rotation around an axis perpendicular to the plane in which the roll-slide or swing-glide movements are being performed, can be added to the movements described.

Mobilization techniques

Glenohumeral joint

The following techniques require mobilization of the humeral head in relation to the scapular glenoid.

Traction

— *Aim:* to test joint play and end feel, to set the cockpit parameters, and to identify specific conditions (the exact point of limitation or pain). To increase the range of movement of the humerus in the glenoid cavity.

— *Patient:* supine. The limb to be examined is positioned in slight flexion and abduction.
— *Therapist:* on the same side as the shoulder to be tested.
— *Hold:* place the hands as close as possible to the humeral head. The caudal hand holds the upper third of the humerus and the proximal hand steadies the scapula and clavicle. The hold should prevent slippage.
— *Execution:* traction should be exerted perpendicular to the glenoid cavity. An intermediate position of the humerus is necessary to test for joint play.
— *Notes:* the humerus may be positioned in internal or external rotation to obtain more specific positions.

The glenoid is orientated in a lateral, anterior and cranial direction, consequently if the aim is to obtain information about joint play, this orientation must be taken into account. Since it is not easy to know how much traction to apply in the anterior, lateral or cranial directions, the more anterior part of the acromion can be used as a reference and traction applied in that direction (Fig. 14.16).

Compression/translation

— *Aim:* this may also be called a provocation test. It is at the same time a mobilization technique: it may be included in the warm-up for treatment or during the recovery period between two therapeutic sessions.
— *Patient:* supine, limb slightly flexed and abducted.
— *Therapist:* on the same side as the shoulder to be treated.
— *Hold:* to have good control over the proximal part of the humerus, the therapist may use two hands to hold the humerus; the outer hand on the outer side of the humerus to apply compression, while the inner hand in the axilla holds the more proximal part of the humerus to encourage translation.
— *Execution:* this technique can help to reproduce the arthrokinematic movements required.
— *Notes:* this technique can also be performed with the patient in a seated position; it is useful in specific positions. It is not recommended if pain is present (Fig. 14.17).

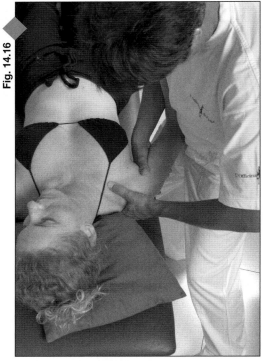

Fig. 14.16

Glenohumeral joint: traction.

Translation

Translation can be performed in the following directions:
— caudal;
— anterior; and
— posterior.

Cranial translation is not normally performed, unless the humeral head is in a very low position; it does not assess joint play but is simply a means of provoking subacromial impingement.

The joint surface of the glenoid should be regarded as being extended by the glenoid labrum, which increases its concavity; consequently, when these manoeuvres are being performed, this orientation must be respected to avoid running up against the glenoid labrum (Fig. 14.15a). Caution is particularly important in caudal and posterior translation.

Anterior and posterior translation tests may become provocation tests (not in the acute phase). In this case, the concavity of the glenoid surface/labrum is not

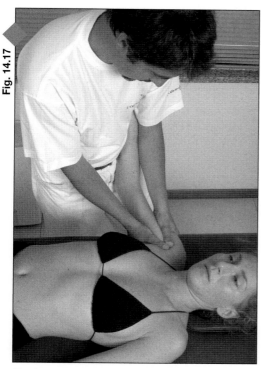

Fig. 14.17

Glenohumeral joint: compression/translation.

respected, but provocation of the glenoid labrum is achieved with a slight thrust.

Translation may be too extensive if glenohumeral joint instability is present.

Caudal translation

— *Aim:* to assess the arthrokinematic component to set the cockpit parameters. To increase joint mobility by the therapeutic technique.
— *Patient:* lateral decubitus.
— *Therapist:* in front of the patient.
— *Hold:* the caudal hand steadies the scapula, while the cranial hand which performs the translation is positioned as close as possible to the humeral head.
— *Execution:* the direction of translation is at a tangent to the joint surfaces, and will thus be anteromedial.
— *Notes:* more specific positions may be used in internal or external rotation or a traction component may be added.

It is important, so as not to run up against the glenoid labrum (particularly in the final phase of the manoeuvre), to give the translation movement a curvilinear trajectory, particularly if performed in a caudal and posterior direction (Fig. 14.18b).

— *Variant in the sitting position:* therapist behind the patient's shoulder. The fingers of the therapist's

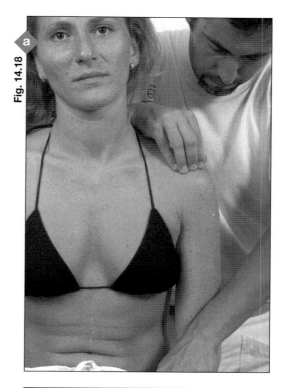

Fig. 14.18

a

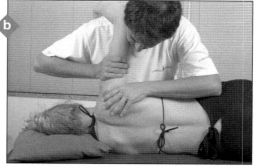

b

Glenohumeral joint. Caudal translation: **(a)** in a seated position, **(b)** in lateral decubitus.

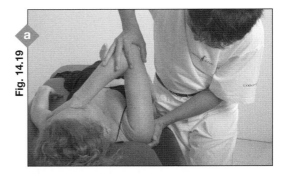

Fig. 14.19

inner hand are positioned in the subacromial space to detect movement of the humeral head. The outer hand applies distolateral thrust to the forearm, just under the elbow (Fig. 14.18b).

Dorsal translation at about 60° abduction

— *Aim:* to increase the passive amplitude of abduction.
— *Patient:* supine, limb abducted as far as the joint restriction, elbow semi-flexed. Neutral rotation of the limb.
— *Therapist:* positioned distal to the limb to be mobilized.
— *Hold:* the lateral hand supports the limb in abduction at the elbow, while the inner hand is placed centrally on the humeral head to perform posterolateral translation.
— *Execution:* posterolateral translation is possible for up to 90° of abduction (for a hypothetical restriction of the posterior part of the capsule) (Fig. 14.19b).
— *Notes:* avoid posteromedial translations to prevent the humeral head impacting on the glenoid labrum.

Dorsal translation in horizontal adduction

— *Aim:* to assess accessory passive movement; to increase the passive amplitude of movement in a specific position.
— *Patient:* supine, limb adducted as far as the movement restriction, elbow flexed.
— *Therapist:* in front of the patient on the side of the limb to be treated.
— *Hold:* with the inner hand placed on the patient's elbow, the therapist's forearm is the extension of the patient's humeral diaphysis; the outer hand steadies the scapula with the thenar and hypothenar eminences.
— *Execution:* the distal hand pushes in the direction of the humeral diaphysis, while the proximal hand steadies the scapula to achieve posterolateral translation (for a hypothetical restriction of the posterior part of the capsule) (Fig. 14.19a).
— *Notes:* avoid posteromedial translation so as not to cause the humeral head to impact on the glenoid labrum (Fig. 14.19).

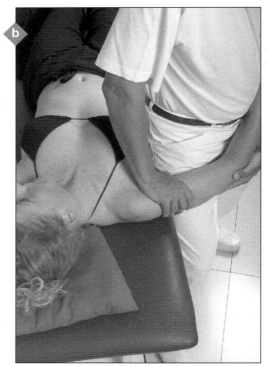

Glenohumeral joint: dorsal translation **(a)** in horizontal adduction, and **(b)** in abduction of the arm.

Caudolateral translation beyond 90° abduction

— *Aim:* evaluation test. Therapeutic technique for the recovery of abduction movement in highly specific positions (extreme degrees).
— *Patient:* seated, limb abducted and externally rotated, elbow flexed.
— *Therapist:* behind and on the side of the limb to be mobilized.

— *Hold:* the outer hand supports the patient's limb, holding the elbow, while the inner hand is placed close to the humeral head.
— *Execution:* while the outer hand places the shoulder in a specific position or abducts the limb (two-component technique: angular movement and translation), the other hand applies caudolateral thrust to the humerus.
— *Notes:* beyond 90° of glenohumeral abduction, an external rotation component must be added (Fig. 14.20a).

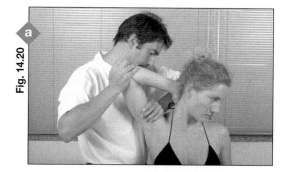

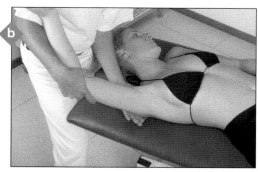

Glenohumeral joint: **(a)** caudolateral translation beyond 90° abduction, **(b)** translation in the final degrees of abduction.

Variant

— *Aim:* evaluation test. Therapeutic technique for the recovery of abduction movement in highly specific positions.
— *Patient:* supine, limb abducted and externally rotated as far as the joint limit, elbow semi-flexed.
— *Therapist:* proximal to the limb to be mobilized.
— *Hold:* the lateral hand supports the limb at the elbow maintaining the selected parameters, while the medial hand is placed in a superior position, close to the humeral head.

— *Execution:* beyond 90° abduction, the thrust applied to the humeral head with the medial hand should be in a caudolateral direction.
— *Notes:* beyond 90° of glenohumeral abduction, an external rotation component must be added.
The direction of the scapular spine indicates the position of the glenoid; caution should be exercised when performing the translation in a caudolateral direction in relation to the position of the glenoid in the space (Fig. 14.20b).

Traction in a specific position (adduction in the horizontal plane)

See Figure 14.21.

Ventral translation at about 90° abduction

— *Patient:* prone (Fig. 14.22).

Posterolateral translation

— *Aim:* evaluation test. Therapeutic technique for the recovery of internal rotation movement in specific positions. Technique for stretching the posterior capsule.
— *Patient:* seated, arm rotated internally, in a specific position while remaining comfortable.
— *Therapist:* on the side of the shoulder to be treated.
— *Hold:* the scapula and clavicle are steadied by the rear hand, and the hand which performs the translation is positioned anterior to the humeral head, and also in this case close to the joint.
— *Execution:* the direction of the translation is at a tangent to the joint surfaces, and the thrust will therefore follow a posterolateral trajectory, with a small caudal component.
— *Notes:* the hand applying the thrust must be positioned correctly on the humeral head and not on the coracoid apophysis.
This technique is not recommended in the presence of posterior impingement, in cases of posterior instability and if it causes pain (Fig. 14.23).

Inferior capsular stretching

— *Aim:* capsular stretching.
— *Patient:* lateral decubitus, limb abducted as far as the non-physiological limit of the PROM (specific position). Comfortable position for the patient.
— *Therapist:* in front of the patient.

Fig. 14.20

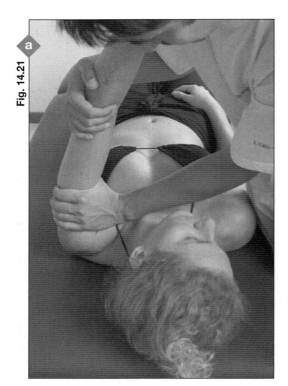

Fig. 14.21

a

b

Glenohumeral joint: traction in a specific position (adduction in the horizontal plane).

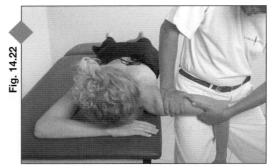

Fig. 14.22

Glenohumeral joint: ventral translation at about 90° abduction.

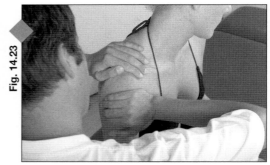

Fig. 14.23

Glenohumeral joint: posterolateral translation.

— *Hold:* holding the humeral diaphysis, close to the glenohumeral joint, the cranial hand supports the arm in a specific position; the caudal hand holds the scapula at the inferior angle.
— *Execution:* the cranial hand causes adduction of the scapula, while the caudal hand keeps the arm in maximum possible abduction.
— *Notes:* This technique is performed in very specific positions, also with an external rotation component added.

Substantial sensitivity and precision are required to perform capsular stretching.

The degree of tissue reactivity should be evaluated before performing the manoeuvre. It is performed by maintaining for 15–20 seconds a position in which the patient perceives a feeling of tension (in the soft tissues stretched). The manoeuvre can be repeated 2–3 times. Care should be taken not to cause pain; the manoeuvre should, therefore, be explained to the patient, along with the importance of patient cooperation. Dynamic techniques should be preferred to passive static stretching.

We propose the following two dynamic techniques:
— *contraction-relaxation:* this technique, which derives from Kabat's principles, involves placing the shoulder in a position close to the maximum possible amplitude of the movement it is intended to develop. The antagonists, in this case the adductors, are then contracted against manual isometric resistance, static contraction is performed for a few seconds, and then the patient is asked to stop contraction rapidly and completely. The relaxation of the muscle is used to gain a few degrees passively in the desired direction; and

— *rhythmic stabilization:* this technique, which is also derived from Kabat, involves placing the shoulder in a position close to the maximum amplitude in relation to that which it is desired to improve. A series of static contractions of the antagonists and then of the agonists of the movement which it is desired to amplify is then performed against maximum manual resistance, and the manoeuvre ends with slight pressure being applied in the chosen direction.

Rhythmic stabilization is followed by a 'hold' (manual static posture, by the therapist, for 15–20 seconds in the desired direction) (Fig. 14.24).

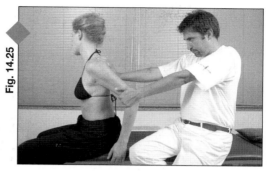

Fig. 14.25

Stretching the anterior capsule.

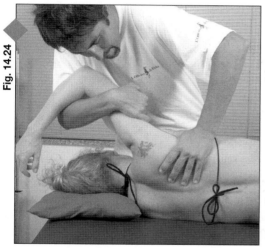

Fig. 14.24

Stretching the inferior capsule.

Stretching the anterior capsule

— *Aim:* stretching the capsule, particularly the anterior part.
— *Patient:* seated.
— *Therapist:* behind the patient, on the side of the shoulder to be treated.
— *Hold:* the medial hand stabilizes the scapula, the outer hand holds the patient's arm close to the elbow.
— *Execution:* the lateral hand extends the shoulder into the specific position desired to stretch the capsule tissue; the medial hand provides anterior thrust to steady the scapula and to keep the patient's trunk in a neutral position (Fig. 14.25).
— *Notes:* as for the previous technique.

Stretching the capsule – anteroinferior part (variant)

— *Notes:* to stabilize the inferior angle of the scapula correctly. The conditions are the same as for the two previous techniques (Fig. 14.26).

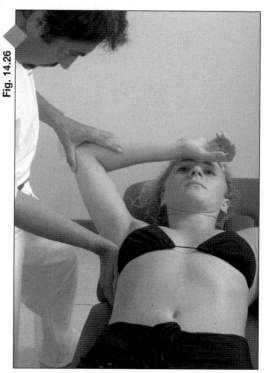

Fig. 14.26

Stretching the anterior capsule (variant).

Stretching the posterior capsule

— *Aim:* stretching the posterior part of the capsule.
— *Patient:* seated, limb abducted at 90° in horizontal adduction of the glenohumeral (in a specific position), in the position in which the scapula begins to abduct.
— *Therapist:* on the side opposite the shoulder to be treated.
— *Hold:* the rear hand placed on the inferior angle of the scapula, the front hand holding the elbow and supporting the patient's limb.
— *Execution:* the rear hand steadies the scapula and the front hand adducts the limb in question.
— *Notes:* This, like all the capsule stretching techniques, must be performed in very specific positions. The procedure is the same as for the other stretching techniques described (Fig. 14.27).

Fig. 14.27

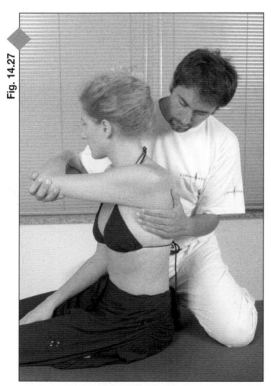

Stretching the posterior capsule.

Attention should be paid to the patient's head: tilting to the opposite side, in the specific position required, will stretch the subscapular nerve.

Variant

— *Notes:* Internal rotation of the limb is induced with one hand, while the other (the outer hand) steadies the elbow correctly. The conditions are the same as for the previous techniques for capsule stretching (Fig. 14.28).

Fig. 14.28

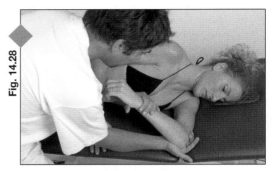

Stretching the posterior capsule (variant).

Scapulothoracic joint

The scapula can perform the following movements: elevation, depression, retraction and protraction (Fig. 14.29).

Fig. 14.29

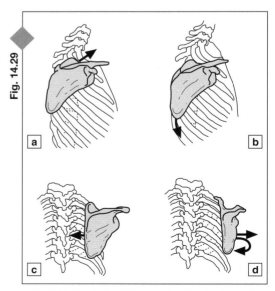

The movements of the scapula: **(a)** elevation, **(b)** depression, **(c)** retraction, **(d)** protraction.

Manipulation

— *Aim:* to free the scapulothoracic joint from possible fibrous adhesions.
— *Patient:* prone.
— *Therapist:* on the side of the scapula to be treated.
— *Hold:* the cranial hand holds the top of the shoulder, while the fingers of the caudal hand, at the inferior angle of the scapula, try to penetrate between the scapula and chest (it is easier to position the caudal hand with a passive inferior glide of the scapula).
— *Execution:* to lift the scapula from the chest, causing distraction, according to a manipulative method. The therapist first tests for the position in which the movement of the scapula is restricted, then tension is increased and it is manipulated in a posterolateral direction, perpendicular to the plan of the scapula on the chest.
— *Notes:* this technique is very useful following long periods of immobilization, which have left sequelae of fibrous adhesions that have formed in the subscapularis muscle and anterior serratus and between the planes of these and the chest.

Crepitation is sometimes felt in the scapulothoracic joint, due to these fibrous adhesions between the scapula and chest.

This technique should not be performed if pain is present or immediately following immobilization (Fig. 14.30).

Mobilization

— *Aim:* to 'free' the scapula.
— *Patient:* lateral decubitus
— *Therapist:* in front of the patient.
— *Hold:* both hands hold the scapula and the caudal hand is placed at the inferior angle, while the cranial hand is positioned very close to the medial rim.
— *Execution:* the therapist looks for the position in which the movement of the scapula is restricted and then 'frees' it: in the posterolateral direction, perpendicular to the plane of the scapula on the chest. (Fig. 14.31).

Gliding

— *Aim:* to mobilize the scapula in retraction and in protraction, proprioceptive training.
— *Patient:* lateral decubitus.

Fig. 14.30

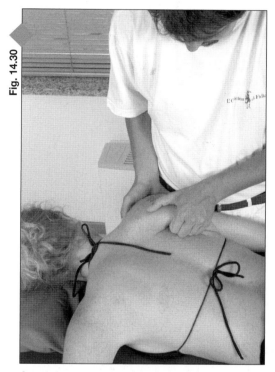

Scapulothoracic joint: manipulation.

Fig. 14.31

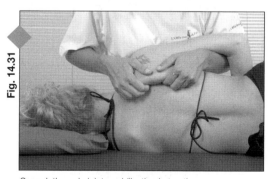

Scapulothoracic joint: mobilization in traction.

— *Therapist:* in front of the patient, with the therapist's caudal arm supporting the patient's arm.
— *Hold:* the cranial hand is positioned above the scapular spine and the therapist uses their own body to steady the scapulohumeral joint; the caudal hand presses on the medial and inferior angle of the scapula.
— *Execution:* both the therapist's hands move the scapula in superior rotation and protraction or inferior rotation and retraction.

Manual therapy in rehabilitation

— *Notes:* movement in protraction may be restricted in patients who have been immobilized for a long period.

Mobilization should take into account the configuration of the glide plane of the ribs-anterior surface of the scapula (rounded surface of the rib cage) (Fig. 14.32).

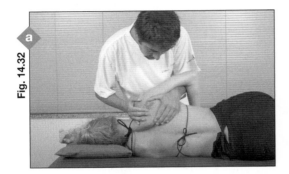

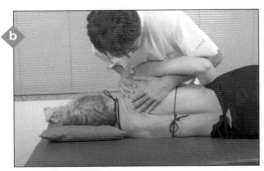

Scapulothoracic joint: gliding in the craniocaudal direction; **(a)** starting position, **(b)** end position.

A dynamic technique can also be performed using the conditions described above, i.e. contraction-relaxation or rhythmic stabilization for proprioception training.

Scapular proprioceptive training

— *Aim:* proprioceptive training. To facilitate the recruitment of the dynamic stabilizers of the scapula (anterior serratus, trapezius, levator scapulae, rhomboid).
— *Patient:* supine decubitus.
— *Therapist:* on the side opposite the scapula.
— *Hold:* with the fingertips in the intercostal space, close to the medial and inferior edge of the scapula (or the superior edge, depending on what is being tested for).

— *Execution:* the fingers push gently against the medial rim of the scapula, and the patient is asked to resist the movement of the scapula.
— *Notes:* vigorous contractions of the muscles should be avoided; the patient should be asked to perform slow, sustained contractions of moderate intensity (Fig. 14.33).

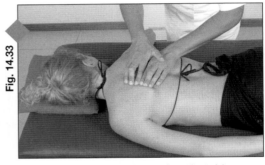

Scapulothoracic joint: scapular proprioceptive training.

Acromioclavicular joint

Although this joint is known to be anatomically variable (Chapter 1), the AC joint rim is generally orientated in a posterolateral direction. The joint surface of the acromion is concave, whereas the distal end of the clavicle has a convex shape. From an arthrokinematic point of view, the movements of the acromion on the clavicle are thus a swing and a glide in the posterolateral direction.

During anterior flexion of the upper limb, the distal end of the clavicle moves as follows:
— through the first few degrees of elevation in a ventral direction;
— in a craniodorsal direction; and
— through the final degrees in a caudal direction.

The distal end of the clavicle can be imagined to move in the shape of a '6' during anterior flexion.

Examination and palpation of the acromioclavicular joint

The landmark for the correct palpation of the AC joint is the spine of the scapula. The scapular spine forms the lateral continuation of the dorsal part of the acromion. It is easy to identify the angle and the anterior part of the acromion at this point. The joint rim can, however, be palpated by following the clavicle from the inner to the outer side, in the direction of the acromion.

Fig. 14.32

Fig. 14.33

Traction

— *Aim:* to evaluate the arthrokinematic movements for setting the cockpit parameters, to treat any joint limitations.
— *Patient:* seated, the back supported against the therapist.
— *Therapist:* behind the patient.
— *Hold:* the therapist holds the lateral third of the clavicle between the index finger and thumb of their inner hand; the thumb of the outer hand rests on the scapular spine, while the index finger presses on the anterior part of the acromion.
— *Execution:* The therapist applies traction in a dorsolateral direction to the acromion with the outer hand, while the inner hand steadies the clavicle.
— *Notes:* the technique involves traction on the acromion backwards and outwards, in line with the joint physiology.

The manoeuvre should be performed correctly on the acromion and the humerus should not be moved in a poster direction in error (Fig. 14.34).

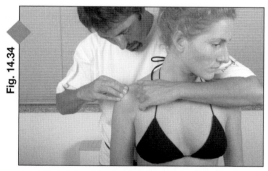

Fig. 14.34

Acromioclavicluar joint: traction.

Posterolateral translation

— *Aim:* to evaluate and treat posterolateral translation movement.
— *Patient:* seated, with the back supported against the examiner.
— *Therapist:* as above.
— *Hold:* as above.
— *Execution:* the medial hand steadies the clavicle (as in the previous technique), while the lateral hand applies translation in a posterolateral direction and an accessory medial end-range component for the morphofunctional characteristics of the clavicle (Fig. 14.35).

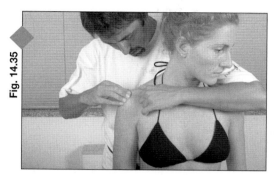

Fig. 14.35

Acromioclavicular joint: dorsolateral translation.

Sternocostoclavicular joint

The sternocostoclavicular joint is saddle-shaped: it has two curves running in opposite directions; it is convex in one direction and concave in the other.

The sternal end of the clavicle:
— is concave in a ventrodorsal direction; and
— is convex in a craniocaudal direction.

The arthrokinematic movements of the sternocostoclavicular joint, in relation to the angular movements, can be described as follows:
— *protraction of the shoulder:* (ventral swing and glide) movement of the sternal end of the clavicle in a ventral direction;
— *retraction of the shoulder:* (dorsal swing and glide) movement of the sternal end of the clavicle in a dorsal direction;
— *elevation of the shoulder:* (cranial roll and caudolateral slide) the rotation movement occurs in the opposite direction to the translation; and
— *depression of the shoulder:* (caudal roll and craniomedial slide) the rotation movement occurs in the opposite direction to the translation.

As with the other joints already examined, the movement of the sternocostoclavicular joint can be limited at any point in the arc of movement, not necessarily at the end of range.

Examination and palpation of the sternocostoclavicular joint

With a finger positioned close to the superior angle of the sternum, on the clavicular side, the movement of the clavicle can be perceived on the sternum by performing protraction and retraction movements of the shoulder, and the joint rim can thus be identified.

Manual therapy in rehabilitation

Traction

— *Aim:* to evaluate the arthrokinematic movements to set the cockpit parameters, to treat any joint limitations.
— *Patient:* seated, with the back supported against the therapist.
— *Therapist:* behind the patient.
— *Hold:* the physiotherapist's lateral hand pinches the proximal third of the clavicle, with the index finger and thumb of the medial hand on the joint rim, the other fingers on the sternum.
— *Execution:* the lateral hand applies traction on the clavicle along its axis (lateral and slightly dorsal direction).
— *Notes:* the technique involves traction of the clavicle backwards and outwards in line with the joint physiology.

The manoeuvre should be performed correctly on the clavicle, and the scapula should not be stabilized in error (Fig. 14.36a), variant in the supine position (Fig. 14.36b).

Caudolateral translation

— *Aim:* to evaluate the arthrokinematic movements to set the cockpit parameters, to treat any joint limitations affecting shoulder elevation and abduction.
— *Patient:* supine, shoulder position in elevation (specific position) at the point of limitation.
— *Therapist:* cranial to the patient.
— *Hold:* the lateral hand is on the clavicle, the thumb on the upper surface of the clavicle close to the joint; the medial hand is supported on the chest, with the thumb supporting the thumb of the opposite hand.
— *Execution:* translation in a caudolateral direction.
— *Notes:* the technique also provides for a combination of the translation movement with the elevation movement (e.g. the lateral hand elevates the shoulder while the thumb of the medial hand encourages caudolateral translation) (Fig. 14.37a); variant: while the outer hand carries out the translation, the fingers of the inner hand palpate the rim, evaluating the movement (Fig. 14.37b).

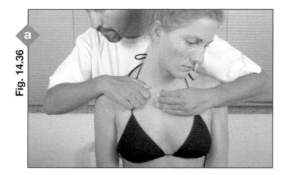
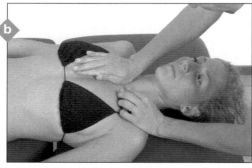

Fig. 14.36

a

b

Sternoclavicular joint: **(a)** traction, **(b)** variant in a supine position.

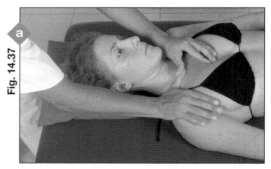
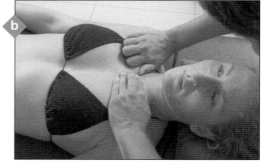

Fig. 14.37

a

b

Sternoclavicular joint: **(a)** caudolateral translation, **(b)** variant.

Craniomedial translation

— *Aim:* to evaluate the arthrokinematic movements to set the cockpit parameters, to treat any joint limitations.
— *Patient:* supine, shoulder in a depressed position (specific position) at the point of limitation.
— *Therapist:* on the side of the shoulder to be treated, orientated in a cranial direction in relation to the patient.
— *Hold:* the thumb of the lateral hand on the anteroinferior surface of the clavicle, in its medial part; the inner hand supported on the chest and the thumb positioned on the back of the other thumb.
— *Execution:* translation in a craniomedial direction.
— *Notes:* this technique also provides for a combination of the translation movement with the depression movement (e.g. the lateral hand depresses the shoulder, while the thumb of the medial hand encourages craniomedial translation) (Fig. 14.38).

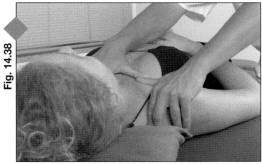

Fig. 14.38

Sternoclavicular joint: craniomedial translation.

Variant

While the outer hand carries out the translation, the fingers of the inner hand palpate the rim, evaluating the movement.

Dorsal translation

— *Aim:* to evaluate the arthrokinematic movements to set the cockpit parameters, to treat any joint limitations due to anteflexion, protraction and horizontal adduction of the shoulder.
— *Patient:* supine, shoulder to be evaluated off the couch.

— *Therapist:* on the side opposite the shoulder to be treated, facing in a cranial direction in relation to the patient.
— *Hold:* the outer hand holds the top of the shoulder — the acromial end — while the middle and ring fingers of the inner hand steady the sternum close to the joint.
— *Execution:* the physiotherapist retracts the shoulder, while evaluating the movement at a sternoclavicular level with the medial hand.
— *Notes:* the shoulder should be sufficiently free to retract to reach the end of the range: this is possible by positioning the top of the shoulder off the couch, or adding a soft layer under the spinal column.

Ventral translation

— *Aim:* to evaluate the arthrokinematic movements to set the cockpit parameters, to treat any joint limitations due to the anteflexion, protraction and horizontal adduction of the shoulder.
— *Patient:* supine, arm abducted at about 90° and in horizontal adduction (specific position).
— *Therapist:* on the side of the shoulder to be treated, facing in a cranial direction in relation to the patient.
— *Hold:* the proximal hand holds the arm — above the elbow — while the distal hand steadies the sternum close to the joint.
— *Execution:* the physiotherapist protracts the shoulder steadying the sternum, or holds the shoulder in protraction and applies force to the sternum in a dorsal direction.
— *Note:* this technique may be painful for the patient.

Conclusions

The examples shown in this chapter provide an overview of situations in which passive treatment may be beneficial in reducing pain or increasing the range of movement of the shoulder complex.

The biomechanical principles underlying mobilization state that, in order for a physiological angular movement (for example, abduction) to occur, a normal arthrokinematic movement must also take place.

The techniques shown are valid for restoring the normal function of a joint.

A knowledge of neurophysiology reveals that lower grades of mobilization (grades 1 and 2) can alleviate pain and improve vascularization, whereas grades 3 and 4 can additionally help to recover the PROM.

Manual therapy in rehabilitation

Mobilization techniques are chosen by the physiotherapist according to the information yielded by the subjective and objective examination, the diagnosis and the guidelines provided by the surgeon. The conditions and contraindications for these techniques are based on a knowledge of pure science and on the correct classification of the clinical case being treated.

Acknowledgements

To all my friends and colleagues at the 'Officina di Fidia' Rehabilitation Centre, and in particular Mauro Scopa, Gianni Secchiari and Cristina Berdini (graduates in Motor Sciences), and Sabina Caciorgna and Luca Ensebi (holders of the ISEF diploma).

Bibliography

Akeson W.H., Amiel D., Abel M.F., Garfin S.R., Woo S.L., 'Effects of immobilization on joints', *Clin. Orthop.* 219: 28–37, (1987)

Akeson W.H., Amiel D., Woo S.L., 'Immobility effects on synovial joints: the pathomechanics of joint contracture', *Biorheology* 17(1–2): 95–110, (1980)

Amiel D., Akeson W.H., Harwood F.L., Mechanic G.L., 'The effect of immobilization on the types of collagen synthesized in periarticular connective tissue', *Connective Tissue Res.* 8(1): 27–32, (1980)

Bang M.D., Deyle G.D., 'Comparison of supervised exercise with and without manual physical therapy for patients with shoulder impingement syndrome', *J. Orthop. Sports Phys. Ther.* 30(3): 126–137, (2000)

Barden J.M., Balyk R., Raso V.J., Moreau M., Bagnall K., 'Dynamic upper limb proprioception in multidirectional shoulder instability', *Clin. Orthop. Relat. Res.* 420: 181–189, (2004)

Bellotti P., Matteucci E., *Allenamento sportive*, UTET, Turin (1999)

Calligaris A., *Le scienze dell'allenamento*, Società Stampa Sportiva, Rome, (1997)

Cohen K.I., McCoy B.J., Diegelmann R.F., 'An update on wound healing', *Ann. Plast. Surg.* 3: 264, (1979)

Evans D., 'The use of human tissue: an outsider's view', NZ. *Bioeth.* J. 3(2): 13–15, (2002)

Frank C., Akeson W.H., Woo S.L., Amiel D., Coutts R.D., 'Physiology and therapeutic value of passive joint motion', *Clin. Orthop.* 185: 113–125, (1984)

Hart D.P., Dahners L.E., 'Healing of the medial collateral ligament in rats. The effects of repair, motion and secondary stabilizing ligaments', *J. Bone Joint Surg.* 69(A): 1194–1199, (1987)

Howell S.M., Galinat B.J., 'Normal and abnormal mechanics of the glenohumeral joint in the horizontal plane', *J. Bone Joint Surg.* 70: 227, (1988)

Israel S., *Grundprinzipien der Bewewungsbedingten Koerpelichen Adaptation*, Koerpererziehungen, pp. 35–37, (1985)

Kellet J., 'Acute ST injuries, a review of the literature', *Med. Sci. Sports Exerc.* 18: 5, (1986)

Kibler B.W., 'Role of the scapula in the overhead throwing motion', *Contemp. Orthop.* 22: 525, (1991)

Kvist M., Jarvinen M., 'Clinical histological and biomechanical features in repair of muscle and tendon injuries', *Int. J. Sports Med.* 3: 12–14, (1982)

Maitland G.D., *Peripheral Manipulation*, 3rd ed. Butterworth-Heinemann, pp. 85–97, (1991)

Myers J.B., Ju Y.Y., Hwang J.H., McMahon P.J., Rodosky M.W., Lephart S.M., 'Reflexive muscle activation alterations in shoulders with anterior glenohumeral instability', *Am. J. Sports Med.* 32(4): 1013–1021, (2004)

Myers J.B., Riemann B.L., Ju Y.Y., Hwang J.H., McMahon P.J., Lephart S.M., 'Shoulder muscle reflex latencies under various levels of muscle contraction,' *Clin. Orthop. Relat. Res.* 407: 92–101, (2003)

Nicholson C.G., 'The effects of passive joint mobilization on pain and hypomobility associated with adhesive capsulitis of the shoulder', *J. Orthop. Sports Phys. Ther.* 6238, (1985)

Pontano O., *Le basi biologiche dell'allenamento*, Libreria dell'Università Editrice, Pescara, (1995)

Poppen N.K., Walter P.S., 'Normal and abnormal motion of the shoulder', *J. Bone Joint Surg.* 58: 195, (1976)

Ricciarelli L., Toccaceli A., *Teoria e metodologia dell'allenamento*, Società Stampa Sportiva, Rome, (1976)

Tipton C.M., James S.L., Mergner W. et al., 'Influence of exercise on strength of medial collateral knee ligaments of dogs', *Am. J. Physiol.* 218: 894–902, (1970)

Vailas A.C., Tipton C.M., Matthers R.D. et al., 'Physical activity and its influence on the repair process of medial collateral ligaments', *Connect Tissue Res.* 9: 25–31, (1981)

Van Wingerden B.A.M., 'Connective tissue in rehabilitation', Scipro Verlag, Vaduz (Liechtenstein) (1995)

Vidik A., 'On the rheology and morphology of soft collagenous tissue', *J. Anat.* 105: 184, (1969)

Von Eisenhart-Rothe R.M., Jager A., Englmeier K.H., Vogl T.J., Graichen H., 'Relevance of arm position and muscle activity on three-dimensional glenohumeral translation in patients with traumatic and atraumatic shoulder instability', *Am. J. Sports Med.* 30(4): 514–522, (2002)

Von Eisenhart-Rothe R., Matsen F.A. 3rd, Eckstein F., Vogl T., Graichen H., 'Pathomechanics in Atraumatic Shoulder Instability: Scapular Positioning Correlates with Humeral Head Centering', *Clin. Orthop. Relat. Res.* 433: 82–89, (2005)

Warner J.J., Lephart S., Fu F.H., 'Role of proprioception in the pathoetiology of shoulder instability', *Clin. Orthop. Relat. Res.* 330: 35–39, (1996)

Warner J.J., Micheli L.J., Arslanian L.E., Kennedy J., Kennedy R., 'Patterns of flexibility, laxity, and strength in normal shoulders and shoulders with instability and impingement', *Am. J. Sports Med.* 18(4): 366–375, (1990)

THERAPEUTIC EXERCISE IN REHABILITATION

CHAPTER 15

F. MUSARRA

A great deal of attention is paid in the literature to therapeutic exercise for painful shoulder. In this chapter we shall try to analyse the intrinsic parameters governing exercises which should be taken into consideration when planning therapeutic exercise for painful shoulder.

We came up against some serious problems when producing this chapter. The scientific literature, which has been expanded in recent decades by many articles about shoulder problems, is not yet sufficiently clear as regards the intrinsic rehabilitation factors underlying therapeutic exercises for painful shoulder. The various articles often analyse different disorders in different populations. It is consequently problematic to compare the various data appearing in the literature.

The paper by Burkhead (1992), for example, shows that conservative treatment is more likely to be indicated in glenohumeral dislocation when atraumatic instability is involved; Brostrom (1992), however, achieved better results using conservative treatment for traumatic shoulder injury. This example clearly shows that the exercise programme recommended is not very different for two different forms of instability and that it is chosen without regard to whether the exercises are suited to the various types of instability. It is, therefore, difficult to evaluate and compare the results obtained from the papers by these two authors.

A further point for initial criticism is the fact that the intrinsic variables of the exercises recommended in the various papers on rehabilitation exercises for painful shoulder are not specified (Allegrucci, 1994; Andersen, 1999; Bang, 2000; Brostrom, 1992; Burkhead, 1992; Davies, 1993; Heiderscheit, 1996; Kamkar, 1993; Kibler, 2001; Russ, 1998; Tortensen, 1994; Van Wingerden, 1997; Wilk, 1993, 2002). Wilk (2002), for example, presents a rehabilitation programme characterized by a functional progression and progressive steps, both clearly justified but, in our opinion, lacking in clarity as regards how to perform the exercise effectively. External or internal rotation exercises of the shoulder with an elastic band can be performed at various speeds, various tensions, different angles of movement, with repetitions, or with more emphasis on eccentric or concentric movement. These variations should not be underestimated because they significantly influence the result of the exercise. The method of performing the exercise determines and depends on the objectives aimed at through a particular exercise.

The inadequate description of exercises leads to the publication of superficial rehabilitation protocols, which do not remedy these shortfalls because they simply suggest a recommended route which is based too often on the authors' interpretations. For example, a comparison of conservative rehabilitation, as proposed by Wilk (2002) and Kibler (2001), shows that they differ significantly from one another. Kibler (2001) proposes a programme involving a functional progression, starting with control of the pelvis, continuing with the trunk and scapula, and ending with the functional control of the glenohumeral joint during throwing. Wilk (2002) adopts a different position for the rehabilitation of painful shoulder in a throwing athlete. While taking into account the importance

Therapeutic exercise in rehabilitation

of functional rehabilitation, Wilk prefers to start with analytical rehabilitation, which places particular emphasis on strengthening the rotator cuff, particularly by external rotation. Both views have their merits, in our opinion, but the starting point, i.e. the strategies and objectives of rehabilitation, are a source of differences between the two.

We would nevertheless like to stress that our aim in making the above comments is to suggest not that these recommendations are invalid, but that they depend on many other factors, not just the disorder in question, and that these factors do not allow a generalized approach to the problem and render a static proto-col irrelevant. The discussion should, in fact, focus on the intrinsic parameters of therapeutic exercise. The lack of scientific evidence currently available in the literature regarding the application of therapeutic exercise in painful shoulder suggests that the literature is lacking in methodology and has a low interpret-ational power (Casonato, 2003; Desmeules, 2003).

The two systematic reviews available in the literature clearly demonstrate this hypothesis (Green, 2003; Philadephia Panel, 2001). The systematic study conducted by the Philadephia Panel (2001) suggests that there is little scientific evidence as regards therapeutic exercise for painful shoulder. The guidelines proposed by the american physical therapy association (APTA) are, according to this study, weak, too vague and not based on a review of the scientific evidence contained in the literature. The positive physiological effects of exercise have not been demonstrated clinically, since insufficient attention has been paid to the type of exercise, adequate intensity and progression (Philadephia Panel, 2001). The systematic review by Green (2003), in a more recent study, shows that therapeutic exercise is effective depending on the duration of the recovery in the short term, and on the functional recovery of rotator cuff injuries in the long term. The combination of therapeutic exercise with manual mobilization has greater benefit, while ultrasound does not improve therapeutic exercise further. The author concludes that the heterogeneous population in the various papers, the small number of groups studied, the methodological quality, the physiotherapy applied and the length of the follow-up of randomized clinical trials were poor, resulting in poor overall evidence. According to the same author (Green, 2003), there is a need in the literature for trials to assess the efficacy of therapeutic exercise, controlling the specific clinical conditions associated with painful shoulder conditions, and the methods of performing the various exercises, both separately and together, not forgetting

to compare them with progress in patients not treated by physiotherapy.

The rehabilitation programmes proposed are mainly based on EMG studies performed on the shoulder (Hinstermeister, 1998) and on studies of isokinetic contractions between healthy volunteers and patients or between the healthy arm and the injured arm. There has been little prospective research, and too few clinical trials have been conducted. This does not mean that the information available in the literature, as already stated, should not be taken into consideration, but that in order to design a valid rehabilitation programme, a methodologically validated structure is needed so that the athlete can return to maximum performance levels.

A careful clinical evaluation, a correct diagnosis and a rehabilitation programme that places the emphasis on monitoring the inflammatory reaction, the recovery of muscle balance, increasing soft tissue flexibility, increasing proprioception, neuromuscular control and resuming specific sport-related activity form the basis for success, according to Wilk (2002). While sharing Wilk's view, we believe not only that a rehabilitation programme should contain these exercise techniques, but also that the intrinsic parameters of the exercises recommended should be taken into consideration.

To ensure that the choice of parameters is valid, it needs to be based on a validated methodology and on the information currently available in the literature. Muscle strengthening may, for example, be suggested for the internal rotators of the shoulder in order to improve their contribution to controlling the stability of the glenohumeral joint; but what are the conditions or, if we wish, according to which parameters should this exercise be performed? Little attention is paid in the literature to these aspects, which express a rehabilitation programme in keeping with the functional progression which has received so much acclaim in recent years.

There has already been discussion of aspects such as postoperative rehabilitation, the role of manual therapy in rehabilitation of the shoulder and the biopsychosocial model proposed by the WHO. We believe that the MLCM, which is a model applicable to rehabilitation based on the WHO proposal (which is based, in turn, on the knowledge that disorders can arise from excessive external load or from a reduction in internal carriability), is a valid solution for utilizing the intrinsic parameters of therapeutic exercise (Bernards, 1994). This model includes all the variables, including individual psychosocial variables. The choice of the type of exercise and functional progression within the programme should take into account personal variables and the individual personal context.

An individual's carriability can be reduced at a local level, for example after a period in plaster, or generally during stress or bereavement. The correct programming of the loads given should take these variables into consideration. The rehabilitation specialist, who administers an exercise with the aim of altering a condition by providing a training stimulus, should be aware that this stimulus will produce an adaptation, and will be effective only if the intensity is in accordance with the individual's carriability. A smaller stimulus, as shown, would not lead to any alteration of the symptoms, whereas a greater stimulus would cause a non-functional adaptation or even an inflammatory reaction. A training stimulus in accordance with carriability will ensure good functional adaptation (Fig. 15.1b). The MLCM is a model that helps the physiotherapist to carry out the physiotherapeutic evaluation, to define objectives and strategies for rehabilitation and to apply the treatment, in accordance with all the variables mentioned.

We shall briefly introduce the MLCM in the next section and shall discuss which of its aspects influence functional progression. We shall finally try to determine the intrinsic parameters of exercises that are relevant for the rehabilitation of painful shoulder.

Multidimensional load/carriability model

The physiotherapist is required to deal daily with patients with various movement incapacity problems (Hagenaars, 2002). The factors responsible for the various disorders are not limited to the locomotor system; they may also include internal and external personal factors. Physiotherapy is aimed above all at dysfunctions, limitations and, only secondarily, the type of damage (Heerkens, 1993). The MLCM focuses on the functional aspect of the disorder. This model provides the physiotherapist with a methodological approach for managing the various disorders of the musculoskeletal system. The comments made in the previous chapter, regarding the biopsychosocial model, have thus been translated into a practical model, which clearly contains a method of evaluating the clinical picture, starting from the medical diagnosis, going on to the physiotherapeutic diagnosis, and ending with planning the rehabilitation treatment (Fig. 15.2). The physiotherapeutic diagnosis has a fundamental role here, analysing the functional deficit present which is to be improved through therapeutic exercise. The model, which was developed from training science, interprets musculoskeletal damage as the result of an imbalance between the external load to which the body, organ or tissue is subjected, and their carriability. An imbalance between the two components may be caused either by an increased external load, such as a trauma, for example, or by a reduction in carriability, such as after a period of immobilization. This reduction in tissue and organ carriability can be caused, in turn, by either a local disorder or 'personal' factors, such as motivation, anxiety or fear (Hagenaars, 2002). The behavioural characteristics of the individual also have a significant influence on the healing process. Bereavement in the family can be a negative prognostic factor, because it can significantly slow this process. The term 'multidimensional' highlights the fact that the reduction in carriability could arise from either local factors or individual, personal factors of various types. Furthermore, adaptation to the external load takes place through a process of adaptation of the body. Adaptation, which forms the basis for all training, is also related to personal factors, i.e. anxiety, motivation, fears, the patient's gender and age, systemic and hereditary diseases, etc. (Bernards, 1999). The clinical history of

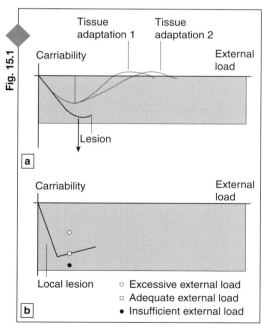

Fig. 15.1

(a) Tissue-specific temporal adaptation. The duration of the recovery after a training stimulus is tissue-specific.
(b) Relation between external load and internal carriability after a local injury (modified from Van Wingerden, 1997).

Therapeutic exercise in rehabilitation

Fig. 15.2

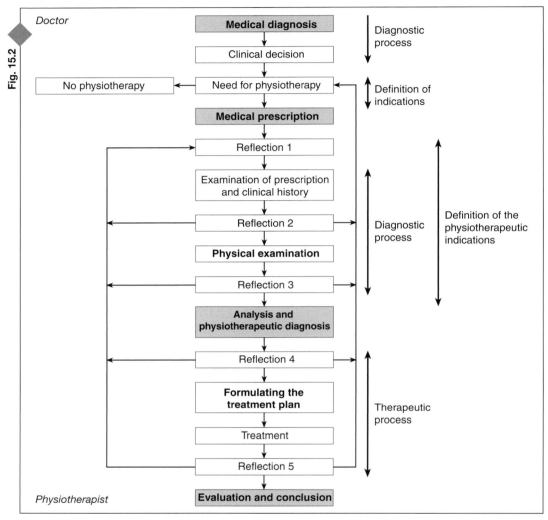

Doctor

Medical diagnosis

Clinical decision

Diagnostic process

No physiotherapy ← Need for physiotherapy

Definition of indications

Medical prescription

Reflection 1

Examination of prescription and clinical history

Reflection 2

Diagnostic process

Physical examination

Reflection 3

Definition of the physiotherapeutic indications

Analysis and physiotherapeutic diagnosis

Reflection 4

Formulating the treatment plan

Therapeutic process

Treatment

Reflection 5

Physiotherapist

Evaluation and conclusion

The physiotherapeutic approach to health profile according to the Royal Dutch Physiotherapy Association – Koninklijke Nederlands Genootschap voor Fysiotherapie (modified from Hagenaars, 2002).

the musculoskeletal systems and its overall condition should also be taken into consideration in this context. The ability to adapt is, moreover, tissue specific and, as it is well known, cartilage tissue has a very different turnover to muscle tissue (de Moree, 1993).

Neglecting these aspects could result in failures and poor adaptation. Recovery that is too hurried, which fails to allow for the phases of healing, for example, after a muscle tear, causes inflexible and dysfunctional scar tissue (Van Wingerden, 1997). The healing process, characterized by the initial inflammatory phase, proliferation and maturing and remodelling, ensures the full recovery of functions only if the adaptation process is not disrupted by the factors mentioned above or by a rehabilitation programme which fails to take into account natural healing times (Jarvinen, 1993; Noonen, 1992; Stanish, 2000).

A further aspect which should not be disregarded is tissue specificity. The exercises recommended should have characteristics that are closely compatible with the sport which the patient wishes to resume. The adaptation process prepares the affected area through the stimuli applied. This means that the rehabilitation programme should evolve as soon as possible towards exercises which are as general and functional as possible. For effective training, it is necessary to understand the carriability of the affected area, to recommend more functional exercises and to determine the external load such that it stimulates the adaptation process in an effective and functional manner.

Therapeutic exercise should help to give the correct training stimulus to tissue, bearing in mind the carriability at that time. The training stimulus for therapeutic exercise is, like any type of training, based on the theory of overcompensation (Fig. 15.1a).

Remember that:

— the MLCM is a practical model for rehabilitation based on the WHO interpretation of health;
— the model provides for application, starting with the evaluation and gathering of data about the problem, and ending with the implementation of the rehabilitation programme;
— therapeutic exercise is only an aid to rehabilitation, which must clearly be carried out according to the criteria of the model; and
— the MLCM grew out of the science of training, which attributes great importance to the process of adaptation of the body and to the conditions of stimulating healing, based on the theory of overcompensation.

Carriability and determining exercise load

In the light of the above considerations, exercise load is determined on the basis of the information gathered from the physiotherapeutic diagnosis which interprets the level of carriability, possible additional functional tests, the factors of the various dimensions which influence it and the objective of the exercise in giving a training stimulus.

The exercise load is determined in advance, during the planning of the exercises and subsequently through continual adaptation during the progression towards the recovery of sport-related activity. It is in these terms that we wish firstly to discuss the exercise load in the light of serious impairments which may influence internal carriability. These data should be combined with the need for an external sport-specific load, (which will be discussed in the section on Psychosocial factors and impairment).

Carriability is the expression of the local and general state of health of the individual. We shall analyse below in greater detail the parameters that are crucial when planning therapeutic exercise, i.e. pain, muscle impairment, impairment of mobility and psychosocial impairment.

Pain as impairment

Our aim in this section is not to analyse the parameter pain from a pathophysiological or diagnostic point of view, but to correlate it with the functional progression in the rehabilitation programme. It is consequently important to know what type of influence pain can have on motor control.

The IASP defines pain as: 'an unpleasant sensory and emotional experience associated with actual or potential tissue damage or described in terms of such damage' (Merskey, 1997). Pain is not, therefore, synonymous with tissue damage, but it can be a warning of potential damage. Therapeutic exercise should not cause pain, because this could indicate further injury to already damaged tissue or have an adverse influence on the adaptation process underlying the improvement in carriability. Hodges (2003) recently presented a review of the influence of pain on motor control (Fig. 15.3), hypothesizing that pain, through various channels such as internal body dynamics, cortical centres, motor planning, proprioceptive input and emotional factors (such as fear, stress and concentration), can alter motor control (Hodges, 2003).

This paper makes two important points: firstly that the proprioceptive deficit and dyskinesia of the scapula, mentioned by many other authors as major aetiological factors in painful shoulder, might then also be secondary factors of subacromial impingement; and secondly that the patient should not feel pain while performing the exercise.

Pain has an adverse influence on the process of adaptation, causing it to be suboptimal. It may lead to muscle imbalances and alter motor control during movement, and this is manifested as an impaired humeroscapular rhythm or a posture with a scapular or humeroscapular deviation (Comerford, 2001; Sahrmann, 2002). The presence of pain during the exercise or an hour or a day later suggests that the workload was probably excessive. The physiotherapist should adapt the exercises, adjusting the internal parameters or changing the exercises themselves.

The adaptation model proposed by Lund (1991) and reported by Hodges (2003) and Sterling (2001) suggests that there is a link between pain and

Therapeutic exercise in rehabilitation

Fig. 15.3

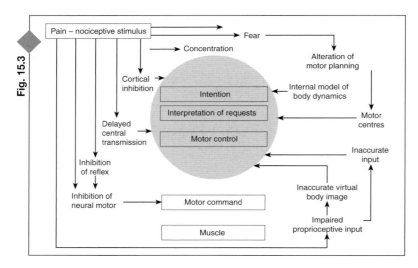

Possible influence of pain on motor control (modified from Hodges, 2003).

parameters such as concentration, fear and stress, confirming once again that the person should be viewed overall.

Functional exercise, which aims to stimulate the healing process, should necessarily take into account the level of reactivity of the shoulder. Any overuse causes an inflammatory reaction, according to Stanish (2000), and inappropriate metabolic adaptation, with the risk that it may lead to a permanently chronic condition. At first the pain is present even at rest, then it is perceived by the patient in the subsequent phases mainly when performing movements or in positions that the patient knows to be painful, such as sleeping on the affected shoulder. Various protocols interpret the absence of pain at rest as a marker indicating that second phase exercises can be started; the absence of pain in daily activities does, in fact, mean that workloads can be increased further, almost to sport-specific loads (Keirns, 1998).

We can conclude that pain is a marker of the patient's carriability.

A functional progression should also respect the natural healing process, which in the literature is usually divided into inflammatory, proliferation and maturation phases (Stanish, 2000).

Finally, we consider it necessary to deduce from the physiotherapeutic diagnosis the levels of reactivity and selectivity, which are a sign of the patient's ability to react effectively to the stimuli of training and type of pain. The type of pain provides us with further information on the origin of the problem. An acute pain is normally sharp, while a chronic pain causes a dull ache. A burning pain is usually the expression of a sympathetic dysfunction, whereas sudden shooting pains often indicate internal joint injury or a partial tear of muscle or tendon tissue in the acute phase. Nocturnal pain suggests an inflammatory problem, while mechanical pain appears mainly at the beginning or end of the day. Classifying pain as an impairment, therefore, helps us to plan exercises in keeping with internal carriability.

Conclusions as regards therapeutic exercise

In the first or inflammatory phase, the primary objective is a reduction in pain. The therapeutic measures mentioned in the literature to achieve this are varied: TENS (Nitz, 1986), hot and cold (Altechek, 2001; Nitz, 1986; Russ, 1998; Wilk, 2002) and injections (Altechek, 2001; Bigliani, 1997); NSAI (Altechek, 2001; Bigliani, 1997); ultrasound (Wilk, 2002; Nitz, 1986), manual therapy (Bang, 2000; Casonato, 2003; Conroy, 1998; Nitz, 1986), rest, and thermal therapy. The randomized prospective study conducted by Bang (2000) shows that manual techniques can relieve shoulder pain due to impingement.

Conroy (1998) also showed, in a randomized trial, that pain in painful shoulder due to primary impingement syndrome can be reduced significantly. Green (2003) maintains that the efficacy of ultrasound, in contrast with NSAI, is poor in painful shoulder, frozen shoulder and tendinitis of the rotator cuff. Laser therapy is, however, more effective than the placebo in frozen shoulder, whereas it is not for rotator cuff tendinitis. Ultrasound and pulsed electromagnetic therapy are capable of reducing pain in calcific tendinitis.

According to the Philadephia Panel (2001), TENS, thermal therapy, therapeutic massage, electrical stimulation and combined rehabilitation techniques are not effective for painful shoulder, whereas ultrasound demonstrates a good level of efficacy in calcific tendinopathy in the first two months, however this result has not been confirmed after five months (Philadephia Panel, 2001).

The randomized study conducted by Ginn (1997) suggests that therapeutic exercise significantly reduces pain in patients with a mechanical shoulder disorder, and becomes more important the nearer the proliferation and maturation phases of healing. Providing stimuli that are functionally useful for the activity the patient has to carry out is vital for achieving adaptation (Van Wingerden, 1997). In chronic painful shoulder, therapeutic exercise is the only way of bringing carriability, and thus functionality, to the desired level.

The type and intensity of the pain, like the presence of pain during functional activity characterized by a specific daily rhythm, are vital for interpreting the patient's state of health.

When analysing the PHP, it is very important to evaluate whether the impairment present is consistent with the resulting dysfunction and level of participation. An excessive loss of participation and functions in relation to the impairment present suggests that the pain perceived is experienced in an excessively negative manner, and that the patient's response to the problem is inappropriate. In these cases, the rehabilitation programme should be suited to the patient, and the patient should be advised how to act, concentrating on not overloading the affected shoulder. An effective and efficient means of analysis is to use the MPQ (Wadell, 2000). This interpretation demonstrates once again how constructing the rehabilitation programme using the PDS model allows each aspect of the individual and their influence on the problem, to be considered.

Loeser's circles (Loeser, 1980) (Fig. 15.4), which demonstrate the different dimensions of pain perceived and in which the size of the circle indicates the importance of the various dimensions, are an excellent way of expressing the characteristics of the pain perceived.

Pain is a fundamental parameter when planning rehabilitation and as well as providing information on the location of the lesion and on local and overall carriability, it shows how current the pain is. These data are very important when planning a therapeutic exercise protocol. It is also important to note how closely

Fig. 15.4

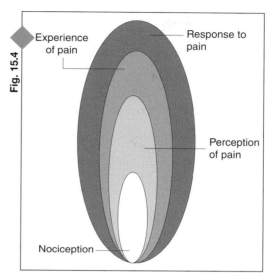

The various components of pain (modified from Loeser, 1980).

the pain is associated with shoulder function. It may, in turn, cause dysfunction of motor control and lead to muscle imbalances which may cause other problems. It is not yet clear, for example, whether an impaired humeroscapular rhythm, also known as scapular dyskinesia, is primary or secondary to subacromial impingement (Matsen, 1990; Warner, 1992). The results obtained by T'Jonck (1998) in his doctoral thesis nevertheless confirm this theory and led him to conclude that the loss of humeroscapular rhythm is a compensatory mechanism for pain relief, induced by the pain present in the acute phase.

There are several electromedical applications for the treatment of pain, and there are as many different medical applications. Therapeutic exercise may act indirectly on pain as an impairment. As mentioned above, therapeutic exercise may indirectly reduce pain, improving its causal factors, for example joint limitation causing subacromial impingement.

Exercise should never be the cause of further pain; consequently, if therapeutic exercise is impossible in the more acute phase, in the presence of severe reactivity, it is often preferable to implement an initial rehabilitation programme without exercise.

Motor control as impairment

Analysis of the various muscle impairments is key to the rehabilitation of painful shoulder. Although studies in the literature formerly analysed muscle activity during a motor movement, owing to the contribution that the muscles made to performing the movement, attention has shifted in the last decade to the motor control necessary to ensure the correct performance of the movement. Various authors have mentioned motor control as an important aetiological factor in musculoskeletal dysfunction (Comerford, 2001; Hodges, 2003, 1999; Lee, 2000; Richardson, 1999; Sahrmann, 2002; Vleeming, 1997). Panjabi (Vleeming, 1997) proposed a conceptual model which describes the various systems responsible for joint stability. This model, proposed initially for the spine, is valid for the whole musculoskeletal system (Lee, 2000). Panjabi defined joint stability as the result of sufficient interaction between inert structures (passive system), the activity of the myofascial system (active system), and the neurological control system (Fig. 15.5). Contact between the two joint surfaces should occur, according to Panjabi (Vleeming, 1997), inside a 'neutral zone', which indicates the centring and stability of a joint. A joint with a point of contact between these joint heads outside the neutral zone is defined as unstable. The three systems mentioned above should control the joint translations occurring at the glenoid level during movements of the arm. See Chapter 2 for the inert ligament and bone component.

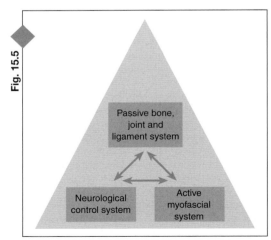

Fig. 15.5

Conceptual model of joint stability (modified from Panjabi, 1992).

In this chapter we shall firstly analyse the role of the myofascial component, and then successively incorporate it in concepts relating to the contribution of neurological control.

The active myofascial system

The myofascial system, which is an anatomical structure, has an important role in the aetiopathogenesis of the shoulder complex. The need for extensive mobility requires stabilization based in particular on the active system and, to a lesser extent, on inert structures. Impingement and joint instability, which can be expressed in different ways and often appear together owing to their aetiopathological association, are the two most frequent causes of painful shoulder in athletes (Gerber, 2000). The myofascial system has an important role, particularly in the mean movement radius, while the inert ligament system is most important at the end of the movement. Maintaining centring between the two joint heads is the decisive factor for minimizing the risks of stress during arm movements (Sahrmann, 2002). Consequently, the muscles not only have to produce movement, they have to do so while maintaining centring. This is not solely the function of the scapulohumeral muscles, but also involves the scapular muscles and the muscles of the trunk and pelvis (Kibler, 2001).

Prior to this development, Jobe (1993) had proposed a division of the shoulder muscles, based on EMG research, into the '4 Ps': protectors (rotator cuff), pivoters (scapular muscles), positioners (deltoid muscle) and propellers (pectoralis major and latissimus dorsi muscles). The resulting rehabilitation proposal was to start with analytical strengthening of the rotator cuff muscles and scapular muscles and then to strengthen the positioner and propeller muscles in the final phase of the rehabilitation process. This method of rehabilitating the shoulder has been largely followed and is reported currently by various authors (Allegrucci, 1994; Amiridis, 1997; Brostrom, 1992; Burkhead, 1992; Donatelli, 2000; Ellenbecker, 1997; Kamkar, 1993; Paine, 1993; Schmitt, 1999; Tata, 1993; Wilk, 2002, 1997).

As an expression of this proposal, Wilk's rehabilitation protocol (2002) initially recommends analytical strength exercises of the rotator cuff in the first and second phase, whereas the use of these muscles in functional exercises is proposed subsequently. The same author also recommends analytical exercises for the scapular muscles.

While sharing the view of the importance of the correct muscle strength of the various muscles involved and making this part of the three pillars which ensure effective stability, we should be aware of the fact that it is the integration of this component with the neurological component that defines its efficacy. An analytical strength exercise with a small functional component also overlaps to some extent with sport-specific activity (Kibler, 2001). The rotator cuff muscles (infraspinatus, teres minor, supraspinatus, subscapularis) produce a combined contraction which allows greater glenohumeral compression and, together with the long head of the biceps and the deltoid muscle (Graichen, 1999), they are seen as primary stabilizers (Wilk, 1997).

Wilk (1997) identifies the anterior serratus, teres major and pectoralis major muscles as secondary stabilizers. The inferior fibres of the rotator cuff muscles also have the task of preventing the contraction of the deltoid muscle translating upwards to the humeral head. The long head of the biceps muscle also helps to prevent the humeral head rising (Karduna, 1996). These two muscle mechanisms should ensure the centring of the humerus on the glenoid during movement.

The arthrokinematics of the glenohumeral joint are currently a subject of great debate (Graichen, 1999; Karduna, 1996; Sharkey, 1995). It can be seen, with reference to Chapter 2, that there is a significant difference between the arthrokinematics of passive and active movements (Karduna, 1996), and that they vary further in the presence of a lesion of the inert structures, particularly the ligaments.

The scapulohumeral muscles are not exclusively responsible for dynamic stability in the glenohumeral joint. The scapular muscles have a key role in the correct functioning of the glenohumeral joint (Kibler, 2001; Rubin, 2002; Sahrmann, 2002). Sahrmann (2002) maintains that shoulder pain develops following a change in scapular movements which adversely influence the centring of the humerus on the glenoid and give rise to accessory joint movements. The scapular muscles should maintain a correct length-tension relationship, guiding the scapula, to ensure efficacy throughout the movement of the arm (Sahrmann, 2002). This also distributes the load better throughout the body during movement of the arm (Rubin, 2002). During a motor movement such as throwing a ball, the whole body is involved in the movement. The kinetic energy, which starts from the feet and travels via the pelvis to the arm, must be transmitted in a coordinated manner by the muscles of the scapula (Rubin, 2002). The upper, lower and middle trapezius muscles, levator scapulae, rhomboids, anterior serratus and pectoralis minor, which act in the movement as agonists or antagonists, are responsible for guiding the scapula during the movement of the arm. The absence of true mutual inhibition causes the continual activation of the various scapular muscles during movement, although they may be antagonists of one another during the movement (Sahrmann, 2002).

The paired movement of the upper trapezius and the anterior serratus muscles is very important. Both muscles cause cranial rotation of the scapula, which is essential during the elevation and abduction of the arm to prevent stress in the glenohumeral joint, while they are antagonists for the adduction and abduction of the scapula, respectively. The levator muscles of the scapula and rhomboids act synergically with the upper trapezius as regards the adduction of the scapula, while they are antagonists for cranial rotation. Excessive activation of these muscles during elevation could create problems in the glenohumeral joint.

The lower trapezius acts synergically with the upper trapezius and the anterior serratus for cranial rotation. This muscle also acts as an antagonist to the pectoralis minor and should, therefore, prevent the pectoralis minor causing anterior tilt of the scapula, significantly reducing the subacromial space (Sahrmann, 2002). An excessive imbalance in favour of the latter is, therefore, believed to increase the risk of impingement lesions in the glenohumeral joint. Dominance by the pectoralis major and the anterior serratus not sufficiently counterbalanced by the subscapularis muscle causes excessive anterior slide of the humeral head (Sahrmann, 2002).

A glenohumeral imbalance between internal rotation and external rotation strength in throwing athletes is accorded great aetiological importance in the literature. Isokinetic analyses have shown that throwers who suffer from impingement frequently exhibit a difference between the strength of the external rotators (ERs) and the internal rotators (IRs) in the throwing arm, compared to the other arm and compared to healthy athletes. According to Wilk (2002), the ratio between ERs and IR should be at least 65% and optimally between 66 and 75%. This is an interesting point to note when planning therapeutic exercises, but requires comment.

The results obtained with the various isokinetic machines are different and difficult to compare. It should furthermore be taken into account that isokinetic muscle strength alters according to the speed of execution (Amiridis, 1997) and according to the scapular plane (Tata, 1993). The position of the scapula influences the length, and thus the strength, of the scapulohumeral muscles. The type of contraction also alters the muscle strength ratio (MSR). Hartsell (1997) identifies 62% as the normal percentage for the MSR_{conc} between ERs and IRs, and this is lower than the value given by Wilk (2002), whereas the ratio for the MSR_{ecc} should be 3/2. Isokinetic training is also not particularly sport-specific.

Amiridis (1997) stated that only concentric isokinetic exercise partly improves eccentric strength too, while eccentric training does not produce an improvement in concentric capacity.

Heiderscheit (1996) demonstrated, on the other hand, that neither isokinetic nor plyometric strengthening improves the throwing capacity of softball pitchers. Isokinetic apparatus is therefore not particularly useful for improving functional capacity and serves principally as a numerical indicator of any imbalance present, allowing us simply to classify numerically the strength deficit existing in that precise setting.

The balance between internal and external rotators provides, according to Wilk (2002), good glenohumeral stability. Baseball pitchers often have greater IRs strength and lower ERs strength in the throwing arm than in the other arm (Wilk, 1993).

Kamkar (1993) makes the point that lack of strength in the rotator muscles can be responsible for possible secondary impingement. This view is shared by Allegrucci (1994) in his paper on the aetiopathogenesis of secondary impingement in swimmers. Lack of correct balance, according to this author, predisposes the athlete to microtraumas due to excessive translation of the humeral head during the athletic movement. Restoring the balance between IRs and ERs strength, particularly by strengthening the external rotators which often seem weaker than normal in athletes with painful shoulder, will improve the quality of movement during throwing.

It should be noted that Kibler (2001) maintains that glenohumeral stability depends on controlling the whole of the muscle chain, starting from control of the pelvis and trunk, and that Sahrmann (2002) considers a lack of balance between agonists, such as the subscapularis, pectoralis major and latissimus dorsi muscles, to be a risk factor for a deficit in glenohumeral control.

The functional representative nature of the isokinetic test is, in any case, very low, since the various muscles express themselves in very variable functional contexts and within a kinetic chain (Kibler, 2001).

Timing and coordination between the various muscles seem to be more important than their absolute strength. For example, we cannot analyse this problem without considering the lumbopelvic region. A structural or functional dysfunction in this region can have a significant influence on shoulder function (Kibler, 2001; Sahrmann, 2002). Poor stabilization of the pelvic girdle and spinal column prevents correct shoulder function. The anterior serratus muscle is also a major stabilizer of the sacroiliac joint, and makes a specific contribution, in synergy with the contralateral gluteus maximus muscle, to the stabilization of the

contralateral sacroiliac joint (Lee, 2000; Vleeming, 1997). Vleeming (1997) further maintains that this stabilization involves the multifidus muscles of the back and the hamstrings of the leg on the same side as the sacroiliac joint to be stabilized. According to the same author, the homolateral fibula muscles of the leg are also involved during walking. During throwing, the transmission of strength from the foot to the hand should be analysed in this context, i.e. bearing in mind that the glenohumeral joint stability will be obtained only if the whole system is working efficiently as a whole.

It is also, in our opinion, worth mentioning studies of lumbar stabilization. They show anticipatory contraction of the transverse abdominal muscle prior to any movement of the arm, which suggests that the pelvic region needs to be controlled before performing shoulder movements (Hodges, 1999), and that there is a link between scapular dysfunction and a lumbopelvic muscle deficit (Young, 1996).

Conclusions as regards therapeutic exercise

It emerges from this discussion that the muscle component has an important role in the management and recovery of motor control. The muscles which should be considered are not just the scapulohumeral muscles, but also the thoracoscapular and thoracohumeral muscles and those of the lumbopelvic region. The muscles are divided according to the contribution they make to motor movements of the shoulder, and rehabilitation protocols have been proposed, based on this division, which give preference to an analytical study of the humeroscapular and scapular muscles in order to include them in more functional exercises.

Other authors place greater emphasis on muscle chain exercise and recommend that exercise should begin with the muscles of the lumbopelvic region and end with the intrinsic muscles of the glenohumeral joint.

Both schools of thought agree, however, on recommending arthrokinematic centring on the glenoid and valid scapular control as the two functions which have most influence on a successful throwing movement without the risk of injury to the shoulder complex. Now, before introducing the methods, we would like to discuss the neurological component of motor control of the shoulder complex.

Neurological control system

Kibler (2001) recently proposed a more global approach to rehabilitation for shoulder problems. Using EMG, Kibler analysed the kinetic chain during throwing movements and came to the conclusion that the scapula has a fundamental role in correct throwing, from the legs to the arm, and that correct function necessarily requires good proximal stability. Good proximal stability was also mentioned by Rubin (2002) for producing a distal movement in effective, risk-free throwing. According to Rubin, good lumbopelvic and scapular stability is, therefore, always necessary to transport kinetic energy from the leg to the arm. A postural deviation, such as lumbar or cervical hyperlordosis, dorsal hyperkyphosis or scapular protraction, may also have an adverse influence on the correct performance of the movement. The axioscapular muscles guide the scapula to prevent compression inside the glenohumeral joint and the humeroscapular muscles remaining at a functional length. This paper aims to rehabilitate primarily the lumbopelvic region and scapular muscles and, only secondarily, the glenohumeral joint.

In supporting this hypothesis, Rubin and Kibler (2002) refer to Hodges (1999), who demonstrated anticipatory contraction of the abdominal transverse muscle before any type of movement with the arm, and described the link between the lumbopelvic region and arm movements. Lumbar exercises in preparation for throwing and scapular exercises are consequently recommended initially, followed only then by integration with the scapulohumeral muscles with functional exercises. These muscles cannot be trained in a functional manner without ensuring correct proximal control. The figures illustrate some of the exercises recommended by these authors (Figs. 15.6–15.8).

A dysfunctional movement derives, according to Sahrmann (2002), from muscle and postural changes

Fig. 15.7

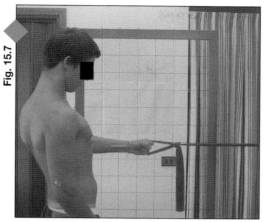

Scapular retraction exercise with the elastic band. Patients are asked to bring their fist to a point in space defined by the orthopaedic chart, improving learning (modified from Kibler, 2001).

Fig. 15.8

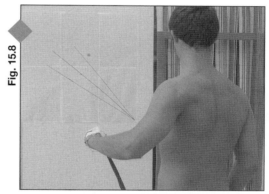

External rotation exercises with control of the scapula. The laser pointer, which provides visual feedback, has been placed on the back of the patient's hand and the patient has to perform the windup phase of throwing, guiding the laser light along the various lines drawn on the wall (modified from Kibler, 2001).

Fig. 15.6

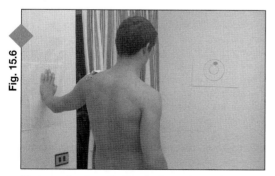

Clock exercise: the patient is asked to perform a clockwise movement with the scapula, keeping the hand on the wall. The laser pointer provides spatiotemporal feedback for the movement and improves learning (modified from Kibler, 2001).

caused by positions held for a long time or specific repeated movements which cause an imbalance between antagonists and agonists. Sahrmann (2002) analyses these muscle imbalances by inspecting posture and active movements in detail. A shortened or lengthened muscle can lead to these dynamic imbalances by altering strength. The exercises recommended are, therefore, analytical movements, and the patient is shown how to perform them by controlling the functional imbalance correctly (Figs. 15.9, 15.10).

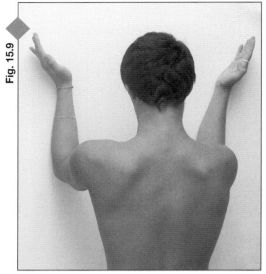

Fig. 15.9

Exercise to raise the arms in external rotation with the forearms against the wall. The exercise aims to train the lower trapezius in a functional manner (Sahrmann, 2002).

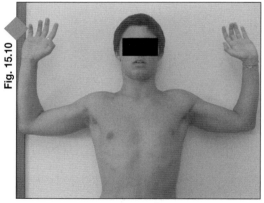

Fig. 15.10

Abduction exercises in external rotation. Contact between the scapulae and the wall provides tactile feedback for scapular movement (Sahrmann, 2002).

Other models for interpreting motor control, or rather movement strategy, derive from movement studies of the spine and distinguish between local stabilizer muscles, global stabilizer muscles and global mobilizer muscles (Comerford, 2001a, 2001b).

Local stabilizer muscles have the task of controlling physiological movements and excessive translation movements between the two joint surfaces. They are characterized by continual activation, capable of ensuring correct centring and correct compacting of the joint during any movement. These muscles anticipate angular movement.

Global stabilizer muscles have the task of controlling stability during rotation movements, by eccentric contractions. It is, therefore, these muscles or muscle fibres that brake movement. Finally, global mobilizer muscles are responsible for producing movement.

It should be further noted that pain, habits and incorrect postures can create dysfunction within the system. The loss of control persists, even after the pain is no longer present (Hides, 1996; Shakespeare, 1985). The patient needs firstly to be taught how to activate the local stabilizer muscles by analytical exercises, and subsequently to integrate the global stabilizer muscles and the global mobilizer muscles with more functional exercises. Trauma, non-mechanical pain, incorrect posture or poor movement habits, according to Comerford (2001a), underlie a movement dysfunction (Fig. 15.11). I believe that this neurophysiological information (Comerford, 2001a, 2001b; Richardson, 1999) should be combined with electromyographic and histological research (Boyd-Clark, 2001, 2002) to which the majority of publications in the literature currently refer. The fibres of the same muscle with a different innervation may belong to a different group, owing to their function (Richardson, 1999). The rotator cuff (scapulohumeral muscles) can be seen as a local stabilizer muscle of the glenohumeral joint, because it is characterized specifically as a muscle responsible for the centring of the humeral head during movement. Furthermore, these same muscles also act as global stabilizers, during motor actions, when they have to contract eccentrically to brake the movement, for example during the final phase of throwing. Sahrmann (2002) states that dominance of the deltoid muscle over the external rotators causes excessive anterior glide. This imbalance can be controlled by a biofeedback system, or by asking the patient to lie down in a supine position and to perform an external rotation, while the therapist palpates any anterior slide (Sahrmann, 2002). This example shows the importance of the neuromuscular contribution to the correct centring of the humeral head.

A further interesting example is the balance between the internal rotators, in which the proportional contributions of the subscapularis muscle (local-global stabilizer), latissimus dorsi (local-global stabilizer) and pectoralis major (global mobilizer) are correct. The thoracoscapular muscles, also known as shoulder pivoters, seem to have a dual function. They can be

Fig. 15.11

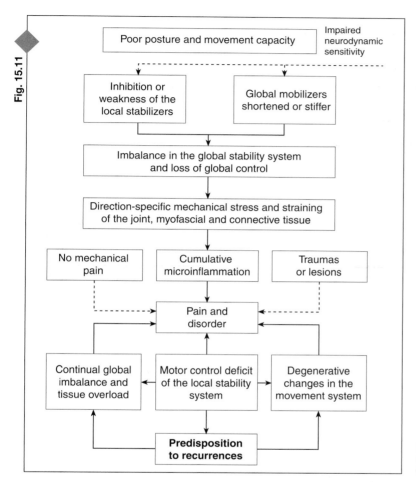

Poor posture and movement capacity — Impaired neurodynamic sensitivity

Inhibition or weakness of the local stabilizers

Global mobilizers shortened or stiffer

Imbalance in the global stability system and loss of global control

Direction-specific mechanical stress and straining of the joint, myofascial and connective tissue

No mechanical pain

Cumulative microinflammation

Traumas or lesions

Pain and disorder

Continual global imbalance and tissue overload

Motor control deficit of the local stability system

Degenerative changes in the movement system

Predisposition to recurrences

Model of dysfunctional movement (modified from Comerford, 2001a).

defined as local stabilizer muscles, since they are responsible for controlling the position of the scapula in relation to the rib cage. These muscles are responsible for controlling anterior scapular tilt in the sagittal plane, scapular winging in the transverse plane and creating a good fixed point for rotation movements of the arm when throwing a ball (Kibler, 2001; Rubin, 2002; Sahrmann, 2002). The second function of the scapular muscles is to guide the scapula so as to ensure a correct ratio between the two joint heads on the glenoid. The scapular muscles behave in this case as global stabilizers which, by means of eccentric co-contraction, guide the movement of the scapula and provide extensive mobility without affecting stability (Rubin, 2002).

The thoracohumeral muscles finally also act as global mobilizers. They are responsible for the production of angular movement and also stabilize the joint in end-range movements in the presence of extreme shear strain forces (Hodges, 1999).

Conclusions as regards therapeutic exercise

To conclude, if we compare the models proposed by Comerford (2001a, 2001b), Sahrmann (2002) and Kibler (2001), we can see that great attention is paid to quality of movement and less to quantity of strength. Analysis of motor movement must necessarily involve the central and peripheral neurological system, which guide movement. Without going into too much detail, we can see that there is a close interaction between the central and peripheral neurological system as regards motor control, and between movement planning, postural control and body dynamics, in which proprioceptive afferences and cortical and

Therapeutic exercise in rehabilitation

spinal activity interact continually. An analysis of athletic movement and the recovery of athletic ability can clearly not be confined to a musculoskeletal analysis, but should include the neurological system. The discussion in the previous section on the role of muscle strength must necessarily be included among these concepts.

This new way of interpreting musculoskeletal problems is perhaps instigating a 'revolution' in therapeutic exercise planning. The protocol proposed by Rubin and Kibler (2002) pays considerable attention to scapular dysfunction and states that it is only in the presence of efficient proximal lumbopelvic and scapular stabilization that effective dynamic stabilization of the glenoid can occur.

Though we share this interpretation, we would like to make three comments:

— In the light of the comments by Comerford, the latest scientific research on lumbopelvic function and research into movement planning, we believe we can say that an effective, risk-free movement needs proximal stabilization. Stabilization occurs not only inside the kinetic chain underlying the movement. Analyses of the role of the myofascial system regarding motor control of the shoulder should also include muscle mobility. There are several factors which can cause joint limitation. Our aim in this section is to analyse only joint limitation caused by the myofascial system, noting that glenohumeral joint posterior capsule retraction causes major functional problems and should be rehabilitated using mainly manual techniques. Lumbopelvic stabilization, for which we refer the reader to the books by Richardson (1999) and Lee (2000), is a system which should be taught initially autonomously and analytically. The patient should first learn how to activate this form of local stabilization. These are analytical exercises, yet they are functional, because they aim to teach the patient anticipatory contraction which controls arthrokinematic centring. These authors initially recommend analytical exercises to teach the patient to contract local stabilizer muscles, after which exercises for the global stabilizer muscles and global mobilizers will progressively be added. We, therefore, believe that it is not sufficient to control the ability to balance on one leg to assess lumbopelvic stability, as maintained by Kibler (2001), and to recommend functional exercises which emphasize the correct position of the pelvis. The stability of a segment or region depends on the correct coordination of the various stabilization levels

within the same segment. It is only after teaching the patient how to control the lumbopelvic region that more specific exercises are indicated.

— Secondly, we should be aware that learning any motor movement depends on the central nervous system. The automation of a movement and the choice of a movement strategy need to be learnt in the first place. We should, therefore, teach patients movements that are initially easy, and subsequently add to them more complex automatic movements. The rotator cuff principally has the task of keeping the humerus centred correctly on the glenoid. Correct scapular function ensures the correct tensioning of these muscles, which should, however, contract in a coordinated anticipatory manner. Without this control, the athlete will have persistent problems. The scapular muscles have a dual task: controlling the position of the scapula in relation to the chest and guiding it during arm movement, to prevent glenoid problems; these actions consequently need to be learned, initially in an analytical manner and only subsequently through a specific kinetic chain. As mentioned above for the lumbopelvic region and also for local glenohumeral and scapulothoracic stabilization, we believe that the activation of muscles that have a local stabilizer function should be learned first. Only then can more functional exercises be combined, such as those proposed by Sahrmann (2002) or Kibler (2001), in which arm movement is incorporated with the movement of the scapula and trunk. If the patient is a throwing athlete, we should include local and global stability in the kinetic chain of the movement in order to obtain an effective, risk-free movement.

— The final comment concerns the neurophysiological background of a motor movement. Movement is based on integration between the peripheral and the central neurological system, and the final movement, with its spatiotemporal parameters, is the expression of this. Movement planning arises from the internal dynamic body model, the external frame of reference, continuous efferent information, body dynamics, cognitive intentions and the interpretation of the request. Proprioceptive information, which has a vital role in refining movement through the spinal reflex and central integration, is equally important in the central planning of movement (Bevan, 1994; Cordo, 1994; Hocherman, 1995; LaRue, 1994; Sainburg, 1993, 1995). It should be kept in mind that an athletic movement results from central programming and that to alter its expression, particularly from a spatiotemporal point of view, it is vital to focus initially on motor learning. The preference for analytical exercises aimed at the local or global stabilizer muscles of the shoulder complex, also called protectors and pivoters, seems obvious from this, and highly functional.

Taking the two sections together, we can say that motor timing (LaRue, 1994; Sahrmann, 2002), neuromuscular control of the movement and its motor sequence are more important in functional progression than parameters of plyometric strength, resistance, etc. These parameters form part of a third-phase sport-specific functional progression. To return to the MLCM, we can then say that neuromuscular control, the correct sequence of the movement and, therefore, coordination form the basis of any functional progression (Sterling, 2001). It is only when the patient has acquired good regional control and a good motor sequence in a kinetic chain, that we can begin to include more sport-specific variables intrinsic to exercise.

Mobility as impairment

Limitation of movement, whether of joint or muscle origin, is important in planning exercise. The origin of movement limitation may be various, and the consequences different. For painful shoulder in an athlete, we consider it important to stress glenohumeral limitation, which is due to retraction of the posterior capsule, modification of muscle length and postural variations which significantly influence mobility inside the shoulder complex.

— Capsule limitation may be present in an anterior, inferior or posterior direction (Conroy, 1998). Glenohumeral joint posterior capsule retraction, mentioned in the literature as an aetiological factor of subacromial impingement in an athlete's shoulder, causes a superior shift of the humeral head, resulting in limitation in internal rotation and adduction and jeopardizing the centring of the humerus on the scapula during dynamic movements (Kamkar, 1993; Matsen, 1990, Tyler, 1999).

By pulling the posterior capsule during surgery on cadavers, Harrymann (1990) found an increase in the superior shift of the humeral head and an increase in anterior and posterior translation during flexion and horizontal adduction of the shoulder. This limitation of internal rotation, which may also be caused by muscle limitation, is often present in throwing athletes

suffering from impingement (Bang, 2000; Warner, 1990). It is not, however, entirely clear whether this adaptation is related to a sport-specific need or whether it is the expression of poor joint adaptation (Ellenbecker, 1996). The importance of a possible imbalance between internal and external glenoid rotation should be interpreted in the light of the overall state of the patient. Manual therapy techniques and stretching exercises seem to be highly indicated to restore the correct movement radius (Bang, 2000; Conroy, 1998).

— Changes in muscle length can be due to poor movement habits, injuries or inappropriate postural attitudes. These pathological adaptations should clearly be included with the neurodynamic mechanisms discussed earlier (Comerford, 2001a). Muscle shortening is caused by keeping the same muscle in a shortened position, and this has a considerable effect on muscle strength at optimal length (Gossman, 1982). Sahrmann (2002) defines this muscle shortening defect as relative stiffness or flexibility. A muscle can be excessively shortened or lengthened and both cause inadequate function. These changes, therefore, give rise to muscle imbalances which may lead to an impairment of movement. An example of a shortened muscle that can create shoulder problems is the pectoralis minor, which causes anterior tilt of the scapula. This tilt can be induced equally by shortened biceps brachii or anterior deltoid muscles. The levator scapulae and the upper trapezius, by contrast, cause cranial migration of the scapula. Shortening of the pectoralis major and the latissimus dorsi may limit external rotation movement, while limitation of the external rotators of the scapula may limit internal rotation movement. A shortened deltoid muscle causes cranial migration of the humerus.

These imbalances can also be interpreted in relation to neurodynamic muscle concepts, in which greater use of the mobilizer muscles, at the expense of inhibition of the global and local stabilizers, causes pathological muscle adaptation (Comerford, 2001a). Sahrmann (2002) proposes restoring muscle balance by means of corrective functional exercises, for example, to improve the radius of movement of the shoulder in elevation, and the performance of the trapezius muscle and the external rotator muscles (Fig. 15.12).

— Mobility may also be impaired by an incorrect posture of the cervical and dorsal spine. These deviations cause a reduction in local mobility in accordance with the mobility of the shoulder

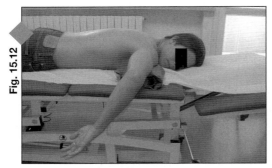

Fig. 15.12

Internal rotation movement. The patient has to perform internal rotation by activating the subscapularis, which should be dominant in relation to the deltoid (Sahrmann, 2002).

complex. The movement of the shoulder complex is distributed between the glenohumeral, acromioclavicular, sternoclavicular and thoracoscapular joints, and between the cervical and dorsal spine. A limitation in one region will consequently cause greater stress in the other joints.

Conclusions as regards therapeutic exercise

Joint mobility is, therefore, an important parameter to be considered when planning exercises. Joint mobility should be restored particularly by manual therapy, while muscle flexibility deficits should be addressed by functional muscle rehabilitation.

Proprioception as impairment

This component is very important. Motor control is produced at two levels: on a spinal level proprioceptive afferences have a decisive role via the spinal reflexes, while on the level of the encephalic trunk the proprioceptive information is incorporated with visual and vestibular information for management of postural control (Lephart, 1994; Radebold, 2001). Accuracy of movement depends on the sensory components of the motor system (Hodges, 2003). Proprioceptive and tactile efferent information contributes, along with vestibular and visual information, to the creation of internal motor and body dynamics and to movement planning (Cohen, 1994; Ivanenko, 2000). Prud'homme (1994) showed that proprioceptive information activates the somatosensory cortex differently depending on the type of movement and on the type of muscle activity. Ghez (1994) maintains that

proprioceptive information updates models within the limb, and thus movement planning.

Proprioception also guides movement timing (Bevan, 1994; Cordo, 1994; Hocherman, 1995; LaRue, 1994; Sainburg, 1993, 1995) by a feed-forward mechanism. It is worth pointing out that the perception of position is more accurate during joint movements and muscle activity. Greater speed of movement also allows a better perception capacity, suggesting that the motor spindles have an important role (Cordo, 2000; Verschueren, 1999).

This supports the claim that exercises should be performed with specific spatiotemporal references and in as functional a manner as possible. Proprioceptive information gives rise to spatiotemporal information in the cerebral cortex. Pain alters proprioceptive information at receptor level, causing a reduced sense of position (Brumagne, 2000; Ghez, 1995; Gill, 1998; Gordon, 1995; LaRue, 1994; Lephart, 1994; Myers, 2002) and modulates proprioceptive information centrally (Capra, 2000). Gandavia (1992, 1994, 1996) considers that proprioception yields information on the position of the joint, on muscle recruitment and on the timing of the contraction. Comerford (2001a) has suggested, on the basis of research conducted by Grimby and Hannerz (1976), that a reduction in proprioceptive afference leads to greater difficulty activating slow motor units, responsible for local stabilization, than fast motor units. The optimal treatment of patients with musculoskeletal problems should include identification of neuromuscular activity, timing of muscle activity with movement and contraction patterns and proprioceptive control (Sterling, 2001).

Conclusions as regards therapeutic exercise

A proprioceptive impairment should be considered in therapeutic exercise. Repositioning tests can be performed using a pointer. The evaluation should be carried out with the eyes covered, but not closed, because eye position could influence the result through the motor spindles of the eye muscles (Rougier, 2003). During the test, the patient is asked to stare forwards. A second point that emerges from this discussion is that proprioception guides and contributes to movement planning. This means that the exercises recommended should where possible have feedback (Fig. 15.13).

The last comment to be made in this respect is that muscle fatigue significantly influences the quality of proprioceptive afferences (Voight, 1996); exercises aiming to improve movement quality should consequently be performed in the absence of muscle fatigue.

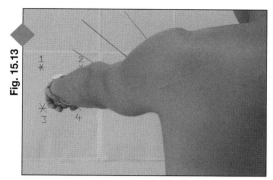

Fig. 15.13

Exercise for sense of position. The patient first feels the positions with eyes closed. The patient then has to bring the laser pointer into the positions requested by the therapist.

Psychosocial factors and impairment

For psychosocial factors, which are important to the therapeutic decision, (see the section on Pain as impairment). Psychosocial differences can have an extreme influence, particularly on recovery times and expectations (Vlaeyen, 1997) since, as already mentioned, motivation, stress and the athlete's ability to manage the problem personally are key aspects of therapeutic training.

Proposals for the future

It is clear from the above that the scientific evidence for therapeutic exercise for painful shoulder is weak. The great variety of problems that can be responsible for painful shoulder and the large quantities of variables intrinsic to the exercises make standardization complex. It is only by analysing the factors intrinsic to exercise and to painful shoulder that we will be able to standardize therapeutic exercise and make it reproducible by all. If, however, we wish to consider the efficacy of therapeutic exercise and to propose a useful, reproducible approach in the literature, we need trials to evaluate the efficacy of physiotherapy with controlled specific clinical conditions associated with shoulder pain, and of different exercise conditions, both separately and together (Green, 2003).

Planning therapeutic exercise, therefore, needs a model for codifying the various parameters which influence the choice and method of exercise. We believe that the load and carriability model, comprising the ICF proposed by WHO, is currently the most appropriate model for constructing a therapeutic programme.

This chapter has addressed the parameters that influence the patient's local and general carriability, whereas the next chapter will focus on sport-specific parameters. Pain has a key role in exercise planning. It is also an expression of the link between the physical damage and the psychological impact of painful shoulder on the individual.

Research in musculoskeletal rehabilitation is focusing increasingly on the neuromuscular aspect. It is no longer the quantitative strength of individual muscles which must guide therapeutic exercise to restore function, but the relationship between the various muscles from the qualitative point of view. There are various rehabilitation models of this approach: Kibler (2001) proposes an approach in which the aim of the exercises is to improve proximal stability, with a view to achieving correct glenohumeral function. This interpretation seems to be largely in line with that proposed by Sahrmann (2002) who, nevertheless, places greater emphasis on muscle imbalances in the muscle chain responsible for the deficit.

According to other authors (Comerford, 2001a, 2001b; Hodges, 1999; Lee, 2000; Richardson, 1999; Vleeming, 1997), the stability of a joint does not simply depend on the correct functioning of the dynamic chain of movement. These authors maintain that anticipatory contraction of local muscles, with the task of maintaining joint centring during dynamic movements, has a key role in joint stability. Proximal stability needs to be learned, initially locally, and then integrated with dynamic movement and with exercises that take into account any imbalances that may be present.

It is our hypothesis that the rotator cuff function is specifically local stability. It should primarily ensure good control of glenohumeral centring. This function is clearly supported by the scapular muscles, which guide the movements of the scapula maintaining the correct centring of the latter on the chest.

We believe that research should investigate these aspects in particular, with the aim of demonstrating this intrinsic function during shoulder movements. There is additionally the need to successfully construct a method of clinical evaluation for the efficacy of local activity.

One option could be to use surface EMG to identify the activity of the rotator cuff muscles during standardized movements. The correct positioning of the electrodes will be very important in this case.

The literature states, furthermore, that exercises should always have spatiotemporal coding which helps the patient to learn the most suitable motor conditions. Therapeutic exercise should, therefore, be coded on the basis of qualitative parameters, paying great

Therapeutic exercise in rehabilitation

attention to neuromuscular aspects. Motor learning is only possible if the patient is offered spatiotemporal and particularly proprioceptive parameters. Functional progression should start with local motor control, arriving progressively at global and sport-specific motor control. Pain disturbs proprioceptive feedback, motor control and movement planning via various mechanisms. All exercises which aim to restore quality of movement should be performed in the absence of pain.

Acknowledgements

To Claudio Massanelli for the photography and to my wife, Federica, with love, for her many recommendations.

Bibliography

Allegrucci M., Whitney S.L., Irrgang J.J., 'Clinical implications of secondary impingement of the shoulder in freestyle swimmers', J. Orthop. Sports Phys. Ther. 20(6): 307–318, (1994)

Altechek D.W., Hobbs W.R., 'Evaluation and management of shoulder instability in the elite overhead thrower', Orthop Clin N Am 32(3): 423–430, (2001)

Amiridis I.G., Cometti G., Morlon B., Van Hoecke J., 'Concentric and/or eccentric training-induced alterations in shoulder flexor and extensor strength', J. Ortop. Sports Phys. Ther. 25(1): 26–33, (1997)

Andersen N.H., Sojberg J.O., Johannsen H.V., Sneppen O., 'Self-training versus physiotherapist-supervised rehabilitation of the shoulder in patients treated with arthroscopic subacromial decompression: a clinical randomized study', J. Shoulder Elbow Surg. 8(2): 99–101, (1999)

Bang M., Deyle G.D., 'Comparison of supervised exercise with and without manual physical therapy for patients with shoulder impingement syndrome', J. Ortop. Sports Phys. 30(3): 126–137, (2000)

Bard C., Fleury M., Teasdale N., Paillard J., Nougier V., 'Contribution of proprioception for calibrating and updating the motor space', Can. J. Phys Pharmacol. 73: 246–254, (1995)

Bernards A.T.M., Haagenaars L.H.A., Oostendorp R.A.B., Warms H.W.A., 'Het meer dimensionale belasting-belastbaarheidmodel: een conceptueel model voor fysiotherapie (The load/carriability model: a conceptual model for physiotherapy)', Ned. T. Fysiother. 109(3): 58–65, (1999)

Bevan L., Cordo P., Carlton L., Carlton M., 'Proprioception coordination of movement sequences: discrimination of joint angle versus angular distance', J. Neurophysiol. 71(5): 1862–1871, (1994)

Bigliani L.U., Ticket J.B., Flatow E.L., Soslowsky L.J., Mow V.C., 'The relationship of acromial architecture to rotator cuff disease', Clin. Sport Med. 10(4): 823–839, (1997)

Boyd-Clark C., Briggs A., Galea M.P., 'Comparative histo-chemical composition of muscle fibers in a pre and post-vertebral muscle of the spine', J. Anat. 199: 709–716, (2001)

Boyd-Clark C., Briggs A., Galea M.P., 'Muscle spindle distribution, morphology and density in longus colli and multifidus muscle of the cervical spine', Spine 27(7): 694–701, (2002)

Brostrom L., Kronberg M., Nemeth G., Oxelback U., 'The effect of shoulder muscle training in patients with recurrent shoulder dislocations', Scand. J. Rehab. Med. 24: 11–15, (1992)

Brumagne S., Cordo P., Lysens R., Verscheuren S., Swinnen S., 'The role of the paraspinal muscle spindles in lumbosacral position sense in individuals with and without low back pain', Spine 25(8): 989–994, (2000)

Burkhead W.Z., Rockwood C.A., 'Treatment of instability of the shoulder with an exercise program', J. Bone Joint. Surg. 74(6): 890–896, (1992)

Capra N.F., RO J., 'Experimental muscle pain produces central modulation of proprioceptive signals arising from jaw muscle spindles', Pain 86 (1-2): 151–162, (2000)

Casonato O., Musarra F., Frosi G., Testa M., 'The role of therapeutic exercise in the conflicting and unstable shoulder', Phys. Ther. Rev. 8: 1–16, (2003)

Cohen D.A., Prud'Homme M.J.L., Kalaska J.F., 'Tactile activity in primate primary somatosensory cortex during active arm movements: correlation with receptive field properties', J. Neurophysiol. 71(1): 161–172, (1994)

Comerford M.J., Mottram S.L., 'Functional stability re-training: principles and strategies for managing mechanical dysfunction', Manual Ther. 6(1): 3–14, (2001a)

Comerford M.J., Mottram S.L., 'Movement and stability dysfunction – contemporary developments', Manual Ther. 6(1): 15–26, (2001b)

Conroy D.E., Hayes K.W., 'The effect of joint mobilization as a component of comprehensive treatment for primary shoulder impingement syndrome', J. Ortop. Sports Phys. Ther. 28(1): 3–12, (1998)

Cordo P., Carlton L., Bevan L., Carlton M., Kerr K., 'Proprioceptive coordination of movement sequences: role of velocity and position information', J. Neurophysiol. 71(5): 1848–1861, (1994)

Cordo P.J., Gurfinkel V.S., Levik Y., 'Position sense during imperceptibly slow movements', Exp. Brain Res. 132: 1–9, (2000)

Davies G.J., Dickoff-Hoffman S., 'Neuromuscular testing and rehabilitation of the shoulder complex', J. Ortop. Sports Phys. Ther. 18(2): 449–457, (1993)

De Moree J.J. Dynamiek van, het menselijk bindweefsel: functie, beschadiging en herstel (The dynamics of connective tissue: function, lesion and healing). 2nd ed. Stafleu Van Loghum, Bohn Houten (1993)

Desmeules F., Côté C.H., Frémont P., 'Therapeutic exercise and orthopedic manual therapy for impingement syndrome: a systematic review', Clin. J. Sport Med. 13: 176–182, (2003)

Donatelli R., Ellenbecker T.S., Ekedahl S.R., Wilkes J.S., Kocher K., Adam J., 'Assessment of shoulder strength in professional baseball pitchers', *J. Ortop. Sport Phys. Ther.* 30: 544–551, (2000)

Ellenbecker T.S., Mattalino A.J., 'Concentric isokinetic shoulder internal and external rotation strength in professional baseball pitchers', *J. Ortop. Sports Phys. Ther.* 25(5): 323–328, (1997)

Ellenbecker T.S., Roetert E.P., Piorkowski P.A., Schulz D.A., 'Glenohumeral joint internal and external rotation range of motion in elite junior tennis players', *J. Ortop. Sports Phys. Ther.* 24(6): 336–341, (1996)

Gandavia S.C., 'Kinesthesia: roles for afferent signals and motor commands', In: Rowell L.B., Shephard J.T. (eds.), *Handbook of physiology*, section 12, exercise: regulation and integration of multiple systems, Oxford University Press, New York (1996)

Gandavia S.C., 'The sensation of effort co-varies with reflex effect on the motoneurone pool: evidence and implications', *Int. J. Industrial Ergonomics* 13: 41–49, (1994)

Gandavia S.C., McCloskey D.I., Burke D., 'Kinaesthetic signals and muscle contraction', *Trends Neurosci.* 15: 62–65, (1992)

Gerber C., Sebasta A., 'Impingement of the deep surface of the subscapularis tendon and the reflection pulley on the anterosuperior glenoid rim: a preliminary report', *J Shoulder Elbow Surg* 9(6): 483–490, (2000)

Ghez C., Gordon J., Ghilardi M.F., 'Impairments of reaching movements in patients without proprioception. II. Effects of visual information on accuracy', *J. Neurophysiol.* 73(1): 361–371, (1995)

Ghez C., Sainburg R., 'Proprioceptive control of interjoint coordination', *Can. J. Physiol. Pharmacol.* 73: 273–284, (1994)

Gill K.P., Callaghan M.J., 'The measurement of lumbar proprioception in individuals with and without low back pain', *Spine* 23(1): 62–65, (1998)

Ginn K.A., Herbert R.D., Khouw W., Lee R., 'A randomised, controlled clinical trial of a treatment for shoulder pain', *Phys. Ther.* 77: 802–811, (1997)

Gordon J., Ghilardi M.F., Ghez C., 'Impairments of reaching movements in patients without proprioception. I. Spatial errors. J. Neurophysiol.* 73(1): 347–360, (1995)

Gossman M.R., Sahrmann S.A., Rose S.J., 'Review of length-associated changes in muscle', *Physical Ther.* 62(12): 1799–1808, (1982)

Graichen H., Bonel H., Stammberger T., Haubner M., Rohrer H., Englmeier K., Reiser M., Eckstein F., 'Three-dimensional analysis of the width of the subacromial space in healthy subjects and patients with impingement syndrome', *AJR* 172: 1081–1086, (1999)

Green S., Buchbinder R., Hetrick S., 'Physiotherapy interventions for shoulder pain (Cochrane review), The Cochrane Library, issue 4, (2003)

Grimby L., Hannerz J., 'Disturbance in voluntary recruitment order of low and high frequency motor units on blockades of proprioception afferent activity', *Acta Physiol. Scandin.* 96: 207–216, (1976)

Hagenaars L.H.A., Bernards A.T.M., Oostendorp R.A.B., *The multidimensional load/carriability model*, Nederlands Paramedisch Instituut, Amersfoort (2002)

Harryman D.T., Sidles J.A., Clarck J.M., McQuade K.J., Gibb T.D., Matsen F.A., 'Translation of the humeral head on glenoid with passive glenohumeral motion', *J. Bone Joint Surg.* 72A(9): 1334–1343, (1990)

Hartsell H.D., Forwell L., 'Postoperative eccentric and concentric isokinetic strength for shoulder rotators in the scapular and neutral planes', *J. Ortop. Sports Phys. Ther.* 25(1): 19–25, (1997)

Heerkens Y.F., 'Zin en onzin van het gebruik van de ICIDH (The sense and nonsense of using the ICIDH)', In: *Fysiopraxis*, vol. 18, (1993)

Heiderscheit B.C., McLean K.P., Davies G.J., 'The effect of isokinetic vs plyometric training on the shoulder internal rotators', *J. Ortop. Sports Phys. Ther.* 23(2): 125–133, (1996)

Hides J.A., Richardson C.A., Jull G.A., 'Multifidus muscle recovery is not automatic after resolution of acute, first low back pain', *Spine* 23: 2763–2769, (1996)

Hinstermeister R.A., Lange G.W., Schultheis J.M., Bey M.J., Hawkins R.J., 'Electromyographic activity and applied load during shoulder rehabilitation exercises using elastic resistance', *Am. J. Sports Med.* 26(2): 210–220, (1998)

Hocherman S., 'Proprioceptive guidance and motor planning of reaching movements to unseen targets', *Exp. Brain Res.* 95: 349–358, (1995)

Hodges P., Moseley G.L., 'Pain and motor control of the lumbopelvic region: effect and possible mechanisms', *J. Electromyography Kinesiology* 13: 361–370, (2003)

Hodges P.W., 'Is there a role for the transverse abdominis in lumbo-pelvic stability?' *Manual Ther.* 4: 74–86, (1999)

Ivanenko Y.P., Grasso R., Lacquaniti F., 'Neck muscle vibration makes walking humans accelerate in the direction of gaze', *J Physiol* 525(3): 803–814, (2000)

Jarvinen M.J., Lehto M.U., 'The effect of early mobilisation and immobilisation on the healing process following muscle injuries. Sports Med', 15(2): 78–89, (1993)

Jobe F.W., Pink M., 'Classification and treatment of shoulder dysfunction in the overhead athlete', *J. Ortop. Sports Phys. Ther.* 18(2): 427–432, (1993)

Kamkar A., Irrgang J.J., Whitney S.L., 'Nonoperative management of secondary impingement syndrome', *J. Ortop. Sports Phys. Ther.* 17(5): 212–224, (1993)

Karduna A.R., Williams G.R., Williams J.L., Iannoti J.P., 'Kinematic glenohumeral joint influences of muscle forces, ligamentous constraints and articular geometry', *J. Orthop. Res.* 14: 986–993, (1996)

Keirns M.A., 'Trattamento conservativo della sindrome da conflitto della spalla (Conservative treatment of shoulder impingement syndrome)', In: Andrews J.R., Wilk K.E. (eds.), *La spalla dell'atleta (The athlete's shoulder)*. Antonio Delfino Editore, Rome, pp. 605–627, (1998)

Kibler W.B., McMullen J., UHL T., 'Shoulder rehabilitation strategies, guidelines, and practice', *Orthop. Clini. N. Am.* 32(3): 527–538, (2001)

Larue J., Bard C., Fleury M., Teasdale N., Paillard J., Forget R., Lamarre Y., 'Is proprioception important for the timing of motor activities?' *Can. J. Physiol. Pharmacol.* 73: 255–261, (1994)

Lee D., 'The Pelvic Girdle: an approach to examination and treatment of the lumbo-pelvic-hip region', 2nd ed. Churchill Livingstone, Edinburgh (2000)

Lephart S., 'Reestablishing proprioception, kinesthesia, joint position sense, and neuromuscular control in rehabilitation', In: Prentice W.E. (eds), *Rehabilitation techniques in sports medicine*, 2nd ed. Mosby, St Louis, pp. 118–137, (1994).

Lephart S.M., Warner J.J., Borsa P.A., Fu F.H., 'Proprioception of the shoulder joint in healthy, unstable and surgically repaired shoulders', *J. Shoulder Elbow Surg.* Nov.: 371–378, (1994)

Loeser J.D., 'Perspectives on pain', In: Turner P. (eds.), 'Clinical Pharmacy and therapeutics' Macmillan, London (1980)

Lund J.P., Donga R., Widmer C.G., Stohler C.S., 'The pain-adaptation model: a discussion of the relationship between chronic musculoskeletal pain and motor activity', *Can. J. Physiol. Pharmacol.* 69: 683–694, (1991)

Matsen F.A., Arntz C.T., 'Subacromial impingement', In: Rockwood C.A., Matsen F.A. (eds.), *The Shoulder*, vol. 2. WB Sauders Company, Philadelphia (1990)

Merskey R., 'Pain terms: a list with definitions and notes on usage', *Pain* 6: 249–252, (1997)

Mink A.J.F., Ter Veer H.J., Vorselaars J.A.C., '*Extremiteiten: functie-onderzoek en manuele therapie* (*Extremities: functional evaluation and manual therapy*)', Stafleu Van Loghum, Houtem/Zaventem Bohn (1990)

Myers J.B., Lephard S.M., 'Sensimotor deficits contributing to glenohumeral instability', *Clin. Orthopaed. Related Res.* 400: 98–104, (2002)

Nitz A.J., 'Physical Therapy management of the shoulder', *Physical Ther.* 66(12): 1912–1918, (1986)

Noonen T.J., Garett W.E., 'Injuries at the myotendinous junction', *Clini. Sport Med.* 11(4): 783–806, (1992)

Paine R.M., Voight M., 'The role of the scapula', *J. Ortop. Sports Phys. Ther.* 18(1): 386–390, (1993)

Panjabi M.M., 'The stabilizing system of the spine. I: function, dysfunction, adaptation and enhancement', *J. Spine Disord.* 5(4): 383–389, (1992)

Peterson D.E., Blankenship K.R., Robb J.B., Walzer M.J., Bryan J.M., Setts D.M., Mincey L.M., Simmons G.E., 'Investigation of the validity and reliability of four objective techniques for measuring forward shoulder posture'. *J. Ortop. Sports Phys. Ther.* 5(1): 34–42, (1997)

Philadephia Panel, 'Evidence-based Clinical practice guidelines on selected rehabilitation interventions for shoulder pain', *Physical Ther.* 81(10): 1719–1729, (2001)

Prud'Homme M.J.L., Kalaska J.F., 'Proprioceptive activity in primate primary somatosensory cortex during active arm reaching movement', *J. Neurophysiol.* 72(5): 2280–2299, (1994)

Radebold A., Cholewicki J., Gert K., Polzhofer B.A., 'Impaired postural control of the lumbar spine is associated with delayed muscle response times in patients with chronic idiopathic low back pain', *Spine* 26(7): 724–730, (2001)

Richardson C., Jull G., Hodges P., Hides J., 'Therapeutic exercise for spinal segmental stabilization in low back pain: scientific basis and clinical approach', Churchill Livingstone, Edinburgh (1999)

Rondhuis G.B., 'Knierevalidatie (Rehabilitation of the knee)', Tijdstroom, Utrecht (1996)

Rougier P., Zanders E., Borlet E., 'Influence of visual cues on upright postural control: differentiated effects of eyelid closure', *Rev. Neurol.* 159(2): 180–188, (2003)

Rubin B.D., Kibler W.B., 'Fundamental principles of shoulder rehabilitation: conservative approach to postoperative management', *Arthroscopy* 18(9): 29–39, (2002)

Russ D.W., 'In-season management of shoulder pain in a collegiate swimmer: a team approach', *J. Ortop. Sports Phys. Ther.* 5: 371–376, (1998)

Sahrmann S.A., 'Diagnosis and treatment of movement impairment syndromes', Mosby, St Louis (2002)

Sainburg R.L., Ghilardi M.F., Poizner H., Ghez C., 'Control of limb dynamics in normal subjects and patients without proprioception', *J. Neurophysiol* 73(2): 820–834, (1995)

Sainburg R.L., Poizner H., Ghez C., 'Loss of proprioception produces deficits in interjoint coordination', *J. Neurophysiol.* 70(5): 2136–2147, (1993)

Schmitt L., Snyder-Mackler L., 'Role of scapular stabilizers in etiology and treatment of impingement syndrome', *J. Ortop. Sports Phys. Ther.* 29(1): 31–38, (1999)

Shakespeare D.T., Stokes M., Sherman K.P., Young A., 'Reflex inhibition of the quadriceps after meniscectomy: lack of association with pain', *Clin. Physiol.* 5: 137–144, (1985)

Sharkey N.A., Marder R.A., 'The rotator cuff opposes superior translation of the humeral head', *Am. J. Sport Med.* 23(3): 270–275, (1995)

Stanish W.D., Curwin S., Mandell S., '*Tendinitis: its etiology and treatment*', Oxford University Press, New York, (2000)

Sterling M., Jull G., Wright A., 'The effect of musculoskeletal pain on motor activity and control', *J. Pain* 2(3): 135–145, (2001)

T'jonck L., 'Functionele evaluatie en revalidatie bij patienten met glenohumerale instabiliteit en subacromiaal impingment (Evaluation and functional rehabilitation in patients with glenohumeral instability and subacromial impingement)', Doctoral thesis in physiotherapy, Leuven (1998)

Tata D.E., NG L., Kramer J.F., 'Shoulder antagonistic strength ratio during concentric and eccentric muscle action in the scapular plane', *J. Ortop. Sports Phys. Ther.* 18(6): 654–660, (1993)

Tortensen T.A., Meen H.D., Stiris M., 'The effect of medical exercise therapy on a patient with chronic supraspinatus tendinitis. Diagnostic ultrasound. Tissue regeneration: a case study', *J. Ortop. Sports Phys.* 20(6): 319–328, (1994)

Tyler T.F., Roy T., Nicholas S.J., Glein G.W., 'Reliability and validity of a new method of measuring posterior shoulder tightness', *J. Orthop. Sports Phys. Ther.* 29(5): 262–274, (1999)

Van Wingerden B.A.M., 'Bindweefsel in de revalidatie (Connective tissue in rehabilitation)', Scipro Verlag, Liechtenstein (1997)

Verschueren S.M.P., Swinnen S.P., Cordo P.J., Dounska N.V., 'Proprioception control of multijoint movement: unimanual cycle drawing', *Exp. Brain Res.* 127: 171–181, (1999)

Vlaeyen J.W., Seelen H.A., Peters M., De Jonge P., Aretz E., Beisiegel E., Weber W.E., 'Fear of movement/(re) injury and muscular reactivity in chronic low back pain patients: an experimental investigation', *Pain* 82(3): 297–304, (1997)

Vleeming A., Mooney V., Dorman T., Snijders C.H., Stoeckart R., 'Movement, stability and low back pain: the essential role of the pelvis', Churchill Livingstone, New York (1997)

Vleeming A., Snijders C.F., Stoeckart R., Mens F.M.A., 'The role of the sacroiliac joint in coupling between spine, pelvis, legs and arms', In: *Movement, stability and low back pain: The essential role of the pelvis*, Churchill Livingstone, New York, pp. 53–71, (1997)

Voight M.L., Hardin J.A., Blackburn T.A., Tippett S., Canner G.C., 'The effect of muscle fatigue on the relationship of arm dominance to shoulder proprioception', *J. Orthop. Sports Phys. Ther.* 23(6): 348–352, (1996)

Wadell G., 'The Back Pain Revolution', Churchill Livingstone, Edinburgh (2000)

Warner J.J.P., Micheli L.J., Arslanian L.E., Kennedy J., Kennedy R., 'Scapulothoracic motion in normal shoulder and shoulder with glenohumeral instability and impingement syndrome: a study using Moire topographic analysis', *Clin. Orthop.* 85: 191–199, (1992)

Warner J.J.P., Micheli L.J., Arslanian L.E., Kennedy J., Kennedy R., 'Patterns of flexibility, laxity and strength in normal shoulders and shoulders with instability and impingement', *Am. J. Sports Med.* 18: 366–375, (1990)

Wilk K., Arrigo A.A., Andrews J.R., 'Current concept: the stabilizing structures of the glenohumeral joint', *J. Ortop. Sports Phys. Ther.* 25(6): 364–378, (1997)

Wilk K.E., 'Current concept in the rehabilitation of the athletic shoulder', *J. Ortop. Sports Phys. Ther.* 8: 365–378, (1993)

Wilk K.E., Andrews J.R., Arrigo C.A. et al., 'The strength charateristics of the internal and external rotator muscles in professional baseball pitchers', *Am. J. Sports Med.* 21: 61–66, (1993)

Wilk K.E., Meister K., Andrews J.R., 'Current concepts in the rehabilitation of overhead throwing athletes', *Am. J. Sports Med.* 30(1): 136–151, (2002)

Young J.L., Herring S.A., Press J.M., 'The influence of the spine on the shoulder in the throwing athlete', *J. Back Musculoskeletal Rehabil.* 7: 5–17, (1996)

CHAPTER 16

PREVENTION AND PHYSICAL AND ATHLETIC TRAINING

A. Fusco
C. Scotton

The meaning of prevention

The word 'prophylaxis' is defined as 'preventing a disease' (Hewitt, 1956), and is derived etymologically from the Greek προφυλασσειν, 'to protect'.

Prevention is defined as the whole range of measures taken to avoid disease and can be primary, secondary or tertiary. Primary prevention aims at avoiding a harmful event, as, for example, a rule designed to avert direct collisions in a sport. Secondary prevention refers to the possibility of mitigating or preventing the serious consequences of a disease by early diagnosis and therapy (*Various Authors*, 1996). The best-known methods include routine examinations or screening tests performed on individuals at risk from specific diseases. The aim of tertiary prevention is to avoid an existing disease becoming worse or potential complications appearing (Rumolo, 1992). Prevention in the case of an overhead athlete involves monitoring the training loads used. To implement effective prevention, the usual basic questions (what?, why?, when?, how?, where? and who?) that characterize a scientific approach should be addressed (Guyatt, 1991; Cartabellotta, 1997).

The literature contains few sufficiently specific and detailed studies of the prevention of shoulder problems, however the work by Pink, Jobe et al., who devote the first chapter of their book to prevention, is worth noting (Pink, 1995).

One of the purposes of this book is to encourage a multidisciplinary approach to the health of athletes (professionals or amateurs). The aim will consequently be to demonstrate that it is possible to adopt prophylactic measures by studying and observing various aspects of athletic training.

It is clear that there is only a narrow margin for preventive measures where acute disorders are concerned.

Measures that are effective to some extent are, however, probably feasible in some chronic problems.

In recent years, as acknowledged by the same authorities, approximately 50% of sport injuries were caused by overload (Santilli, in La Torre, 1999) and many accidents are due to overload injury, related to increased training load (La Torre, 1999).

An attempt at the prevention of chronic pathology could be hypothesized in this respect if an aetiological intervention were possible. A starting point could be the analysis of aspects of workloads on a general level and subsequently an examination of the balance of local loads.

The aspects of athletic movements that potentially predispose towards injury have already been examined (Section II, Chapter 3), and the biomechanical characteristics that are decisive in terms of athletic technique have been identified. A classification of sports which can be used as a reference by the various professionals is given below. The next part will deal with aspects of prophylaxis identifiable in planning (see the section on Periodization and monitoring of athletic training) and methodology of athletic training (see the section on Methodology and objectives of athletic training).

It should be kept in mind that training comprises aspects of athletic preparation and training (proper) varying in manner and quantity depending on the discipline and level of performance. These aspects are related to the objectives of the training known as organic, muscular and neuromuscular ability (see the sections on Organic and muscular objectives of

Prevention and physical and athletic training

athletic training and Neuromuscular objectives of athletic training).

It will become apparent how a prophylactic measure can be identified in the structure of the training (planning, periodization) or its contents (methodology, athletic technique). Such a measure requires retrospective and prospective monitoring, enhancing the importance of the evaluation.

The subject of prevention will conclude, in the next section, with a way of observing recurrent errors in the structuring of athletic training and in technical performance.

Athletic training and classification of sports

'Athletic training is a complex educational teaching process, based on bioethics, which takes place over long periods of time, [...] which is achieved through systematically organized physical exercise, repeated in quantity, and of an intensity and level of efficacy so as to produce loads that are always diversified [...], that can stimulate the body's biological processes of adjustment, adaptation and overcompensation [...] in order to reasonably increase, consolidate and enhance its competitive performance' (Bellotti, 1999).

Training is based on the principles of biological adaptation to a stimulus and on the principle of overcompensation: the body reacts to an adequate motor stimulus with a state of fatigue; it then overcompensates, increasing its future ability to respond to the same stimulus (see Figs. 14.1 and 14.5).

Training requires planning, periodization, the use of a methodology, setting objectives and monitoring.

Physical exercise or load is generally divided into general exercise, specific exercise and competitive exercise. The purpose of general exercise is to achieve general development and it is carried out through movement, with and without equipment, and also through various sport disciplines. Specific exercise aims to improve specific requirements through performing elements of competition. Competitive exercise involves elements of full or virtually full competition from the point of view of technical complexity and psychological involvement.

There are many sport disciplines which involve extensive use of the shoulder joint. If this study were to be limited to Olympic disciplines, it would already be a very difficult task to examine their characteristics with the aims of this book in mind (evaluation, treatment and prevention).

Furthermore, a study of this type would run the risk of excluding very many artistic and athletic

activities which require specific use of the shoulder, as well as of becoming rapidly obsolete owing to the constant evolution and introduction of codified sports.

It is difficult when analysing athletic movements performed by the shoulder to classify sport disciplines which require the predominant use of this joint.

A recent classification reported in the literature is rather complex yet not exhaustive (Table 16.1).

Table 16.1

Definitions of technique and sport equipment (Scotton, 2003)

Definition of technique

Technique means selecting and performing sport-related motor skills which have become fairly automatic, and carrying out predominantly mental activities, applying the laws of physics and biology to humans in order to achieve the optimal result while keeping within the rules.

Definitions of sport equipment

Definition of sport equipment

We define 'sport equipment' as equipment specified by the rules and essential for performing a discipline.

Definition of propulsion equipment

We define 'propulsion sport equipment' as equipment which, when performing a discipline, aids the movement of the participant in space.

Definition of impulsion equipment

We define 'impulsion sport equipment' as equipment which, when performing a discipline, is subject to one or more impulses applied by the participant and does not act as an aid to movement.

Definition of equipment not subject to incident forces

We define 'sport equipment not subject to incident forces' as equipment which, though essential and not optional when performing a discipline, does not have essential characteristics associated with forces exerted on or through it (cards, chess).

Definition of accessory equipment

We define 'accessory sport equipment' as equipment used when performing a sport, the use of which is permitted and not imposed by the rules, and, therefore, not crucial to technique (wrist straps, gloves, life-jackets).

Such a classification can help health workers determine the requirements of athletes in terms of ability; it should not, however, be seen as a decision-making algorithm for therapeutic or prophylactic purposes.

There are at least three factors which seem to support a classification:

— the multidisciplinary character at which this chapter is aiming, in the hope of being able to contribute to creating a common language;
— the quantitative and qualitative evolution of sport disciplines, which means that any reference limited to sports practised today rapidly becomes obsolete; and
— the identification of similarities and differences between athletic movements, the environments in which they are performed and the equipment used for evaluation.

An attempt at classifying techniques based on a number of recognizable characteristics may perhaps make this book useful for those interested in 'minor' sports, while at the same time creating a cultural resource of references for adherents of 'new' motor activities.

To return to the feasibility of a classification, various problems stand out, as mentioned above.

First of all, there is little in the international literature with a multidisciplinary content covering the fields of medicine, sport technique and motor sciences.

Medical literature scarcely meets the technical specifications that are typical of and necessary to the world of motor sciences, particularly as regards terminology.

Sport literature, moreover, contains classifications based on the technical content of the discipline (sports of degree, positional sports, strength sports, etc.) (Harre, 1972) which will rapidly become obsolete owing to the constant evolution of the world of sports.

Bioenergy and biomechanics studies are peripheral disciplines.

Although bioenergy studies use mainly biochemical terminology and biomechanics studies predominantly mathematical language, they represent a point of linguistic and scientific convergence.

Studies in the field of biomechanics have up to now been limited to a few areas (analysis of segmental movement, analysis of walking). Chapter 2 of this book, which refers to 3D studies of movement, makes an outstanding contribution in this respect.

The biomechanical aspects of the shoulder joint constitute one of the most difficult areas to study owing to its unique versatility in sports as a result of phylogenetic adaptations in human beings, i.e. the change in the shoulder joint in humans who, over 'a few' thousand years, have evolved from quadrupedalism (locomotion function) to upright stature (relation function), probably passing through a quadrumanism phase (including a suspension function).

The practice of sports, viewed from the perspective of prevention, involves various aspects which can be grouped, for clarity, as technical and biomechanical aspects (technique and physiology of movement), and functional aspects (muscle and organic ability, neuromotor ability). It is worth identifying the professional figures interested in the different aspects, and to note that it is presumably difficult for the various professionals involved to use a common language:

— the fundamental aspects of technique and aspects deriving from these (actions, rules, tactics, methodology) concern technicians, but cannot be disregarded by athletic trainers, physiotherapists and sport injury doctors ('technique' is defined in Table 16.1);
— the biomechanical aspects concern the scientific world and rehabilitation professionals, but motor sciences and technicians also have an interest (in Italy; the Italian national olympic committee or (CONI)). It is clear that there are planning, financial and practical difficulties linking the scientific aspect, laboratory research and application in the practice of sport. Nevertheless, the arthrokinetic and arthrokinematic studies undertaken seem to offer particular interest as regards practical performance;
— aspects relating to muscle and organic (or conditional) abilities prevalent in a given discipline, in the realm of the motor sciences, concern physiotherapists and sport injury doctors as well as technicians (motor science graduates, athletic coaches, trainers and instructors – in Italy – of CONI);
— aspects relating to the neuromotor (or coordination) abilities prevalent in a given discipline, concern technicians, physical trainers, physiotherapists, sport injury doctors and sport psychologists to a varying extent; and
— neurophysiological aspects primarily concern medical research; however, the results of some studies have practical repercussions for the work of physiotherapists, technicians, athletic trainers and sport injury doctors.

The technical classification of sport disciplines referred to (Scotton, 2003) can be used to determine aspects of sport disciplines that involve the use of the shoulder.

Sport-related motor ability can, therefore, be:

A1: (stereotyped): technical execution generally refers to a theoretical model which is reproduced by the athlete under similar conditions, called closed skill. The objective of a closed skill is frequently an absolute performance, such as throwing the javelin;

A2: (non-stereotyped): technical execution is determined by unpredictable factors (opponents, environment), consequently the movement is implicitly variable (open skill); examples are combat sports or team games;

B: one or more muscle and organic (or conditional) capacities have a decisive role;

B1: (muscle resistance): the technical execution of the disciplines in which this ability is prevalent often requires cyclic movements, with a predominant rhythm, which can undergo temporary variations; this is the case with swimming and rowing;

B2: (speed, but according to other authors, velocity): the technical execution of the disciplines in which this ability is prevalent often involves throwing small 'projectiles'; an example is baseball (the role of the pitcher);

B3: (force): the ability involved in the majority of ballistic disciplines (in which the throwing movement is used) in its various forms; the explosive force or velocity may vary according to the different weights or dimensions of the projectile;

C: based on the presence of a special decisive coordination ability in sports 'with prevalent non-stereotyped motor abilities' (e.g. water polo, volleyball and tennis), conditions imposed by the rules must be taken into account: these conditions result in adaptations of actions due to feedback varying according to the sport; in volleyball, the presence of the net means for the hitter that the involvement of the antagonist muscles will be greater to avoid touching it; in water polo, throwing in the water involves the need for proximal-distal stabilization of the body; and

D: joint biomechanics, an intrinsic and unique aspect of any athletic movement, may in turn be influenced by the environment in which the sport is played and by the equipment used. These factors may increase local load (shoulder joint) or disturb the optimal arthrokinematics.

Based on the predominant method of use of the upper limb, a number of distinctions can be made in relation to the osteokinematic position of the shoulder in space, the existence of a constraint at the end of the limb, the use of equipment, and the type of muscle contraction.

The following are examples of athletic movements:

D1: above 90° of abduction (e.g. swimming styles, throwing in track and field) or below 90° of abduction (e.g. golf, rowing);

D2: in an OKC, in which the upper limb has a predominantly relational function (e.g. throwing). In a CKC in which the upper limb has a predominantly locomotion-support function (e.g. gymnastics and climbing);

D3: with impulsion equipment (racquets, clubs) or without impulsion equipment (e.g. throwing) (sport equipment is defined in Table 16.1);

D4: with propulsion equipment (e.g. windsurfing or water-skiing);

D5: predominantly involving plyometric contraction, or preliminary acceleration of the projectile (throwing in general, also in team sports), but also in gymnastics (in particular the rings, beam and asymmetric bars).

Relation between load and carriability: overuse syndrome and overtraining

The biopsychosocial model (Jones, 2002) (Section IV, Chapter 12) provides a guide to prevention in the various areas, i.e. biological, psychological and social, in which the subject may show signs of altered homeostasis. The MLCM (Hagenaars, 2002) (Figs. 14.2 and 15.1) suggests two different locations of overuse, i.e. local and general.

An athlete is an individual exposed to the risk of disorders due to overuse; consequently each of the three aspects (biological, psychological and social) deserves examination in detail, since each is capable of triggering a vicious circle, regardless of whether it is caused by motivational, sociocultural or biological aspects, and their reciprocal influences, together with environmental and personal factors.

In an athletic context, we can assume that the general level corresponds to overtraining (OT), and the local level to overuse syndrome.

Psychosocial factors have been linked in the literature to general and local problems.

Reference is made in general to the body's metabolic and cardiovascular conditions: the literature shows that symptoms of overtraining are highly individualized, for athletes of all levels. That would suggest aiming preventive measures at the biological (organic) level at which the dysfunction is occurring. Psychological disturbances, however, increase in proportion to the training load and return to normal faster the further the individual is from the point of overreaching (Rossi, 1999); this would suggest the need for monitoring of mood in athletes in order to prevent OT (see the section on Periodization and monitoring of athletic training).

Reference is made on a local level to the biological conditions of tissues and organs; epidemiological studies have been conducted (Harkness, 2003) into shoulder disorders and have found that intrinsic and extrinsic factors such as young age, male gender and the number of years of participation, can cause a higher incidence of painful shoulder (Berlusconi, 1990).

It should also be noted that for athletes, a small anatomical injury (impairment) can significantly limit competitive activity (participation problem), leading to a psychological attitude detrimental to solving the problem.

Both levels also interact in both directions with psychological aspects which are sometimes neglected, particularly for 'local' problems.

It can be hypothesized, in the light of the above, that professional athletes are exposed more to OT than amateurs, since they are subjected to greater overall training load volumes, with more frequent and intense effort and, as a result, less time for recovery. Amateur athletes may, however, also be exposed, though to a lesser extent, to overuse syndrome, since they undergo training that is less planned, less varied in content, and less directed at general carriability and consequently more repetitive and 'stressful' at a local level.

There are comments in the literature about the term overtraining, which has for some time been part of the language of sport medicine. Training exercises for participation in sport cause a state of fatigue; under physiological conditions, fatigue is a crisis phase, followed by the process of recovery during which the physical and mental energy reserves used to perform the exercise are not only restored but actually increased (principle of overcompensation). If the ability to recover is exceeded or the physiological conditions are disturbed, this constitutes overreaching; the parameter most useful for assessing this seems to be recovery time, which should be between 72 hours and 15 days after maximum physical effort (Kentta, 1998).

The situation in long-term overtraining seems to be rather complex; the interaction of more than one factor should be considered, and physical, psychological, social, immunological, endocrine and other aspects come into play.

The symptoms of OT can be varied and highly individualized, and may affect athletes at all levels; the main symptom in common seems to be a decline in performance. The hypotheses that most deserve further examination include the dysregulation of the nervous system.

This dysregulation is believed to be the result of prolonged 'stressful' stimuli, to which the body is no longer able to respond optimally.

The greatest difficulty is to identify the threshold between training and overreaching, since it is a continuum. It should be kept in mind that prolonging borderline overreaching will eventually place the organism in a condition of unbalanced adaptation, which culminates in overtraining syndrome, otherwise known as staleness syndrome, a sensation of being drained and refusing to continue training.

It currently seems possible to base a diagnosis of OT on laboratory tests, such as ACTH (Meeusen, 1995; Meeusen, 2003), but this has a certain latency; consequently, such a diagnosis is reached in practice by exclusion, in the presence of a prolonged decline in performance.

As regards overuse, the literature data suggest that the damage is caused by irritant stresses, repeated in cycles for prolonged periods, or at high intensity on various sites or tissues (Mondardini, 1999).

The concept of overuse can be seen, in relation to the MLCM (Section IV, Chapter 12), as a combination of high (abnormal) levels of stress applied repeatedly to normal tissue, or as the effect of normal stresses applied to structures with reduced carriability (due to intrinsic factors such as age, gender or race, or extrinsic factors such as fatigue, nutrition, anxiety, etc.).

Overuse can be defined as the result of microlesions due to repeated strains (Section II, Chapter 4) which lead to polymicrotraumatic clinical pictures such as impingement disorders (Jobe, 1991).

The harmful effects of functional overuse and its related clinical manifestations can appear in any formation of the musculoskeletal system, but the sites most affected are the tendons, with their appendages, and the joint cartilages (Candela, 1998).

Repeated, persistent microtraumatic action on tendon tissue does not allow adequate repair of the damage it undergoes in the course of functional effort, in the context of the anabolic process. The initial response of the tendon to irritant stimuli generally involves the appearance of acute inflammation which, if the trigger persists, develops into tissue degeneration and chronic inflammation.

Joint cartilage has a similar fate to tendons, aggravated by the lack of cell turnover. Excessive functional stresses can give rise to the appearance of a lesion which, after undergoing the phases of softening, fissuring, fibrillation and surface erosion, may eventually involve exposure of the subchondral bone, thus resulting in a picture similar to osteoarthritis. Harmful phenomena can be summarized as compression, slow stretching and rubbing.

This scenario does not always have precise anatomical evidence, since inflammatory or degenerative alterations do not commonly occur in an incapacitating state (for example, histochemical lesions of structures subjected to traumatic action). The various pathological pictures are, therefore, defined simply using topographical rather than gross pathological terms (Colombo, 1987); thrower's shoulder is an example.

The prevention of overuse therefore appears to be connected to identifying firstly the damaging mechanism, and secondly the intrinsic or extrinsic predisposing conditions which lead to the internal tissue resistance being exceeded.

Referring to the MLCM (Chapter 12, Section IV), it seems clear that overuse can also be the result of reduced carriability (incorrect or inadequate training).

The possible prevention strategies include the early identification of risk factors (Inklaar, 1994):

— intrinsic factors, such as physical and mental state of health and individual characteristics (joint mobility, muscle stiffness, laxity, functional stability, previous lesions); and

— extrinsic factors, such as participating in a sport (exercise load, contact with opponents).

Athletic movements can in turn increase the risk of an incident, as shown in Chapter 3, Section II (Fig. 3.1). The aim of evaluating technique and training planning is to identify the aspects of each factor that can be modified for preventive purposes.

Periodization and monitoring of athletic training

Periodization of training is understood to mean dividing up the entire training cycle into periods, each having specific characteristics and different objectives. The overall duration of periodization varies according to the level of competition, ranging from four-yearly for the highest levels (for example, for preparing an Olympic performance), to annual cycles for national levels. Periodization usually involves a division of training into macrocycles, mesocycles and microcycles. These divisions correspond to general preparation, special preparation and competition; mesocycles can correspond to a month and microcycles to a week.

When planning training, sport technicians should take into account technical and personal factors concerning the athlete.

Technical factors include the rules and their implications for technological development, technique and its evolution; personal factors include motor and tactical capacity and psychological characteristics.

The necessary premise for the optimal use of the progress obtained in training is the appropriate determination of work loads, the principal parameters of which are quantity, intensity and density, as well as regional distribution combined with organized progression.

The periodization of training can, and should, result in planning the athlete's career programme. Although it is true that shoulder disorders begin at a young age, but are usually manifested after a number of years of participation (eight or nine according to some authors) (Berlusconi, 1990), individual performance should be assessed cautiously in order to optimize the athlete's performance throughout their entire career.

Monitoring seems to be a useful tool for gaining access to a database of individual and group subjective and objective data, relating to athletes. Monitoring can be carried out on a team and individual level, using simple methods.

At a team level, epidemiological monitoring will provide technical staff (primarily athletic coaches and trainers) with a remarkable tool for the correct management of athletic preparation in both pre-competition and competition phases, as well as describing the personal, temporal and spatial characteristics of injuries, and any sequelae (descriptive epidemiology). Analytical epidemiology can identify the predictive factors and factors associated with the injury. It should be kept in mind that in Italy, only a small percentage of injuries is regularly reported to the sport insurance body. Insurance claims are not made in particular for injuries considered to be minor and for athletes competing at lower levels (Lanzetta, 1993).

A method of individual/subjective monitoring has been suggested to counteract the effects of OTS, using several variables (Rossi, 1999):

— *monitoring the indicators of stress occurring during a performance:* control of the more rapidly variable biochemical and psychological parameters and study of the conditions and times of appearance and any associated causes, assessing the correlation between subjective sensations and objective findings in the athlete;

— *monitoring mood:* psychological disturbances increase in proportion to the training load and return to normal faster the further away the point of overreaching (section on Athletic training and classification of sports). A rating scale like the Hamilton depression rating scale (HAMD) can easily be adapted to the needs of an athlete;

— *identification of factors influencing an athlete's ability to adapt:* i.e. duration, repetitiveness, degree of risk, physical effort, associated stress, individual and natural qualities; and

— *organization of all the phases of the recovery process:* redesigning the training plan by correctly managing training loads, modifying goals by 'modulating' both the number of competitive events and early optimization of recovery, personalizing the exercise : rest ratio, providing adequate psychological support, analysing dietary requirements and supplementing the diet with specific antioxidants.

The data for monitoring can be gathered retrospectively or prospectively. The retrospective form seeks the cause of the disturbance of the athlete's homeostasis, by asking questions such as: 'What happened that was negative?'. The prospective form aims to identify the signs and symptoms of OT.

Monitoring should, therefore, yield data that are useful for quantifying work objectively (quantitative data), but above all for evaluating how the athlete perceives the work; some of the items could be: work load (volume and intensity), enjoyment of work, muscle soreness, physical well-being, mental well-being, and the intensity of the training day (Foster, 1997). It seems important to suggest enhancing the athlete's capacity for self-assessment (by means of a personal diary or periodic sessions). This procedure may help to evaluate the individual perception of fatigue by the athlete, to recognize overreaching early, and to measure the individual's capacity for recovery.

It should be kept in mind, as regards overtraining, that many athletes train more than once a day and a third daily training session has recently been introduced for some disciplines. The questions to be asked in these cases concern the balance between training and recovery and evaluation by the athlete of normal recovery. It is also important to recommend that OT be assessed by means of more than one exercise, and at maximum exercise levels (McKenzie, 1999).

Turning to individual monitoring, its fundamental value also lies in its ability to allow optimal adjustment of individual programming over several years or collective programming. If an athlete is transferred to another team and has their personal data for the previous season, it is easier to make qualitative and quantitative adjustments of training loads. From the biopsychosocial point of view, the 'stressful' aspects represented by a new environment, new responsibilities, and the new trainer, should not be disregarded.

Prevention advice relates to the use of adequate physical preparation which takes into due consideration the organic, muscular and neuromuscular objectives important for the sport in question, based on an evaluation of general and local carriability, through a regular programme.

Methodology and objectives of athletic training

The methodology of training can be defined as a knowledge of how to use the contents of training.

The phrase 'training method' means the use of specific exercises performed and organized according to biophysiological principles, to achieve a given aim.

The use of a single method to achieve a specific motor capacity seems to be less effective than a combination; this assumption leads to a conclusion that is only apparently paradoxical: in order to adapt better, you should never need to adapt.

As regards the prevention of shoulder disorders, the majority of training programmes identify the following as making the most important contributions to the organic and muscular, and neuromuscular objectives:

— achieving and maintaining the organic and muscular capacities for strength, resistant strength and joint mobility; and

— achieving and maintaining neuromotor qualities, i.e. perception and coordination qualities.

These objectives are considered necessary for combining the effective performance of an athletic movement with correct joint function.

Organic and muscular objectives of athletic training

The organic and muscular objectives of athletic training for prophylaxis concern strength, resistant strength, joint mobility and muscle extendibility.

Muscle strength

An improvement in strength may, but does not always, imply an improvement in performance. However, the role of muscle strength as a guarantee of joint stability has already been discussed. Some authors, including Kerlan and Jobe, have focused on identifying certain muscles as glenohumeral 'protectors'. This role arises from a functional view, according to which muscles are divided into motors and stabilizers.

We have seen (Section II, Chapter 3) that the muscle strength requirement in overhead sports is variable and depends on several factors. Technicians should, therefore, carefully assess the amount of the strength and muscle contraction type required by the sport and

Prevention and physical and athletic training

adjust training (training methods) and monitoring accordingly. The types of muscle contraction are concentric, eccentric, isometric and plyometric. Plyometric contraction is a sequence of intense eccentric contraction followed by maximal concentric contraction, performed with variable loads. The medical literature regards plyometric contraction as a variant of eccentric contraction.

The various sport training methods for improving strength should be well known to technicians in order to exploit their benefits to the full, but also to be able to foresee their side effects, such as delayed onset muscular soreness (DOMS) which we shall discuss shortly.

We have also seen that the onset of shoulder pain is early in many cases; it has been hypothesized that this depends on quantitative or qualitative muscle insufficiency. It consequently seems appropriate to provide an adequate muscle strengthening programme for young athletes taking part in overhead sports.

The essential methodological principles for strength training in young athletes are the following: initial individual evaluation, compensation for any deficiencies identified, 'centrifugal' training, constant monitoring of the co-existence of muscle requirements (strength, resistant strength), joint requirements (joint mobility and muscle elasticity) and coordination requirements (neuromuscular control).

The maximum repetition method is suggested for monitoring strength, adjusting the method for young athletes by testing for a maximum from 10 repetitions at most instead of from maximum repetition. Roy Sinclair's well-known predictive table may be useful in this respect (Harre, 1972).

Starting from the assumption that muscle tension is an important factor in itself in increasing muscle strength during training, the fact that higher tensions can be obtained in eccentric actions (Tesch 1990) than in concentric or isometric actions would suggest that this type of training is preferable. Isolated animal skeletal muscle has the ability to produce approximately 100% more strength eccentrically than isometrically (Horstmann, 2001).

But it is important to note that eccentric actions differ from concentric and isometric actions in other ways too, such as electromechanical efficiency: the same level of strength can be produced in eccentric action as in concentric action, but with lower EMG activation. Studies by Komi (2000) show that the maximum eccentric moment was greater than the concentric moment at all velocities.

The existence of a mechanism regulating tension that prevents the development of maximum strength in situations of very high tension, to protect the musculoskeletal system from lesions which could occur if muscles were allowed to be activated completely, can, therefore, be hypothesized. It should also be noted, however, that the EMG in eccentric activity does not alter with the increase in velocity, confirming the hypothesis that tension does not increase in eccentric action at increasing velocities. The capsule receptors, free nerve endings in the muscle, pain receptors and Golgi organs are believed to be responsible for the feedback of this mechanism (Westing, 1990).

Some studies suggest that strength training optimizes muscle hypertrophy by eccentric actions and preserves the increase in fibre volume obtained after not training for a month for a very long period; it also minimizes DOMS (Hather, 1991). DOMS is not the same as common fatigue; it is believed to reflect structural damage and may occur when skeletal muscle is subjected to unusual exercise. A high level of fitness does not seem to protect against muscle overuse, since it even occurs in elite athletes. Unusual exercise very probably causes muscle pain, if it involves eccentric muscle action (Golden, 1992) and high strength peaks.

The process of recovery from exercise-induced muscle damage is slow and studies suggest that a complete recovery of strength may take more than a week (Donnelly, 1992).

A second exercise session, performed five days after the first session, does not reduce the rate of recovery of damaged muscles, but does reduce pain and symptoms, showing that some adaptation has already taken place.

Practical implications

In order to draw practical conclusions, the following should be stated:
— the most effective training programmes for increasing strength and muscle mass seem to be those which include both concentric and eccentric contractions;
— training programmes including only eccentric contractions do not seem to cause significant hypertrophy, only neural adaptations. It is possible that normal training protocols are insufficient to fatigue the muscle with eccentric contractions and, therefore, insufficient to cause hypertrophy;
— muscle has a very high fatigue index (FI) in eccentric contraction: it is more difficult for it to become fatigued and it develops lower concentrations of lactic acid and ammonium, at least in medium to high velocity contractions;

— although muscle succeeds in developing higher tensions in eccentric contraction than in concentric and isometric contraction, a smaller number of muscle fibres is activated; these fibres develop greater strength than that obtained in concentric or isometric contraction, with virtually complete activation; it seems useful, in an exercise consisting of a concentric phase and an eccentric phase, to overload the latter with resistance greater than that applied in the concentric phase; this will produce a greater increase in strength, even if it is exclusively in the eccentric phase;

— the use of eccentric contractions causes the phenomenon of DOMS, which does not have positive effects. The symptoms of DOMS are similar to those inflammation, although with some differences from the conventional definition;

— DOMS causes a reduction in structural strength, that is not dependent on the sensation of pain, and recovery is spontaneous;

— adaptation to exercise can occur, in which the repetition of the same exercise which had caused DOMS, after an interval of 15 days, no longer causes symptoms or, if it does, they are far less severe. Adaptation persists for a variable length of time, based on the various parameters considered, for example, the effect on plasma CK concentration may last for six months; and

— a considerable advantage of using eccentric contraction is the possibility of performing exercise in sectors of the ROM that cannot be reached in concentric contraction owing to a muscle deficit. The participant can be helped to reach the end of the ROM and allowed to return actively to the starting position in eccentric contraction.

Resistant strength

Resistant strength is the ability to express high tensions for a relatively long time.

It is also the ability of a muscle group or the entire organism to resist fatigue in actions in which prolonged and repeated muscle effort is required (Fiorini, 2003).

In the 1970s, Morehouse was one of the first authors to identify strength as an essential quality for the performance of high-level swimmers. At a time when prejudice against strengthening through overloading was widespread, his proposal of muscle strengthening in swimmers, athletes for whom the ability to swim and cover distance seemed to be sufficient, was rather perplexing. What he was referring to was resistant strength; his comments related, in fact, to a decline in

performance, which many athletes exhibit in the second part of the competitive season.

A few years later, significant analogies were found between 'inexplicable' declines in the performance of athletes and the declines in performance caused by the occurrence of joint disorders which were minor and often unrecognized, yet capable of having a detrimental effect on performance.

A deficit in resistant strength in an overhead athlete is, in fact, capable of disturbing correct glenohumeral and perhaps scapulothoracic joint centring, secondary to a proprioceptive impairment. Voight (1996) has documented that proprioception (understood as joint repositioning ability) is significantly disturbed by muscle fatigue.

The quantity of training may be directly related to the occurrence of muscle imbalances, which will be discussed as pathogenetic conditions; these imbalances may be present, though less marked, but already configured, in asymptomatic athletes (McMaster, 1993).

It may, therefore, be useful to include a test of resistance as part of monitoring to evaluate the behaviour of antagonists at the onset of fatigue, using a dynamometer. The reference value can be the fatigue index, expressed as a percentage of the maximum strength peak.

Joint mobility and muscle extendibility

Joint mobility is identified, in the fields of motor sciences and sport technology, as the ability to perform movements of the whole body or individual body segments through the maximum amplitude permitted by the anatomical structures forming the joints involved in the movement, or in any case acting on these, with the aim of achieving as useful a result as possible.

The concept of joint mobility is often associated with that of muscle extendibility, even in the medical field, and are both covered by the term flexibility.

This is acceptable owing to the importance of muscle extendibility among the factors limiting joint mobility. The other factors currently considered are: tendon and ligament stiffness, the shape of bone epiphyses (or joint heads), and contact with interposed bone or soft tissue.

As regards shoulder mobility, it is worth noting that rehabilitation studies demonstrate the importance of joint mobility of the chest, dorsal spine and cervicothoracic junction (Crawford, 1991).

In the field of medicine, the two concepts of joint mobility and muscle extendibility are different. Joint mobility is frequently referred to as ROM, and is expressed in degrees. Muscle extendibility is generally considered in the context of myofascial retraction which is intrinsically negative. Prolonged inactivity is known to cause a reduction in the extendibility of connective and muscle tissue. This phenomenon is the outcome of a lack of adaptation to altered physiological conditions. Retraction of myofascial tissue concerns connective tissue primarily and to a greater extent than muscle tissue. The stressing of connective tissue due to sudden traction is also known to cause it to thicken, reducing its functionality.

It should be noted that greater external rotation of the dominant arm at 90° abduction is often observed in throwing athletes, with reduced internal rotation (kvitne sign). A study of healthy professional baseball players compared the mobility and laxity of the dominant and non-dominant limb. Mean external rotation with the limb abducted at 90° was greater and internal rotation smaller in the dominant limb, regardless of the role of the player. Pitchers exhibited an ROM in both limbs that was on average greater in anterior elevation and in external rotation and a level of internal rotation that was on average smaller. As regards the degree of laxity, this was significantly smaller in pitchers compared to positional players (Bigliani, 1997).

Muscle extendibility and elasticity are also sometimes used as synonyms, however, they refer to functionally different concepts.

Elasticity is the characteristic whereby muscle, after being stretched returns to its original length when the stimulus ceases: the velocity of the phenomenon is a quantitative factor which qualitatively characterizes the elasticity.

The elasticity of muscle seems to be a predictor of risk of injury (Pope, 1999).

Extendibility is the property of soft tissue which allows it to stretch following appropriate stimulation; the extent of the stretch, i.e. its quantitative measurement, indicates the quality of muscle extendibility, regardless of the time necessary to achieve it or the size of the stimulus.

From the physical point of view, the elongation of an elastic material is proportional to the force applied. The relation between the elongation and the force applied is a straight line. The slope of the line is called the elasticity constant (k), and the inverse of this constant is compliance (c).

The elongation of an element will depend on its resting length and its section:
— the greater its initial length, the greater its elongation with equal force applied; and
— the greater its section, the greater the force needed to obtain the same elongation (Hooke's law).

In the field of sport technology, the same stresses are applied to try to increase or maintain joint mobility and muscle extendibility. The various known methods have arisen in order to increase muscle elasticity, since this is assumed to be useful in athletic performance. These methods, generally known as stretching, are traditionally divided into active and passive. The most widely used active methods are proprioceptive neuromuscular facilitation (PNF), contract-relax-antagonist-contract (CRAC), and the ballistic method (dynamic exercises performed closed to the limit of joint mobility). Passive methods vary according to the time for which the stretch is held.

The view is currently held that increasing the extendibility of the myotendinous unit can increase performance and reduce the epidemiological incidence of musculoskeletal problems.

Stretching exercises are consequently often included in the warm-up and warm-down phase of many athletes.

There is, however, no incontrovertible evidence in support of these assumptions.

Stretching has, in fact, been associated with a temporary deficit in strength for up to an hour afterwards (Kokkonen, 1998); for this finding to be assessed as positive or negative with regard to performance, the organic and muscular qualities required for each sport need to be identified.

Some authors, including Wilson (1988), have found that muscle elasticity training is appropriate before performance-enhancing training; the authors maintain, however, that the gain in terms of performance is minimal.

This part of the book nevertheless concerns the relation between elasticity or muscle extendibility and prevention of disorders.

The methodological quality of studies of the possible preventive implications of stretching is generally poor and these studies do not reach conclusions based on scientific evidence (Murlow, 1987).

The literature data suggest that stretching increases shoulder mobility, with some evidence in favour of the PNF method, although there is still some disagreement about this (Lucas, 1984).

The upper limb tension test (ULTT) (Coppieters, 1999) (Chapter 8) has aroused interest in the world of musculoskeletal therapy. The rationale underlying the evaluative test also seems to be valid for treatment or exercise to improve the extendibility of the neuroconnective structures.

Practical implications

Joint mobility and muscle extendibility have not as yet been investigated in detail by either sport or rehabilitation studies. The quality of the studies available is often unsatisfactory since almost all studies of the relation between stretching and injury prevention concern the lower limbs.

We report the 'state of the art' which is evidently not of a sufficient level to advocate increasing muscle extendibility as a means of prevention.

There is some evidence that flexibility increases performance (Lucas, 1984), but the results are not shared by all (Nelson, 2001); the data seem, moreover, to vary according to the areas of the body considered and types of performance.

It has been shown that the efficacy of stretching on postexercise muscle pain, DOMS, (Buroker, 1989) is not significant.

As regards prevention of injury, some authors believe that there is a significant effect (Ekstrand, 1983; Cross, 1999), while others do not (Shirer, 1999).

It seems that some of these contradictions can be explained by considering the different types of sport (Ettema, 2001). Explosive sports require the myotendinous unit to be sufficiently elastic (compliance) to store and provide a high quantity of elastic energy. Consequently, when the number of stretch-shortening cycles is large, elasticity and extendibility seem to be important for the prevention of musculoskeletal injuries.

On the other hand, when sports do not require stretch-shortening cycles, or require predominantly concentric contractions, all the muscle work must be converted into external work. In these cases, the elasticity of the myotendinous unit is less necessary and stretching seems to have no influence on the prevention of musculoskeletal injuries (Gleim, 1997; Witvrouw, 2003).

The same terms in current use, such as flexibility, extendibility and elasticity, do not seem to be used in an entirely relevant way; the anatomical and functional differences which characterize the various periarticular structures will require further multidisciplinary investigation in the future.

Neuromuscular objectives of athletic training

The neuromuscular objectives of athletic training are principally to achieve and maintain the perceptive and coordination abilities required to ensure the dynamic stability of the shoulder, particularly in overhead activities.

We shall, therefore, discuss proprioception, muscle balance and coordination; as we shall see, muscle balance cannot be understood simply as a quantitative aspect of the strength of the motor muscles of the shoulder, since they control coordination.

In ballistic actions, optimization of muscle drive is more important than the amount of strength the muscles succeed in recruiting. The principle of the chronological coordination of individual impulses (Hochmut, 1974, quoted in Gatta, 1996) and harmony explains why it is only through the dynamic work of the major muscle chains and the participation of all the joints, during movement or while fixed, that great quantities of impulses are obtained.

Proprioception

Proprioception is the body's ability to transmit the sense of position, to interpret the information and to respond consciously or unconsciously to stimuli, by appropriate changes in posture and movement (Houglum, 2001).

Proprioception may be defined as neuromuscular control (Wilk, 1993), which some authors attribute to a continual interaction between afferent and efferent impulses. The most significant afferent component is probably kinaesthesia; kinaesthesia can be defined as the ability to distinguish joint position, the relative weights of body parts and joint movements, including direction, amplitude and velocity (Newton, 1982).

As regards the shoulder, kinaesthesia and coordination capacity are necessary to select the appropriate voluntary muscle contractions which can stabilize the joint and alter joint position to prevent excessive displacement of the humeral head.

The ability to control the shoulder during active movement is also called neuromuscular reactive control and it is believed to be more important, for normal shoulder function, than joint position or repositioning ability (Wilk, 1993).

Neuromuscular reactive control describes the individual's ability to integrate proprioceptive information and motor control to react to the information.

Some neuromuscular dysfunctions, including loss of perception of muscle tension or sense of position, could be due to eccentric exercise; this phenomenon could be partly responsible for the postexercise reduction in strength and joint ROM. A study by Saxton (quoted in Seger, 1998) has shown that the amplitude of baseline tremor increased both immediately and 24 hours after eccentric exercise, but its frequency remained unchanged; the proprioception of strength and articular angle was impaired, causing tension and the angle produced to be overestimated, although the tension required (expressed as a percentage of maximum tension) was correct, considering the maximum value that could be expressed that day. In other words, if a muscle expresses a strength of

100, after eccentric exercise which halves its strength, the nervous system will respond to a further request for effort equal to 50 with only 25.

Muscle balance and joint stability

A thrower's shoulder needs to be fairly lax to permit extreme external rotation, but fairly stable to prevent symptomatic subluxations of the humeral head; it consequently requires a delicate balance between functional stability and mobility. This is what is meant by the 'thrower's paradox' (Wilk, 2002).

The muscle balance conditions necessary for movements of the upper limb in throwing can be divided into global and regional.

At a global level, the effector kinetic chains of the shoulder girdle, i.e. the thoracoappendicular and spinoappendicular muscles, should be balanced between a stabilizer and effector function (Saha, 1983; Jobe, 1988; Kibler, 1991).

These effector chains should, in turn, be supported by the normal function of the pelvic girdle, which consists largely of its stability.

At a regional level, i.e. as regards effector function, balance should be guaranteed between agonist and antagonist chains. As regards the glenohumeral joint, this factor seems to be crucial to correct function, on the basis of studies suggesting that imbalance is primarily or jointly responsible for impingement syndrome (Bernard, 1996; De Carli, 1991; Giombini, 1991; McMaster, 1991; Warner, 1990; Wilk, 1993). The combined effect of the synergic action of the rotator cuff creates compression in the glenoid, which is the key component for joint stability. The term 'balance of forces' between deltoid and cuff, therefore, seems more appropriate than 'pair relation of forces' (Wilk, 1997).

By means of comparative evaluations of healthy individuals and patients, the literature has identified the importance of muscle balance in the shoulder between internal rotator and external rotator muscle groups and between humeral adductors and abductors. The balance values, recommended by studies conducted using isokinetic dynamometers, indicated an internal to external rotation ratio of 1.3:1. Subsequent studies nevertheless reported asymptomatic athletes with muscle balance values significantly different from those recommended.

This situation can probably be explained firstly by an intercurrent relation between proprioception, joint repositioning ability and muscle fatigue (Voight, 1996), and secondly by the presence of these imbalances in asymptomatic athletes (McMaster, 1993).

Specificity of athletic training

The adaptation responses of the body to training stimuli are specific; for the effect of training to be significant, it needs to produce an effect that is functional for the sport for which the athlete is training.

Many studies have investigated the concept of the specificity of training and have observed adaptations specific to factors such as training method, muscle length and rate of muscle shortening. An additional factor which may result in training having specific effects is the type of muscle action used, i.e. whether training consists of isometric, concentric or eccentric muscle actions, or a combination of these (Seger, 1998). A specific, targeted working methodology, which takes into account the use of strength in the various sports disciplines, can prove useful in preventing injuries.

Specificity in training posture has also been observed: following maximal eccentric training in an upright position, increases in strength were no longer visible in a supine position (Porter, 1997).

Dynamic posture, or rather the morphofunctional characteristics of the cervicothoracic spine, is very important as regards eye-hand coordination training, specific to throwing disciplines. This ability is the result of integration of visual information with movements (or adjustments of movements) of the upper limb, in order to reach a predetermined objective (for example, the opponents' goal), with appropriate force, velocity, amplitude, timing, etc. Since the cephalic position is dependent on the cervicothoracic position and correct cervicothoracic functionality is essential for adequate shoulder function, it seems advisable to supervise the functional efficiency of these structures in the context of the specificity of training for overhead sports.

Acknowledgements

The authors wish to thank the following for their contributions to this chapter: Gianni Brignardello, UC Sampdoria trainer, Rehabilitation Gymnasium, Lavagna (GE), former trainer of the Italian national water polo team; Mimmo Barlocco, chair of the National Association of Swimming and Water Polo Trainers (ANAN); Michel Bosch, Fédération Française d'Athlétisme, independent professional, Cagnes sur mer (FRA); Francesca Coaro, independent professional, Vicenza.

Bibliography

Various Authors, 'Dizionario Oxford della Medicina I', Gremese, Rome (1996)

Bellotti P., Matteucci E, 'Allenamento sportivo', UTET, Turin, pp. 5–86, (1999)

Berlusconi M., 'La spalla dolorosa del nuotatore: inquadramento epidemiologico, clinico e strumentale', In: Proceedings of the XVI ANAN convention, Rapallo (GE), pp. 29–37, (1990)

Bernard P.L., Fagot P.H., Codine P. et al., 'Evaluation isocinétique et prévention des déséquilibres musculaires de l'épaule du sportif', J. Réadapt. Méd. 16: 67–76, (1996)

Bigliani L.U., Codd T.P., Connor P.M. et al., 'Shoulder motion and laxity in the professional baseball player', Am. J. Sports Med. 25: 609–613, (1997)

Buroker KC., Schwane J.A., 'Does postexercise static stretching alleviate delayed muscle soreness?' Phys. Sportmed. 17: 65–83, (1989)

Candela V., Dragoni S., Traumatologia dello sport, Rhône Poulenc Roerer, Milan, p. 87, (1998)

Cartabellotta A., for the Italian Evidence-Based Medicine Group (GIMBE), 'Verso un'assistenza sanitaria basata sulle evidenze scientifiche: strumenti, competenze, ostacoli', Rec. Prog. Med. 88: 435–438, (1997)

Colombo C., Paletto A.E., Maggi G. et al., 'Trattato di chirurgia', Minerva Medica, Turin, p. 102, (1987)

Coppieters M.W , Stappaerts K.H., Evaraert D.G. et al., 'A qualitative assessment of shoulder girdle elevation during the upper limb tension test I', Man. Ther. 4: 33–38, (1999)

Cramer J.T., Housh T.J., Evetovich T.K., Johnson G.O., Ebersole K.T., Perry S.R., Bull A.J., 'The relationship among peak torque, mean power output, mechanomyography and electromyography in men and women during maximal, eccentric isokinetic muscle actions', Eur. J. Appl. Physiol. 86: 226–232, (2002)

Crawford H.J., Jull G.A., 'The influence of thoracic form and movement on range of shoulder flexion', Physiother. Theory Praxis 9: 143–148, (1991)

Cross K.M., Worrel T.W., 'Effects of a static stretching program on the incidence of lower extremity musculotendineous strains', J. Athl. Train 34(I): 11–14, (1999)

De Carli A., Ferretti A., 'La riabilitazione isocinetica della spalla', In: Roi G.S., Della Villa S. Isocinetica 90. Ghedini, Milan, p. 98, (1991)

Donnelly A.E., Clarkson P.M., Maughan R.J., 'Exercise-induced muscle damage: effect of light exercise on damaged muscle', Eur. J. Appl. Physiol. 64: 350–353, (1992)

Ekstrand J, Gillquist J., 'The avoidability of soccer injuries', Internat. J Sports Med. 4: 124–128, (1983)

Ettema G.J.C., 'Muscle efficiency: the controversial role of elasticity and mechanical energy conversion in stretch-shortening cycles', Eur. J. Appl. Physiol. 85: 457–465, (2001)

Fiorini G., Coretti S., Bocchi S., 'Corpo libero', Petrini, Turin, pp. 160–166, (2003)

Gatta G., 'La catena biocinetica degli impulsi', In: Various authors: 'Corso per allenatori di pallanuoto di primo livello' FIN. I. FIN, Rome (1996)

Giombini A., Colombo G., Lupo S., 'La spalla del nuotatore', La tecnica del nuoto 4: 87–90, (1991)

Gleim GW , McHugh MP: 'Flexibility and its effect on sports injury and performance', Sports Med. 24 (5): 289–299, (1997)

Golden C.L., Dudley G.A., 'Strength afterbouts of eccentric or concentric actions', Med. Sci. Sports Exerc. 24: 926–933, (1992)

Guyatt GH., 'Evidence-based medicine', ACP Journal Club A-16, (1991)

Hagenaars L.H.A., Bernards A.T.M., Oostendorp R.A.B., The multidimensional load/carriability model, Nederlands Paramedisch Instituut, Amersfort, pp. 1–5, (2002)

Harkness E.F., MacFarlane G.J., Nahit E.S. et al., 'Mechanical and psychosocial factors predict new onset shoulder pain: a prospective cohort study of newly employed workers', Occup. Environ Med. 60(11): 850–857, (2003)

Harre D., Teoria e metodologia dell'allenamento, SSS, Rome, pp. 3–94, (1972)

Hather B.M., Tesch P.A., Buchanan P. et al., 'Influence of eccentric actions on skeletal muscle adaptations to resistance training', Acta Physiol. Scand. 143: 177–185, (1991)

Hewitt R.M., Miller E.C., Sanford AH., The American illustrated Medical Dictionary, 22. Saunders Co., Philadelphia (1956)

Horstmann T., Mayer F., Maschmann J. et al., 'Metabolic reaction after concentric and eccentric endurance exercise of the knee and ankle', Med. Sci. Sports Exerc. 33: 791–795, (2001)

Houglum P.A., 'Therapeutic exercise for athletic injuries', Human Kinetics, Richmond, p. 268, (2001)

Inklaar H., 'Soccer injuries: aetiology and prevention', New Zeal Sports Med. 18(2): 81–93, (1994)

Jobe F.W. et al., Operative techniques in upper extremity sport injury, Mosby Year Book inc., pp. 3–15, (1995)

Jobe FW , Pink M., 'Shoulder injuries in the athlete: the instability continuum and treatment', J. Hand Ther. 4: 69–73, (1991)

Jones M., Edwards I., Gifford L., 'Conceptual models for implementing biopsychosocial theory in clinical practice, Man. Ther 7(1): 2–9, (2002)

Kentta G, Hassmen P., 'Overtraining and recovery. A conceptual model', Sports Med. 26: 1, (1998)

Kokkonen J.A., Nelson G., Cornwell A., 'Acute muscular stretching inhibits maximal strength performance', Res. Q. Exerc. Sport 69: 411–415, (1998)

Komi P.V., Linnamo V., Silventoinen P. et al., 'Force and EMG Power Spectrum During Eccentric and Concentric Actions', Med. Sci. Sports Exerc. 32: 1757–1762, (2000)

Lanzetta A: Manuale di traumatologia dell'apparato locomotore, I edizione. Masson, Milan, pp. 188–196, (1993)

La Torre G., Giattino G., 'Epidemiologia degli infortuni in ambito sportivo e la legge 626/94 sulla sicurezza della salute dei lavoratori', Med. Sport. 52: 21–28, (1999)

Lucas R.C, Koslov R., 'Comparative study of static, dynamic and proprioceptive neuromuscular facilitation stretching techniques on flexibility' Percept. Mot. Skills 58: 615–618, (1984)

McKenzie DC., 'Markers of excessive exercise', Can. J. Appl. Physiol. 24: 66, (1999)

McMaster W.C., Long S.C., Caiozzo V.J., 'Isokinetic torque imbalance in the rotator cuff of the elite water polo player', AJSM 19: 72–75, (1991)

Prevention and physical and athletic training

McMaster W.C., Troup J., 'A survey of interfering shoulder pain in US competitive swimmers', *AJSM* 1: 67–70, (1993)

Meeusen R, Piacentini MF., 'Exercises and neurotransmission', *Sports Med.* 20(3): 160–188, (1995)

Meeusen R., Piacentini M.F., Busschaert B. et al., 'Hormonal responses in athletes: the use of a two bout exercise protocol to detect subtle differences in (over)training status', *Eur. J. Appl. Physiol.*: 121–130, (2003)

Mondardini, 'P. News and views', *Alfa Wassermann* 11(3): 3, (1999)

Nelson A.G., Kokkonen A., Elredge C. et al., 'Chronic stretching and running economy', *Scand. J. Sports* 11: 260–265, (2001)

Newton R.A., 'Joint receptor contributions to reflexive and kinesthetic responses' *Phys. Ther.* 62: 22–29, (1982)

Pink M., Murlow C.D., 'The medical review article: state of the science', *Annal. Int. Med.* 106(3): 485–488, (1987)

Pope R.P., Herbert R.D., Kirwan J.D. et al., 'A randomized trial of pre-exercise stretching for prevention of lower limb injury', *Med. Sci. Sports Exerc.* 32(2): 271–277, (1999)

Porter M.M., Vandervoort A.A., 'Standing strength training of the ankle plantar and dorsiflexors in older women, using concentric and eccentric contractions', *Eur. J. Appl. Physiol.* 76: 62–68, (1997)

Rossi R., Parisse I., Tassi C. et al., 'Superallenamento (Overtraining syndrome) e radicali liberi', *Med. Sport.* 52: 159–163, (1999)

Scotton C., 'Classification tecnica delle specialità sportive', Calzetti e Mariucci, Perugia, pp. 12–63, (2003)

Seger J.Y., Arvidsson B., Thorsthensson A., 'Specific effects of eccentric and concentric training on muscle strength and morphology in humans', *Eur. J. Appl. Physiol.* 79: 49–57, (1998)

Shirer I, 'Stretching before exercise does not reduce the risk of local muscle injury. A critical review of the clinical and basic science literature', *Clin. J. Sports Med.* 9: 221–227, (1999)

Tesch P.A., Dudley G.A., Duvoisin M.R., Hater B.M., Harris T.A., 'Force and EMG signal patterns during repeated bouts of concentric or eccentric muscle actions', *Acta Physiol. Scand.* 138: 263–271, (1990)

Voight M.L., Hardin J.A., Blackburn T.A. et al., 'The effect of muscle fatigue on and the relationship of arm dominance to shoulder proprioception', *J. Orthop. Sports. Phys. Ther.* 23: 348–352, (1996)

Warner J.J., Micheli L.J., Arslanian L.E. et al., 'Patterns of flexibility, laxity, and strength in normal shoulder and shoulder with instability and impingement', *AJSM* 21: 366–375, (1990)

Westing S.H., Seger J.Y., Thorstensson A., 'Effects of electrical stimulation on eccentric and concentric torque-velocity relationships during knee extension', *Man. Acta Physiol. Scand.* 140: 17–22, (1990)

Wilk K.E., Andrews J.R., Arrigo C.A. et al., 'The strength characteristics of internal and external rotator muscles in professional baseball pitchers', *AJSM* 21: 61–66, (1993)

Wilk K.E., Arrigo C.A., 'Current concepts in the rehabilitation of the athletic shoulder', *J. Orthop. Sports Phys. Ther.* 18: 365–378, (1993)

Wilk K.E., Arrigo C.A., Andrews J.R., 'Current concepts: the stabilizing structures of the glenohumeral joint', *J. Orthop. Sports Phys. Ther.* 25: 364–379, (1997)

Wilk K.E., Meister K., Andrews J.R., 'Current concepts in the rehabilitation of the overhead throwing athlete', *Am. J. Sports Med.* 30(1): 136–51, (2002)

Witvrouw E., 'Stretching and injury prevention: an obscure relationship', *Abstract book of the International Physiotherapy Congress*, Maastricht (NL), 11–13 December: 62, (2003)

A. Fusco,
R. Zuccarino

PREVENTION AND TECHNICAL ATHLETIC EVALUATION

CHAPTER 17

Evaluation and technical athletic observation

Sport technicians and medical professionals should evaluate the athlete by making observations and measurements of individual physical and technical abilities.

Qualitative and quantitative variables can be used for the evaluation.

Quantitative analysis normally uses measurable variables, which allow the calculation of even very complex derived measurements and of indices. This evaluation can determine organic and muscular capacities, such as strength and speed.

Quantitative evaluations have a primary role in the planning and periodization of athletic training, constituting reference frameworks for selecting, confirming or changing its methodology.

Qualitative variables, however, can consist of judgments such as good, sufficient or poor, or descriptions of attitudes and positions such as upright, flexed or rotated. These variables can be used to construct ordinal scales (e.g. on three levels): very flexed, slightly flexed, or extended; the reference can be external (e.g. the perpendicular for the trunk), in relation to another body segment (angle between trunk and arm), or linear (hand over head, at shoulder or sternum height, according to the type of throwing) (Carbonaro, 1988; Merni, 1986).

The statistical procedures for data analysis can be used in both cases, though in different ways, bearing in mind that non-parametric methods must be used for qualitative variables (Merni, 1991).

It is worth attempting to examine the evaluation of throwing by qualitative variables, given the large number of components involved in a kinetic chain which is, in itself, extremely complex.

It seems advisable to use multiple item rating scales, such as the functional throwing performance index (FTPI) (Davies, 1993) or other similar scales for an objective quantification of qualitative variables.

Two aspects appear to be particularly important for shoulder movements to be effective and, at the same time, to be in keeping with the physiology; these are optimal use of the kinetic chain, and the presence of a rotatory component in the technical action (Fig. 17.1).

Evaluation and functional observation

The functional observation of the athlete with a view to preventing shoulder disorders requires the observation of some of the elements already mentioned in Chapter 8.

Such an observation should be carried out, or at least evaluated, in an interdisciplinary session to confirm that the necessary technical requirements are met and the ratio of ergonomics to effectiveness is correct.

The key points of the observation are as follows:
1. Analysis of overall movement: relation between the position of the feet, pelvis, and spine, the action of the shoulder, the role of the chest, and the role of cervicothoracic movement.
2. Analysis of the movement of the shoulder: direction, amplitude, speed, strength.
3. Body alignment and posture.
4. Analysis of movement in automatic actions.
5. Identification of dysfunctions present.

Prevention and technical athletic evaluation

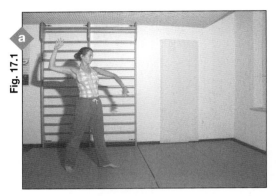
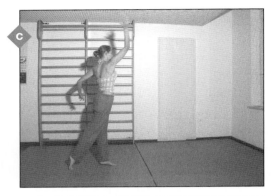
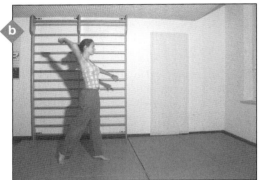
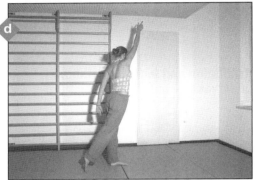

Fig. 17.1

Ventral rotation test in semi-dynamic mode. The test requires a throwing action, demonstrating the dynamic movement of the axis around which the agonistic action occurs. Correct execution of the test requires the body to be continuously aligned around the instant axis and dynamic balance to be maintained by means of the harmonic rotation of the body around the same axis.

6. Identity of the person and their role in the group.
7. Evaluation of the individual's level and skill.
8. Adaptation and compensation (normal and pathological).
9. Bodily, mental and social awareness.

Points 1 and 4 require observation and, if possible, evaluation of neuromuscular or, more simply, coordination capacity, which include agonistic, antagonistic and stabilizing muscle actions. Points 2 and 3 require observation and, if possible, evaluation of organic and muscular capacities. Point 5 refers to the need for a clinical evaluation performed by a medical professional (Section II, Chapters 6 and 8).

Points 6 and 9 refer to the need for a biopsychosocial evaluation (Section IV, Chapter 12).

Points 7 and 8 require observation of the athletic action, in order to detect errors and any compensation.

Identification of limits in athletic training

Training requires planning, periodization, use of a methodology, setting objectives and monitoring.

When planning athletic training, sport technicians need to take into account technical and personal factors relating to the athlete and to the team.

The technical factors will include the rules and their implications for technological development, technique and its evolution; the personal factors will include motor abilities, tactical abilities and psychological characteristics.

The classification of sports presented (Section IV, Chapter 16) can be used to determine the skill requirements of the athlete, depending on the type of activity performed, in order to identify the objectives of training.

The aim of the individual and team evaluations and monitoring is to check that the training is appropriate and to demonstrate any limits. Such limits may predispose towards or facilitate the appearance of disorders, ranging from overtraining syndrome (OTS) to overuse and specific disorders.

Identification of limits in the periodization of training

The necessary premise for the optimal use of the progress obtained in training is the appropriate determination of workloads, the principal parameters of which are quantity, intensity and density. Correct periodization is essential for determining an organized progression of workloads which is, in turn, a prerequisite for adaptation of the organism.

It is, therefore, necessary to check that:
— the periods into which the programme is divided (single sessions, microcycles, mesocycles, macrocycles) are of sufficient duration to meet their objectives;
— the planned calendar of both competitions and training is adhered to as closely as possible;
— sudden changes in competition dates (e.g. postponement of an official competition) correspond to a change in the team's schedule (e.g. friendly match);
— regular training is a feature for the team and for individuals;
— irregular attendance at training by an athlete results in an individually-tailored adjustment of the team programme;
— the transition from one period to the next, involving an increase in workload, is preceded by direct or at least indirect checks (monitoring) on the intermediate results achieved and the athlete's carriability;
— the recovery time necessary between periods is observed at both individual and team level, particularly as regards periods of maximum work intensity; and
— the quality of recovery is sufficient (time required for travelling, quality and quantity of nocturnal rest, alternation between sport and work, sport and study, and sport and recreation).

Identification of limits in the training methodology

The training methodology can be defined as an understanding of how to use the contents of training. The phrase 'training method' is understood to mean the use of specific exercises, performed and organized according to biophysiological principles, to achieve a given aim.

The methodological limits in the training of a throwing athlete might be the following:
— the sameness of methods and tools (multilaterality deficits);
— premature specialization by the athlete;
— deficits in how the content of the session or period is structured;
— the presence of technical errors in the exercises and in the technique; and
— a lack of checks or checks that are not relevant to the specific capacities.

An inappropriate environment, or the use of unsuitable clothing or defective equipment, which do not need to be examined further here, can also be mentioned.

The use of a single method and of few, repetitive training tools runs counter to the need to pursue diverse objectives in relation to the athlete's intrinsic factors (age, gender, race) and extrinsic factors (personal situation, level, capacity).

By using varied methods and tools as part of a correct programme, training can be multilateral, which is one of the recommendations for avoiding OTS and overuse. Multilaterality is characterized by the amplitude and multiplicity of the training methods and means used, and by the ratio of general to special training (Thiess, 1980).

The problem of multilaterality in sport, even from the viewpoint of an elite athlete, should be considered critically. Athletes can attain peak performances only if they specialize at the right time.

However, at the right time does not mean early, in the sense of early specialization (Weineck, 2001).

Any sport science researcher who cares about their professional reputation will state that the training of children and adolescents should be multilateral, insofar as the concept of training itself is admissible in this context (Hagedorn, 1993).

As regards the structuring of a cycle or session, the technician needs to have the contents clearly ranked in relation to the objectives that the athlete is to achieve and the tools to be used.

A common methodological error when planning macrocycles is to assign inappropriate levels of importance to the objectives of the training. The organic and muscular capacities necessary for a throwing athlete should reach an optimal balance between strength and mobility. Coordination capacities should allow effective centrifugal action.

Prevention and technical athletic evaluation

It will consequently be appropriate to suggest the use of qualitative checks on organic, muscular and neuromuscular abilities, while acknowledging the unreliability and poor reproducibility of these checks.

An error that frequently goes unnoticed when planning microcycles or sessions is an incorrect preliminary evaluation of the workload recommended by the technician.

It may be interesting to calculate or to estimate as closely as possible the internal or external load to which the athlete is subjected (Figs. 17.2–17.6). Internal load is calculated indirectly, by recording heart rate (HR). The maximum theoretical heart rate is used to calculate the threshold HR (by means of a VO_{2max} test or application of an empirical formula) (between 87 and 93% of max HR) and the reserve HR (max HR − resting HR). As regards external load, reference has previously been made to Roy Sinclair's table for predicting the maximum load for strength. Recovery in exercises to increase strength, i.e. performed with a substantial load, using up to 3 repetitions or lasting 20 seconds, for a small number of series (1–4), should be full, i.e. from 3 to 5 minutes. Recovery in exercises to increase resistant

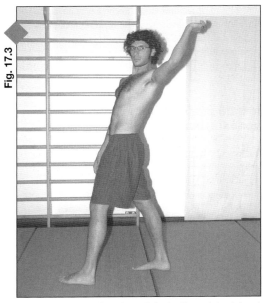

Fig. 17.3

Possible error in cocking phase 2. Lack of homolateral dorsal rotation, with compensation in the form of forced external rotation of the arm. A possible acromioclavicular dysfunction, incorrect scapulothoracic rhythm and a pelvic mobility deficit should be evaluated.

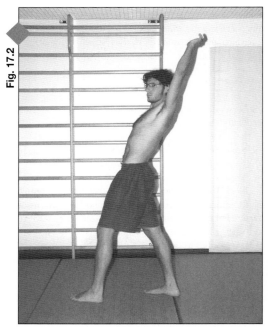

Fig. 17.2

Possible error in cocking phase 1. Lack of homolateral dorsal rotation, with compensation in the form of lumbar hyperlordosis. Scapulothoracic rhythm, rotation of the pelvis and extension of the cervicothoracic spine should be evaluated.

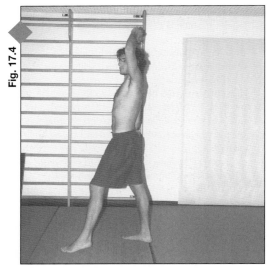

Fig. 17.4

Possible error in cocking phase 3. Limitation in the extension-rotation of the cervicothoracic spine in scapular adduction and in glenohumeral extension. Compensation by the extrinsic muscles of the neck, which carry out excessive elevation of the scapula, a potential requirement for impingement. The limitation is evident in the position of the elbow, which is anterior to the shoulder.

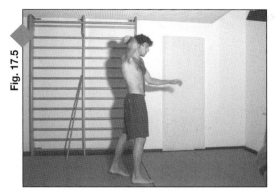

Possible error in the acceleration phase. Incorrect proximodistal recruitment with insufficient production of strength by the proximal muscle chains, resulting in overload of the scapulohumeral structures.

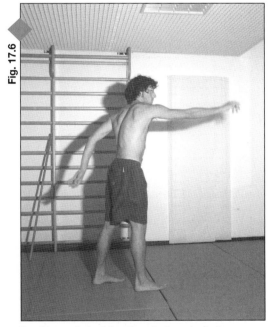

Possible error in the follow-through phase. Ineffective antagonistic muscle action of the athletic movement with compensation by flexing the trunk. This is a possible consequence of an incorrect acceleration phase, with excessive distal muscle recruitment.

in the cause-effect dynamics, in particular in high intensity training or training with excess loads (Bellotti, 1978). The interval between exercises depends on the type of quality to be developed, the method of performing the exercise and the load used.

Technical limits, however, should be divided into aspecific or specific training exercises; aspecific exercises are connected indirectly to competitive technique, while specific exercises concern the limits of the technique (or action) which form part of the competitive technique. The term 'error' is used when the imperfections have become established and interfere in some way with the effectiveness of the movement (Visintin, 1996).

From the methodological point of view, it should be kept in mind that indiscriminate repetitions do not get rid of defects, rather they consolidate them. It will consequently be appropriate to suggest the use of qualitative checks on athletic actions, while acknowledging the unreliability and poor reproducibility of these checks.

Identification of limits in organic and muscular capacities

For athletic actions to be effective and safe, some organic and muscular capacities need qualitative observation to establish an appropriate level; these are joint mobility, muscle extendibility and agonistic and antagonistic muscle strength.

An examination of the above aspects can give an indirect indication of the load to which the individual joint, periarticular and muscular components are subjected. The correct division of the amplitude of the action between all the body segments seems to be a prerequisite for an equal distribution of the load.

It would appear that the agonistic kinetic chain should be as extensive as possible, that is it should comprise as many body segments as possible, using maximum joint amplitude, in accordance with the environment and the rules under which the action is being performed (support, elevation, immersion, etc.). The rationale for these conditions refers primarily to the sum of a greater number of muscles in play, and secondly to the use of a greater 'power arm' and finally, but no less importantly, to the condition of the greater supply of strength by the muscle corresponding to the condition of elongation (see Fig. 17.1).

Shoulder mobility should be observed in the four joints which form the shoulder girdle and in the proximal regions of the body (Crawford, 1991), i.e. the spine, and the connections between the trunk and the

strength, i.e. performed with a moderately low load, using up to 30 repetitions or lasting 20 seconds, for a middle number of series (6–9), should be intermediate, i.e. from 2 to 3 minutes. Recovery is the basic element

Prevention and technical athletic evaluation

lower limbs should be observed, particularly if they have a propulsive function, as well as the extendibility of the muscles involved in movement, particularly agonistic movement.

ULTT (see Chapter 8) may be useful for evaluation of muscle extendibility, with reference to local carriability. The authors describe three such tests, one for the median nerve, one for the radial nerve and one for the ulnar nerve. It should be noted that this procedure has been validated exclusively for the median nerve (Coppieters, 1999).

We describe below a suggestion for the observation and qualitative evaluation of joint mobility and muscle extendibility. The method suggested allows a qualitative assessment of joint mobility and muscle extendibility. The model proposed takes as its starting point the study of movement developed by Noro over the last 20 years, as part of a method which has taken his name (www.kinomichi.com). The joint mobility and muscle extendibility required for throwing amount, from a static point of view, to two positions which recall the culminating moments of late cocking and the follow through, respectively. These moments visually resemble a continuous line with a diagonal and spiral path, around which the kinetic chain develops its action. Maintaining these positions correctly for a few seconds will also provide information on the athlete's level of proprioception.

The tests involve assuming the positions illustrated, starting from an upright stance (Figs. 17.7, 17.8). An interruption in this line is easily identifiable and can be used to identify an increase in load or the presence of compensation in one or more regions of the body. Such an interruption could be due to a deficit of muscle extendibility, joint mobility or both.

Such a defect should be corrected by specific exercises, and the deficit should then be evaluated once again.

Strength should be evaluated quantitatively in the muscle groups, and this evaluation is considered by the technician and health workers to be key to performance and to the prevention of problems.

The muscle chains will, moreover, be examined from a functional point of view, with particular regard to the efficiency of their general and local stabilizing action which may be agonistic, antagonistic or synergic in relation to a given action. This will confirm the presence of the predominant type of muscle contraction necessary for the action: isometric for stabilizing action, plyometric for agonistic action, and eccentric for antagonistic action. The efficiency of the muscles should be evaluated in the specific type of action required by each sport.

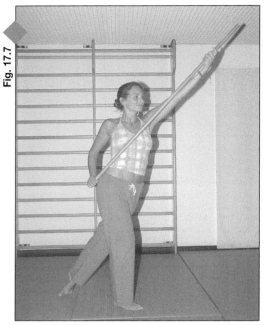

Fig. 17.7

Diagonal test with ventral rotation. The test corresponds to the phase of throwing known as follow through. The direction of the wooden stick identifies the axis of rotation around which the movement is being carried out, which has a diagonal and spiral path, in keeping with the ideal line of the oblique muscle chain. The athlete's weight is predominantly borne by the anterior support, while the posterior support provides anterosuperior thrust.

If limits are identified in aspects of the organic and muscular capacities, these should be evaluated, and remedied as part of the individual athlete's monitoring and training programme.

Identification of limits in neuromuscular capacities

The requirements for guaranteeing the dynamic stability of the shoulder in overhead activities are muscle balance and coordination, the latter being closely connected to proprioception.

The muscle balance conditions necessary, in relation to the movements of the upper limb during throwing, can be divided into global and regional. At a global level, the agonistic muscle chains, which take their movement from the lower limbs, have to guarantee coordinated action in time and space, which will lead to the upper limb via the trunk. The pelvic girdle

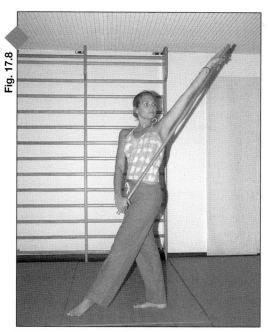

Fig. 17.8

Diagonal test with dorsal rotation. The test corresponds to the late cocking phase. The spiral movement, in its rotation and extension components, starts from the foot and ends at the fingers. The anterior foot, on the same side as the throwing limb, produces the axial action around which the joint 'opening' and muscle pretensioning movement develops. The direction of the wooden stick identifies this axis, which has a diagonal and spiral path. The posterior path supports most of the weight, with the knee adopting a semi-flexed position.

must be in a functional state for this to happen, and this is represented largely by its dynamic stability and the correct action of the antagonistic muscle chains.

At a regional level, the effector kinetic chains of the shoulder girdle, i.e. the thoracoappendicular and spinoappendicular muscles, have to rely on proximal stability to ensure a balance between stabilizing and effector function (Jobe, 1988; Kibler, 1991; Saha, 1983).

At a local level, balance is achieved by a low requirement for local effector action, owing to the kinetic chain which carries action of proximal origin. The dynamic stabilization of the glenohumeral joint is then readily provided by the rotator cuff (Lee, 2000; Otis, 1994), leading to a reduction in mechanical stresses on the same joint (An, 1997).

To summarize, the presence of a rotatory component in the technical movement on a global and local

level would appear to provide the best compromise between efficacy and control of physical balance.

We describe below a suggestion for the observation and qualitative assessment of coordination and chronological sequence. The method suggested allows a qualitative assessment of stabilizing and effector muscle action, agonistic and antagonistic coordination, and the temporal sequence of muscle recruitment.

The models proposed take as their starting point the study of movement developed by Noro (www.kinomichi.com).

The capacity for coordination and producing strength according to precise conditions can be studied by the simulation, in sequence, of the phases of throwing; the test can be performed in semi-dynamic mode, i.e. by maintaining the same support base, or in dynamic mode, i.e. by varying the supports. It is also possible to distinguish the sequence in ventral rotation corresponding to the throwing movement from the sequence in dorsal rotation.

Ventral rotation test in semi-dynamic mode

The test involves a throwing action, demonstrating anterointernal movement of the dynamic axis around which the action occurs (see Fig. 17.1). Correct execution of the test requires the body to be continuously aligned around the instant axis and dynamic balance to be maintained by means of the harmonic rotation of the body around the same axis. A description follows of the principal movements corresponding to each phase of throwing.

— *Wind-up and cocking phase.* The athlete extends and rotates the trunk and head dorsally, adducts and rotates the scapula internally, rotates externally, flexes and abducts the arm, extends the elbow, supinates the forearm, and flexes the wrist dorsally to increase the amplitude of the movement for the acceleration phase. In particular, the shoulder is abducted, extended and rotated externally, the scapula is adducted and rotated, and the thoracocervical spine extended and rotated. The action of the shoulder during the wind-up phase should be minimal (Gowan, 1987).

— *Acceleration phase.* The athlete moves into the propulsive phase of the projectile by means of proximodistal muscle recruitment to accelerate the throwing limb, keeping the pelvis stable. The importance of starting the movement from the pelvis is emphasized in this phase.

— *Deceleration.* The athlete ends the agonistic phase of throwing, by completing the whole arc of movement and modulating the action by means of the antagonistic muscle chains.

— *Follow-through phase.* This phase demonstrates antagonistic and stabilizing muscle action, providing an indicator of neuromuscular control. If the 'laboratory' action is performed correctly, the athlete will end the movement while still having the option of pushing off from the ground with the rear foot.

Dorsal rotation test in semi-dynamic mode

The test involves the backhand action in racquet sports, demonstrating posterolateral movement of the dynamic axis around which the action occurs. The starting position, for this test, is an upright stance with legs slightly apart sagittally, the weight mainly on the anterior limb, and the knee semi-flexed; the athlete carries out dorsal rotation, bringing the weight onto the posterior limb, until the position corresponding to the diagonal in dorsal rotation is reached.

Ventral rotation test in dynamic mode

The starting position is the same as for the semi-dynamic test.

The athlete moves and rotates in a ventral direction through 360°, by taking a step forwards with one leg, an about turn, then a step backwards with the other leg (rotation technique for putting the shot). The pelvis thus rotates as continuously as possible through 360°. During the rotation the athlete performs the throwing action in its various phases. At the end of the rotation, the athlete completes the throwing simulation, as in the semi-dynamic test, ending in the position shown in Figure 17.9, while balance is provided by the antagonistic and stabilizing muscle chains (Hodges, 1997).

Dorsal rotation test in dynamic mode

This test starts with the body in an attitude of flexion and internal rotation, with the upper limb adducted.

The athlete moves and rotates in a dorsal direction through about 270°, by taking a step backwards, an about turn, then a further rotation of the pelvis in the same direction, keeping the last points of support stable. The pelvis thus performs a rotation as continuously as possible through about 270°. During rotation, the athlete extends their body and performs the tennis backhand action. The similarity with the technique of throwing the hammer can be seen.

The test assesses the coordination of the agonistic and antagonistic muscle chains and the temporal sequence of recruitment. This sequence must be in a proximodistal direction: the scapulohumeral motor units are recruited only in the final phases of the arc of movement, while the motor units of the lower limbs and of the shoulder girdle and pelvis are recruited predominantly in the initial phase (Gatta, 1996).

If neuromotor (proprioceptive or coordination) limits are identified in the athletic action, these should be evaluated by a medical professional by means of a regional functional examination to demonstrate compensation and its consequences. Such a functional examination constitutes the premise for taking appropriate measures.

Identification of limits in ballistic actions

Optimizing the muscle thrust is more important in a ballistic action than the amount of strength that the muscles can recruit. The principle of the chronological coordination of individual impulses (Hochmut, quoted by Gatta 1996) and harmony explains why it is only through the dynamic work of the major muscle chains and the participation of all the joints, moving or fixed, that large quantities of impulses are obtained.

Having described the predominant use of the muscles of the lower part of the body by professional throwing athletes, this is often neglected by amateur throwers, who try to throw 'from the shoulder'. The muscles, which initially work eccentrically, suddenly change to concentric contraction, particularly in the immediate transition from cocking to acceleration (Fig. 17.10).

Recommendations for the evaluation of limits in technical actions

Some technical limits occur frequently. We shall look at some which may predispose towards disorders:

— *Possible error in cocking phase 1.* Lack of homolateral dorsal rotation, with compensation in the form of lumbar hyperlordosis. Scapulothoracic rhythm, pre-thrust rotation of the pelvis and extension of the cervicothoracic spine should be evaluated (Fig. 17.2);

— *Possible error in cocking phase 2.* Lack of homolateral dorsal rotation, with compensation in the form of forced external rotation. A possible acromioclavicular dysfunction, incorrect

Fig. 17.9

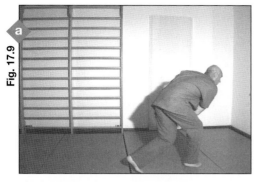

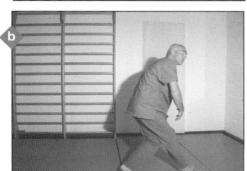

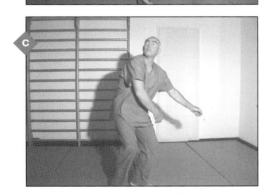

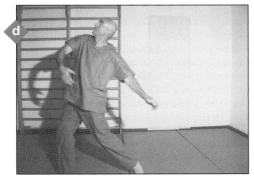

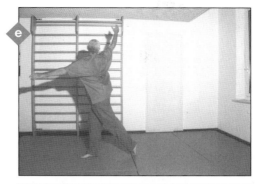

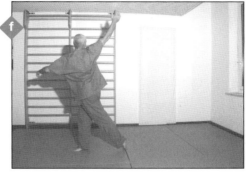

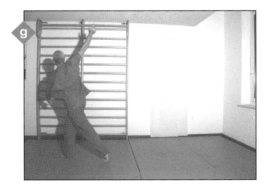

Dorsal rotation test in dynamic mode. Execution sequence of dorsal rotation. It is used as a dynamic evaluation of both the quality of the technical action and neuromotor coordination capacity, with particular emphasis on proximodistal recruitment. It is noted in this respect that the scapulohumeral motor units are recruited only in the final phases of the arc of movement, while the motor units of the shoulder girdle and pelvis are predominantly recruited in the initial phase.

Prevention and technical athletic evaluation

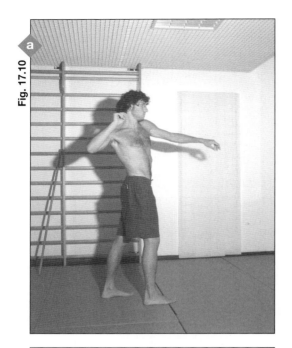

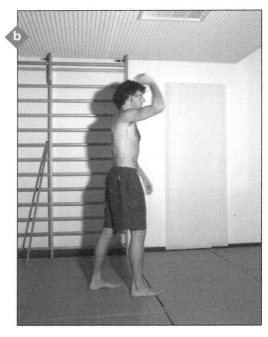

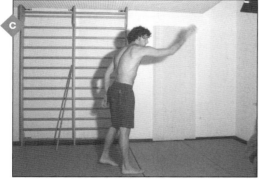

Possible error in a technical action (attack in volleyball): cocking **(a)** is incomplete and imperfectly distributed between the body regions. The acceleration phase **(b)** is predominantly distal and the participation of the lumbopelvic complex and the lower limbs is limited. The deceleration phase **(c)** shows how difficult the athlete finds it to stabilize the upper limb and the whole body.

scapulothoracic rhythm and a pelvic mobility deficit should be evaluated (Fig. 17.3);

— *Possible error in cocking phase 3.* Limitation in the extension-rotation of the cervicothoracic spine in scapular adduction and in glenohumeral extension. Compensation by the extrinsic muscles of the neck, which carry out excessive elevation of the scapula, a potential requirement for impingement. The limitation is evident in the position of the elbow, which is anterior to the shoulder (Fig. 17.4);

— *Possible error in the acceleration phase.* Incorrect proximodistal recruitment with insufficient production of strength by the proximal muscle chains, resulting in overload of the scapulohumeral structures (Fig. 17.5);

— *Possible error in the follow-through phase.* Ineffective antagonistic muscle action of the athletic movement with compensation by flexing the trunk. This is a possible consequence of an incorrect acceleration phase, with excessive distal muscle recruitment; this results in problems for the stabilizing and antagonistic muscles in the technical action (Fig. 17.6).

The term 'error' is used when the imperfections have become established and interfere in some way with the effectiveness of the movement (Visintin, 1996).

From the methodological point of view, it should be kept in mind that indiscriminate repetitions do not get rid of defects, rather consolidate them. It will consequently be appropriate to suggest the use of qualitative checks on athletic actions, while acknowledging the unreliability and poor reproducibility of these checks.

Acknowledgements

Roberta Franzi, independent professional, Studio Fusco, Genoa; Pasquale Greco, of the Institute of Sport Medicine of Genoa; Gino Repetto, doctor of chemistry and pharmaceutical technology (CTF), for the images in this chapter; Stefano Rubini; Tamara Orsi of Studio Fusco, Genoa; and Marco Demelato.

Bibliography

An K.N., Chao E.Y., Kaufman K.R., 'Analysis of muscle and joint loads', In: Mow V.C., Hayes W.C. (eds.) *Basic Orthopaedic Biomechanics* 2. Lippincott-Raven, Philadelphia, (1997)

Bellotti P., Benzi G., Dal Monte A. et al., 'Classificazione degli sport e determinazione dei mezzi di allenamento. Atleticastudi', 3–4: 29–46, (1978)

Carbonaro G., 'La valutazione nello sport dei giovani', SSS, Rome, (1988)

Coppieters M.W., Stappaerts K.H., Evaraert D.G. et al., 'A qualitative assessment of shoulder girdle elevation during the upper limb tension test', 1. *Man. Ther.* 4: 33–38, (1999)

Crawford H.J., Jull G.A., 'The influence of thoracic form and movement on range of shoulder flexion', *Physiotherapy, Theory Praxis* 9: 143–148, (1991)

Davies G.J., Dickoff-Hoffman S., 'Neuromuscular testing and rehabilitation of the shoulder complex', *J. Ortop. Sports Phys.Ther.* 18(2): 449–457, (1993)

Gatta G. 'La catena biocinetica degli impulsi', In: Various Authors (eds.), 'Corso per allenatori di pallanuoto di primo livello', Fin 1. Fin, Rome, p. 148, (1996)

Gowan I.D., Jobe F.W., Tiborne J.E. et al., 'A comparative electromyographic analysis of the shoulder during pitching: professional versus amateur pitchers', *Am. J. Sports Med.* 15: 586, (1987)

Hagedorn G., 'La multilateralità in allenamento e in gara. Scuolainforma suppl. a SdS', 28–29: 36, (1993)

Hodges P.W., Richardson C.A., 'Feedforward contraction of transversus abdominis is not influenced by the direction of arm movement', *Exper. Brain Res.* 114: 362–370, (1997)

Jobe F.W., Bradley J.P., 'The diagnosis and nonoperative treatment of shoulder injuries in athletes', *Clin. Sport Med.* 8: 419–439, (1989)

Kibler W.B., 'The role of the scapula in the overhead throwing motion', *Am. Contemp. Orthop.* 22: 525–532, (1991)

Lee S.B., Kim K.J., O'Driscoll S.W. et al., 'Dynamic glenohumeral stability provided by the rotator cuff muscles in the mid-range and end-range of motion', *J. Bone Jt. Surg.* 82: 849–857, (2000)

Merni F., *Il bambino e la corsa*, SdS, IV: 5, (1986)

Merni F., 'La valutazione delle tecniche sportive', SdS 22(suppl.): 38, (1991)

Otis J.C., Jiang C.C., Wickiewicz T.L. et al., 'Changes in moment arm of the rotator cuff and deltoid muscles with abduction and rotation', *J. Bone Jt. Surg.* 76: 667–676, (1994)

Saha A.K., 'Dynamic stability of the glenohumeral joint', *Acta Orthop. Scand.* 42: 491–505, (1971)

Thiess, Schnabel, Baumann., 'Allenamento dalla A alla', Z. 253, SSS, Roma (1980)

Visintin G., 'La tecnica e l'errore', In: Various Authors (eds.), 'Corso per allenatori di pallanuoto di primo livello', Fin 1. Fin, Rome, p. 314, (1996)

Weineck J., *L'allenamento ottimale. Calzetti e Mariucci*, Perugia, p. 493, (2001)

Wilk K.E., Meister K., Andrews J.R., 'Current concepts in the rehabilitation of the overhead throwing athlete', *Am. J. Sports Med.* 30(1): 136–151, (2002)

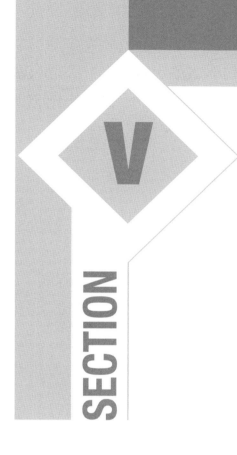

SECTION V

CURRENT TRENDS IN SURFACE ELECTROMYOGRAPHY

SURFACE ELECTROMYOGRAPHY

R. MERLETTI

In a 1997 review, C.J. De Luca likened EMG to a siren, tempting the operator with the extreme ease with which electrodes can be applied to a muscle and an electrical signal observed. The technique is within the reach of many by virtue of its simplicity, but useful to few owing to the complexity of producing and interpreting traces. If this is combined with the lack of training offered by European universities in this sector, it becomes apparent that the method has been used incorrectly and confusedly, in the absence of standards or, at least, a methodological consensus. The European concerted action, surface electromyography for non invasive assessment of muscles (SENIAM), only recently published recommendations for the sector (Hermens, 1999).

Most scientific studies of the EMG signal relate to contractions carried out under isometric conditions, and this has been criticized by many who maintain that isometric conditions are too far removed from the conditions of sports. However, the EMG signal recorded under dynamic conditions is almost invariably distorted by artefacts generated by the movement of the muscle under the skin. Isometric conditions constitute a bench test which allows characteristics of the muscle which cannot be readily observed under dynamic conditions to be observed and documented, and in any case this type of test yields a substantial amount of information. The information obtained under dynamic conditions mainly concerns the activation intervals of various muscles, whereas it is difficult to observe myoelectric signs of fatigue or to document the properties of individual motor units.

Many European projects have focused on the interpretation of the cutaneous EMG signal, mainly in ergonomics and occupational medicine applications (SENIAM, PROCID, NEW), and five important papers have been published in recent years (Cram, 1998; Hermens, 1999; Kasman, 1998; Merletti, 2000, 2004), following the classic paper by Basmajan and De Luca in 1985. This is indicative of a growing body of knowledge in the sector, though unfortunately not yet the subject of academic teaching in Italy.

It can be assumed, with the rapid improvement in sampling, modelling and interpreting techniques, that in a few years the fields of application and advantages of the non-invasive method will be comparable with those of the traditional method using needles, although the methods have their differences.

Many muscles act on the shoulder joint and each one contributes, to an extent that cannot yet be measured, to momentum produced in the joint. Not all these muscles are equally susceptible to EMG analysis. While it is not possible to measure the contribution of each one to the force or total momentum, it is possible to measure the EMG signal of many of them. It is often wrongly believed that the amplitude of the EMG signal (quantified using one of the traditional means of estimation, such as average rectified value (ARV) and root mean square value (RMS), etc.) is proportional to the force produced by the muscle and therefore represents its contribution to the total force (isometric conditions). This belief is incorrect because:

— the amplitude of the EMG signal is attenuated by the width of the subcutaneous signal, which differs between muscles and between individuals;
— deeper motor units in the muscle yield EMG contributions of lower amplitude, and force contributions that are not dependent on depth

and, therefore, cannot be correlated with the amplitude of the EMG signal.

For the same reasons, since the amplitude of the EMG signal increases with the increase in the force produced by a muscle, it is not possible to define a relation between the two variables which is applicable to all muscles or to all individuals. Nevertheless, in cases in which a muscle is successfully activated selectively, this reaction can be 'calibrated' by taking a simultaneous measurement of EMG and force (both generated by the same muscle) for various contraction force values. This relation is used in subsequent measurements to estimate the force produced based on the amplitude of the EMG signal.

Considerable attention has been paid in the last 10 years to the electromyographic analysis of the shoulder muscles in relation to occupational neuromuscular diseases. The trapezius in particular has been studied in great depth for a better understanding of the myalgia that typically affects this muscle. The studies were conducted using either thin wire electrodes or surface electrodes, sometimes with measurements of intramuscular pressure. The many papers which, though addressing aspects of ergonomics, describe a methodology that can be transferred to the sport sector, are of particular interest (Attebrant, 1995; Farina, 2002a; Hagberg, 1981; Jensen, 1993; Madeleine, 2002; Mathiassen, 1995; Palmerud, 1995, 1998).

The surface EMG signal: basic concepts

A physical dimension that is variable in time and space constitutes a signal which can be plotted on a Cartesian graph of the physical dimension, as a function of time or space. A 1- or 2D signal in space may move, following the motion of its source. For example, the halo of light generated on the surface of the water by an under-water lamp follows its movement and fluctuations in intensity in both space (surface of the water) and time. A snapshot of this signal can be imagined which describes its course in space at a particular instant in time. Its course can alternatively be imagined as a function of time at one or more fixed points in space. Finally, there can be a temporospatial description of the signal which describes the intensity at each point and at each instant. In the specific case of the EMG signal, the water in the above example is the conducting volume, consisting of the tissue between sources and electrodes; the surface of the water is the skin and the individual source is a depolarized zone of a muscle fibre. Figure 18.1 shows the distribution of the lines of current and of surface tension for a punctiform electrical source and a double source (a dipole, e.g. a battery). The case of a depolarized zone of a muscle fibre, described in Figures 18.2 and 18.3, is far more complex.

Figure 18.3, in particular, shows the membrane currents according to a tripole model (Rosenfalk, 1969). This model provides a simple illustration of the extinction of the tripole at the musculotendon junction, where the end of fibre phenomenon is generated. This is a short-lived phenomenon of tension due to the conversion of the tripole into a dipole, which does not move and which generates a temporary, more intense electrical field, responsible for part of the phenomenon of crosstalk (Farina, 2002b).

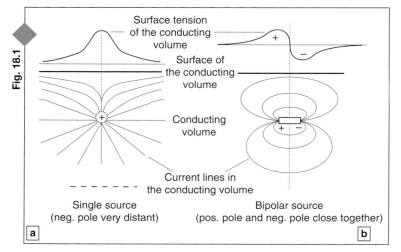

Fig. 18.1

Surface tension of the conducting volume

Surface of the conducting volume

Conducting volume

Current lines in the conducting volume

Single source (neg. pole very distant)

Bipolar source (pos. pole and neg. pole close together)

a

b

(a) Distribution of the current and surface potential lines produced by a punctiform electrical source immersed in a conducting volume. The distribution of potential is similar to the distribution of light which appears on the surface of the water above an immersed source of light; **(b)** distribution of the current and surface potential lines produced by a double electrical source (dipole), for example consisting of two poles of a battery immersed in a conducting volume.

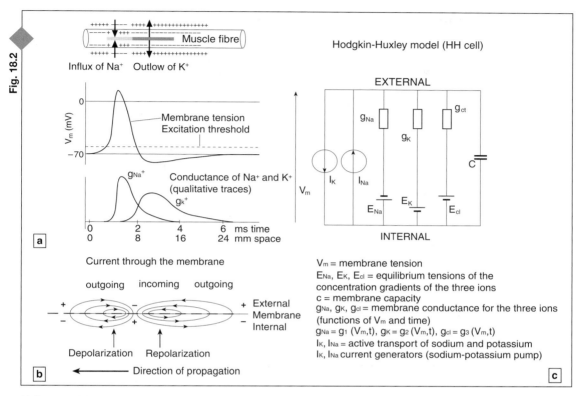

Fig. 18.2

(a) Generation of the action potential in a muscle fibre. The membrane tension evolves in space and in time generating a current, distributed according to the lines shown in (b), characteristic of a tripole source. The Hodgkin-Huxley model in (c) describes the membrane phenomena underlying the mechanism generating the action potential, the active transport of sodium and potassium, the tensions which balance the concentration gradients and the ion channel conductances which depend on the membrane tension V_m. Owing to this dependence, a change in membrane tension above a threshold level, induced for example by a neurotransmitter such as acetylcholine, triggers an action potential.

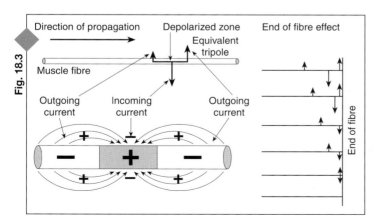

Fig. 18.3

Diagram of membrane currents. The depolarized zone is represented as a current tripole. The tripole is propagated from the innervation zone at the end of the fibre, where it becomes a dipole (with a more intense electrical field which generates the end of fibre effect) and is progressively cancelled out. In the extinction phase, the tripole does not move and constitutes an electrical source variable over time, but substantially invariable in space.

Surface electromyography

Fig. 18.4

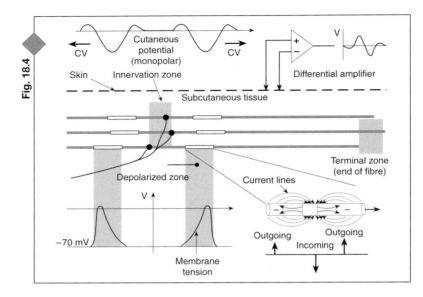

Generation of the motor unit action potential (MUAP) as an accumulation of the contributions of single fibres of the MU. Example of differential (or bipolar) acquisition. It is obvious that a pair of electrodes arranged symmetrically in relation to the innervation zone will acquire a signal that is virtually zero. In the terminal zone, the depolarized zones are extinguished by generating the end of fibre potential which does not move.

Figure 18.4 illustrates the cutaneous signals generated by a motor unit (MU) which, in the example, consists of only three fibres. The cutaneous potentials generated by single fibres of an MU accumulate, generating the motor unit action potential (MUAP) which arises in the IZ and propagates towards the tendons (with a velocity of approximately 4 m/s), where it is extinguished, generating an end of fibre potential (not shown in Fig. 18.4), consisting of the total contribution of the various fibres (described in Figure 18.3).

Figure 18.5a shows a series of differential signals, acquired between contiguous pairs of electrodes in an array of 16 contacts applied to a biceps brachii. Numerous motor units can be distinguished, all innervated under pair 7. The two lines identify an MU and their slope represents the propagation velocity of the MUAP. Figure 18.5b represents differential signals, reconstructed from the previous signals, between non-contiguous electrodes. It is clear that signals acquired between two electrodes in a symmetrical position in relation to the innervation zone are of small amplitude and do not contain much information, since the contributions of the depolarized zones that propagate in opposite directions are cancelled out. These signals are sensitive to small movements of the electrodes and are accordingly not reproducible on successive occasions, whereas signals acquired with both electrodes from the same part of the IZ are of wider amplitude and are more reproducible.

Figure 18.6 shows a differential trace, obtained with an array of electrodes positioned on a biceps brachii. Three MUAPs belonging to three different MUs can be seen. The propagation velocity can be calculated globally using channels 1, 2 or 3, which show unidirectional propagation, and not using channels 4 to 8 which have bidirectional propagation. The conduction velocity of each MU can be calculated, however, after separating the respective MUAPs. These calculations require dedicated software.

Variables and parameters of the EMG signal

The information contained in the EMG signal can be synthesized in some variables, whose course over time yields information on the course of physiological or pathological phenomena that take place in the muscle. Piper observed, as early as 1912, a progressive 'slowing' of the EMG signal with the fatiguing of the muscle. This slowing can today be quantified by the spectral analysis of a signal, based on development in Fourier series (Fourier analysis).

A detailed description of this technique lies outside the scope of this chapter and further information can be obtained from *Elementi di elettromiografia di superficie* by Merletti (2000).

The more widely used variables of the EMG signal can be classified as follows: amplitude variables, spectral variables (both obtained from a single signal),

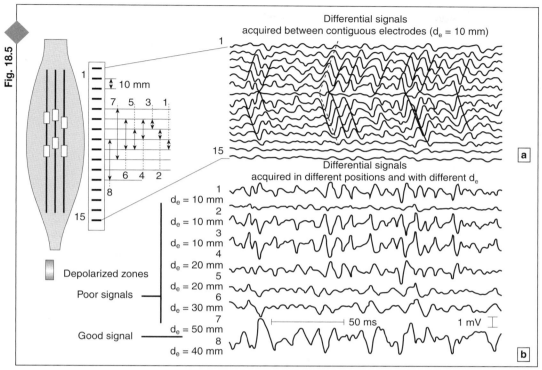

Fig. 18.5

Differential signals acquired between contiguous electrodes (d$_e$ = 10 mm)

10 mm

1

15

a

Differential signals acquired in different positions and with different d$_e$

Depolarized zones

Poor signals

Good signal

1
d$_e$ = 10 mm
2
d$_e$ = 10 mm
3
d$_e$ = 10 mm
4
d$_e$ = 20 mm
5
d$_e$ = 20 mm
6
d$_e$ = 30 mm
7
d$_e$ = 50 mm
8
d$_e$ = 40 mm

50 ms   1 mV

b

A series of equidistant electrodes forms a linear array. A series of differential amplifiers, similar to that shown in Figure 18.4, yields outgoing signals as shown in **(a)**. A great deal of information can be obtained from these signals. The action potentials (MUAP) of numerous MU are identifiable and the propagation velocity can be estimated from the ratio of the interelectrode distance to the delay between signals from contiguous channels (or from the slope of the broken lines). Part **(b)** shows that the EMG signal differs depending on the position and distance between two electrodes. Pairs of electrodes that cover the IZ yield signals that are very sensitive to the position of the electrodes themselves and are affected by the bidirectional propagation of the sources. Signals acquired with two electrodes both on one side of the IZ have a wider amplitude and are more repeatable and reliable.

d$_e$ = interelectrode distance.

(From Merletti R., Rainoldi A., Farina D., 'Surface electromyography for non-invasive characterisation of muscles', *Exercise and Sport Sciences Reviews* 29: 29–25, 2000).

conduction velocity and correlation coefficient (both of which require at least two signals).

The amplitude variables yield information on the amplitude of the signal, defined as the mean value of the rectified signal (negative waves turned positive), calculated in a specific range (usually 0.25–2 sec.), or as an effective value (square root of the mean quadratic value calculated in a range, usually 0.25–2 sec.). These variables are generally known by their English acronyms: ARV and RMS. They are substantially interchangeable and yield similar information.

The spectral variables are the mean frequency (MNF) and the median frequency (MDF) of the spectrum of the EMG signal. The MNF represents the barycentric line of the power spectrum; the MDF

represents the line that divides this spectrum into two equal areas. The global conduction velocity (CV) is obtained by estimating the delay between two EMG signals acquired from two electrode systems (e.g. two pairs or two triplets) and calculating the ratio of the distance between the two systems to this delay. The value obtained is more reliable, the more similar the two signals are. The degree of similarity is given by the correlation coefficient (CC). Figure 18.7 shows a diagram of the system for acquiring and calculating these variables, using the classic configuration of four bar electrodes.

If an array with more than four electrodes is used, the variables calculated according to the method described in Figure 18.7 can relate to electrodes 1–4,

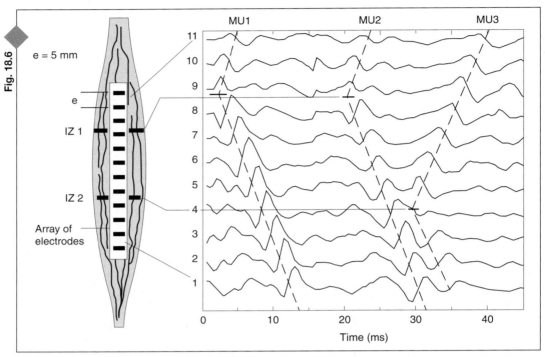

Fig. 18.6

MUAPs from three different MUs innervated in two different zones, IZ 1 and IZ 2, one innervated under electrode pair 4 and two between pair 8 and 9. The slopes of the broken lines represent the propagation velocities of the depolarized zones of the respective MUs.

2–5, 3–6, etc. of the array. A triplet of differential signals is obtained for each group of four electrodes and the courses of the respective variables are observed as a function of time. Alternatively the values of the variables in question can be observed for each triplet along the array, at each point in time. Figures 18.8 and 18.9 show a set of signals acquired using a commercially available system and the EMG variables as a function of time for triplet 2, respectively.

The traces shown in Figure 18.9 provide a further summary of information by using the regression line. The line in relation to which the mean quadratic deviation from the ordinates of the experimental points is least (regression line) is defined for each reasonably linear trace. The value of the intercept of this line with the ordinate is defined as the 'initial value' of the variable, while the slope of the line is defined as the 'rate of variation of the variable' or simply the 'slope'. The ratio of the slope to the initial value constitutes the normalized slope, expressed as %/sec (percentage

of the initial value per second). The initial value and slopes (absolute or normalized) constitute the 'parameters' of the EMG signal variables.

Myoelectric signs of fatigue

The traces shown in Figure 18.9 show that during an isometric contraction at constant force, sustained for 30 seconds, the EMG signal variables undergo changes over time, reflecting a series of physiological phenomena, which take place before mechanical signs of fatigue appear. The EMG variables alter from the start of the contraction, indicating electrophysiological variations in the muscle fibre membranes, which experience an accumulation of metabolites and changes in ionic concentrations as a result of cell metabolism and the generation of repeated action potentials. All these changes together are known as 'myoelectric signs of muscle fatigue'.

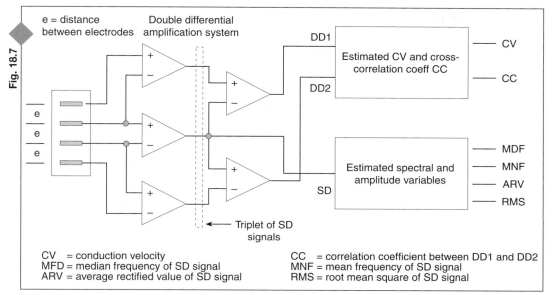

Fig. 18.7

Four-contact system for acquiring the EMG signal. The central single differential signal (SD) is used to calculate the spectral and amplitude variables, and the two double differential signals (DD1 and DD2) are used to calculate conduction velocity (CV). The correlation coefficient provides an indication of the degree of similarity between the two signals used to estimate CV. Double differential signals are preferable to single differential signals for estimating CV because they are affected less by either non-propagating components or common mode disturbances.

One way of facilitating comparison between various variables (such as MNF and CV or ARV) is to plot the percentage variations in these against the initial value. This type of graph, which is called a 'fatigue plot' or 'fatigue diagram', has become a frequent feature of the recent literature. The majority of studies concern the biceps, vastus medialis and lateralis, anterior tibialis and trapezius. There are currently no papers available using this technique on the shoulder muscles. Different myoelectric signs of fatigue and fatigue plots are observed in different muscles, conditions and individuals.

Figure 18.10 shows two fatigue plots of the biceps brachii muscle in two different subjects, both healthy, during isometric contraction sustained for 30 seconds at 70% of maximal voluntary contraction. The measurement was repeated nine times for each subject, to obtain statistical confirmation of the differences observed. It is clear that the two muscles exhibit different myoelectric signs of fatigue and thus have different characteristics, while both sustain the contraction without any mechanical signs of fatigue.

Figure 18.11 shows the fatigue plots of the biceps brachii of two subjects, one young and one older,

representing two study groups (Merletti, 2002). The fact that elderly individuals show a reduction in the myoelectric signs of fatigue correlates with the fact that their type 2 fibres are reduced in number and size (Merletti, 2002). This could be the reason for the differences observed between the two subjects, as shown in Figure 18.10. The correlation between myoelectric signs of fatigue and histological muscle structure has been confirmed by studies in animals (Kupa, 1995). The study of these correlations as regards the shoulder muscles represents a major area of on-going research. The documentation of a possible correlation between fibre type and myoelectric signs of fatigue, suggested by many recent studies, would open up areas of research of great relevance to sport medicine.

Figure 18.12 shows the course of an amplitude variable (ARV) and a frequency variable (MNF) of the EMG signal of the anterior deltoid muscle during a fatiguing contraction lasting 300 seconds in which the subject supports a load of 500 g at the level of the shoulder, with the arm raised in front of the body and the elbow flexed. The downwards course of the mean frequency and the upwards course of the amplitude

Fig. 18.8

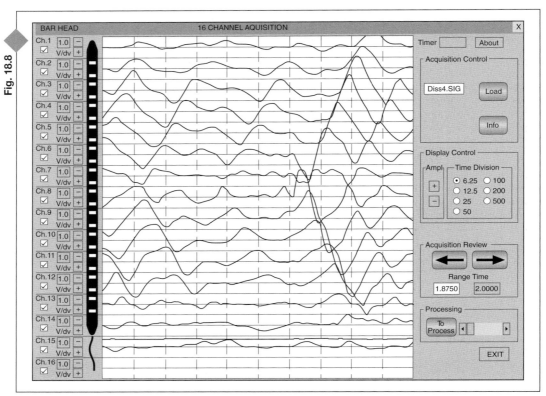

EMG traces obtained with an array of 16 electrodes arranged on the biceps brachii muscle during an isometric contraction. Single differential (bipolar) acquisition with an interelectrode distance of 10 mm.

are evident, demonstrating the onset and progression of muscle fatigue during an isometric contraction at constant force.

Conclusions

This chapter has shown the following that:
- the EMG signal is an extremely rich source of information for both the peripheral system (muscle), and the central nervous system;
- this information can be obtained using electrodes;

- the acquisition of the signal is highly critical and requires specific skills and the correct manual positioning of the electrodes. Incorrect positioning leads to incorrect interpretations and conclusions; and
- acquisition techniques using matrices of electrodes and signal production techniques will, in the next few years, allow documentation of the behaviour of single motor units and will probably allow non-invasive forms of determining the distribution of type I and II fibres.

The state of the art and likely future developments are described extensively in Merletti (2004).

Fig. 18.9

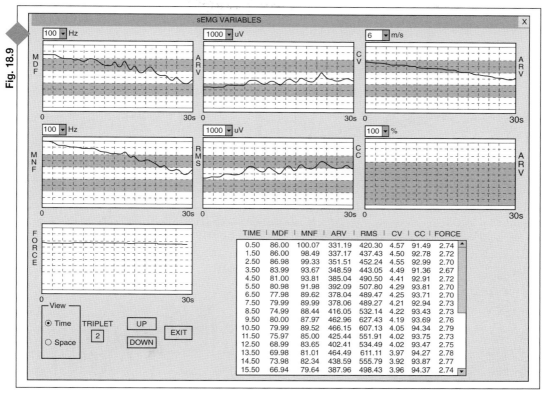

Traces of variables of the EMG signal (triplet 2, see Fig. 18.8) and force as a function of time.

Fig. 18.10

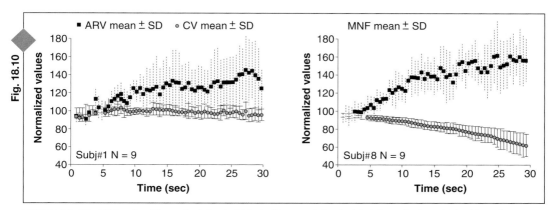

Fatigue plots of two biceps brachii muscles in two individuals. Means and standard deviations of values obtained from nine measurements per subject. It is clear that the two muscles exhibit different myoelectric signs of fatigue and thus have different characteristics, while both sustain the contraction without any mechanical signs of fatigue. (From Rainoldi A., Gorlandi G., Maderna L., Comi G., Lo Conte L., Merletti R., 'Repeatability of surface EMG variables during voluntary isometric contractions of the biceps brachii muscle', *J. Electrom. and Kinesiol.* 9: 105–119, (1999).)

Surface electromyography

Fig. 18.11

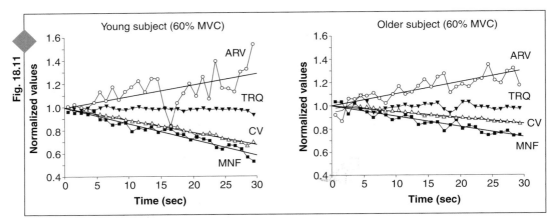

Fatigue plots of the biceps brachii in a young subject (<35 years) and an older subject (>65 years). The graphs show fewer myoelectric signs of fatigue in the older subject (reproduced from Merletti et al., (2002)

Fig. 18.12

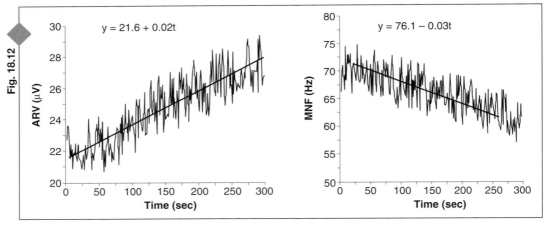

Traces of the mean frequency (MNF) and average rectified value (ARV) of the EMG signal. Fatiguing isometric contraction lasting 300 seconds of the anterior deltoid muscle; the subject supports a 500 g weight with the arm raised to shoulder level and the elbow flexed. The graphs show the lines interpolating the trace of the experimental points in time.

Bibliography

Attebrant M., Mathiassen S., Winkel J., 'Normalizing upper trapezius EMG amplitude: comparison of ramp and constant force procedures', *J. Electrom. Kinesiol.* 5: 345–350, (1995)

Basmajan J., De Luca C., *Muscles alive: their function revealed by electromyography*, 5th ed., Williams and Wilkins, Baltimore (USA), (1985)

Cram J., Kasman G., *Introduction to Surface Electromyography*, Aspen Publications, Gaithersburg (USA), (1998)

De Luca C.J., 'The use of surface electromyography in biomechanics', *J. Appl. Biomech.* 13: 135–163, (1997)

Farina D., Madeleine P., Graven-Nielsen T., Merletti R., Arendt Nielsen L., 'Standardising surface electromyogram

recordings for assessment of activity and fatigue in the human upper trapezius muscle', *Eur. J. Appl. Physiol.* 86: 469–478, (2002a)

Farina D., Merletti R., Indino B., Nazzaro M., Pozzo M., 'Surface EMG crosstalk between knee extensor muscles: experimental and model results', *Muscle and Nerve* 26: 681–695, (2002b)

Hagberg M., 'Electromyographic signs of shoulder muscular fatigue in two elevated arm positions', *Am. J. Phys. Med.* 60: 111–121, (1981)

Hermens H., Freriks B., Merletti R., Stegeman D., Blok J., Rau G., Disserlhorst-Klug C., Hagg G., 'European recommendations for surface electromyography', *Roessingh Research and Development*, Enschede, NL (1999)

Jensen C., Vasseljen O., Westgaard R., 'The influence of electrode position on bipolar surface EMG recordings of the upper trapezius muscle', *Eur. J. Appl. Physiol.* 67: 266–273, (1993)

Kasman G., Cram J., Wolf S., *Clinical applications in surface electromyography*, Aspen Publications, (1998)

Kupa E., Raoy S., Kandarian S., De Luca C., 'Effects of muscle fiber type and size on EMG median frequency and conduction velocity', *J. Appl. Physiol.* 79: 23–32, (1995)

Madeleine P., Farina D., Merletti R., Aarendt-Nielsen L., 'Upper trapezius muscle mechanomyographic and electromyographic activity in humans during low force fatiguing and non fatiguing contractions', *Eur. J. Appl. Physiol.* 87: 327–336, (2002)

Mathiassen S., Winkel J., Hagg G., *Normalization of surface EMG amplitude from the upper trapezius muscles in ergonomic studies – a review, J. Electrom. Kinesiol.* 5: 197–226, (1995)

Merletti R., *Elementi di Elettromiografia di Superficie*, CLUT-Politecnico di Torino, (2000)

Merletti R., Farina D., Gazzoni M., Schieroni MP., 'Effects of age on muscle functions investigated with surface electromyography', Muscle Nerve 25: 65–76, (2002)

Merletti R., Parker P., *Electromyography, physiology, engineering and non invasive applications*, J. Wiley and IEEE Press, New Jersey (2004)

Palmerud G., Sporrong H., Herberts P., Jarvholm U., Kadefors R., 'Voluntary redistribution of muscle activity in human shoulder muscles' *Med. Biol. Eng Comp* 38: 806–815, (1995)

Palmerud G., Sporrong H., Herberts P., Kadefors R., 'Consequences of trapezius relaxation on the distribution of shoulder muscle forces: an electromyographic study', *J. Electrom. Kinesiol.* 8: 185–193, (1998)

Piper H., *Electrophysiologie. Menschlicher Muskeln*, Springer Verlag, Berlin (1912)

Rosenfalk P., 'Intra- and extracellular potential fields of active nerve and muscle fibers. A physico-mathematical analysis of different models', *Acta Physiol. Scand.* 321(Suppl.): 1–168, (1969)

ATLAS OF THE INNERVATION ZONES OF THE SUPERFICIAL MUSCLES OF THE SHOULDER

A. RAINOLDI
R. BERGAMO
A. MERLO

Hundreds of papers have been published in the last 15 years based on an analysis of the amplitude of surface EMG signals. Although the use of EMG signals is particularly widespread in both research and clinical practice to evaluate muscle activity during movement, only a few authors have correctly addressed the problem of positioning electrodes (Hogrel, 1998; Jensen, 1993; Merletti, 2001; Rainoldi, 2004); the problem has been ignored in the majority of cases. In an analysis of 144 recent articles, Hermens et al. (2000) identified 352 different descriptions for positioning electrodes. The first recommendations for standardization by Zipp (1982) advised applying the electrodes parallel to the fibres and symmetrical with the centre, where possible. More recently, in both isometric and dynamic contractions, investigators have placed electrodes on the muscle belly (Gamet, 1993), on the motor points (Duchateau, 1991) or generally half-way along the muscle, without considering the effects that this choice would have on estimates of signal variables. Many clinical manuals, including Cram 1998, base positioning on anatomical landmarks, without justification by recommended standards.

The use of linear electrode arrays makes numerous channels available and increases the quality and usefulness of the information available. In contrast with the signal obtained with a single pair of electrodes (traditional bipolar technique), single motor unit action potentials (MUAP) can be identified along with the position of the innervation zone (IZ), the estimated mean conduction velocity, and single MUAPs and their firing pattern. The mean (or median) frequencies of the signal spectrum and the muscle conduction velocity also differ according to the position of the electrodes on the skin. Figure 19.1 shows estimates of the three variables

(average rectified value, ARV; mean frequency of the spectrum, MNF; and conduction velocity, CV) and of the correlation coefficient (CC which provides a measure of the similarity between two adjacent signals and thus of the reliability of the estimated CV) over 13 cms of skin surface, 1 cm apart during a contraction of the biceps brachii.

It is clear that, according to the position of the electrodes in relation to the IZ and to the tendon endings, the estimated variables are polarized. To minimize this artefact and to make the repeated measurements comparable, the IZ needs to be identified in the muscle and the electrodes applied distally (laterally) or proximally (medially) from this position between the IZ and the tendon ending.

This type of information can be readily obtained if a multichannel system is available; if not, an atlas of optimal positioning available to all users seems particularly beneficial and necessary (Rainoldi, 2004). Such an atlas is obviously valid only in cases where the IZ is located in a standard position for all subjects.

The muscles which act on the scapulohumeral joint have, therefore, been mapped, and 15 have been selected which are accessible to the surface technique (for a taxonomic description, see the following list):
• *Muscles stabilizing the scapula*
— upper trapezius (accessible);
— middle trapezius (accessible);
— lower trapezius (accessible);
— anterior serratus (accessible);
— pectoralis minor (not accessible because covered by the pectoralis major);
— greater rhomboid (accessible);
— lesser rhomboid (accessible).

Atlas of the innervation zones of the superficial muscles of the shoulder

Fig. 19.1

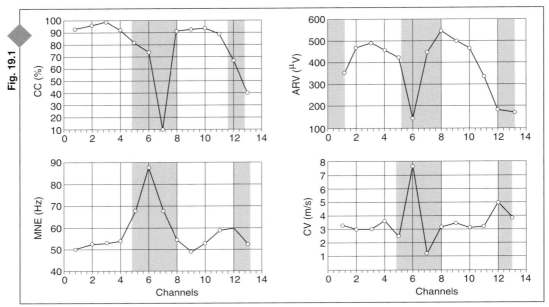

Pattern of estimated EMG signal variables along the array of electrodes (i.e. along the muscle). It is evident that the MNF and CV are overestimated above or close to the innervation zone (IZ), while the ARV and CC are underestimated owing to the generation of MUAPs in the IZ and by their extinction at the tendon endings (the shaded rectangles represent the zones where electrodes should not be positioned). Biceps brachii muscle, interelectrode distance: 10 mm. ARV = average rectified value, MNF = mean frequency of the signal spectrum. CV = conduction velocity of the muscle fibres, CC = correlation coefficient between adjacent channels (this indicates the quality of the estimated CV).

- *Muscles that act on the humerus*
Elevators
— anterior deltoid (accessible);
— middle deltoid (accessible);
— posterior deltoid (accessible);
— biceps: long head (accessible);
— biceps: short head (accessible).
- *Depressors and rotators of the humerus*
— supraspinatus (not accessible because covered by the middle and upper trapezius);
— infraspinatus (accessible);
— subscapularis (not accessible because covered by the pectoralis major);
— teres major (accessible);
— teres minor (superficial but small and difficult to distinguish from the infraspinatus);
— latissimus dorsi (accessible);
— pectoralis major (accessible).

Ten subjects were studied to determine whether, where and to what extent the IZ of these muscles could be uniformly located. Figure 19.2 shows the coefficients of variation (given by the ratio of the

standard deviation to the mean value) of the position of the IZ in the muscles assessed as 'good quality'. Low values (=10%) indicate muscles innervated in a very similar way in different subjects; generalizations can certainly be made for these subjects. High CV values (>20%) indicate great variability in the position of the IZ between different subjects and identify muscles which require previous evaluation for each subject before application of electrodes.

If this information relating to the uniformity of the location of the IZ is combined with the ability to record good quality signals and to estimate the CV with physiological values, it can then be concluded that the anterior deltoid, teres major, upper trapezius, middle trapezius, greater rhomboid, lesser rhomboid, biceps brachii long head and biceps brachii short head muscles are the most suitable for study by surface EMG.

The following charts were obtained from 10 different subjects who were asked to exert effort against isometric resistance (see section: Direction and intensity of the movement asked of the subject) in order to generate an EMG signal without altering the relative position of

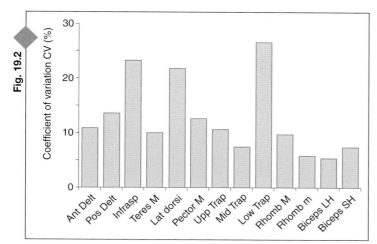

Fig. 19.2

The coefficient of variation of the distance of the IZ from an anatomical landmark for each of the muscles studied is represented here as a measure of the degree of uniformity of the distribution of the innervation zone in 10 different subjects. The lower the CV, the more uniform the position of the IZ will be in different subjects. The IZ cannot be identified in the middle deltoid (lateralis) and the CV cannot be estimated. The IZ cannot be identified in the anterior serratus, but the CV can be estimated using physiological values. The CV can be estimated using physiological values in all the other muscles reported (including in the range 2–8 m/s).
Coefficient of variation CV (%)

the sampling electrodes and the underlying muscle. This can prevent errors in estimating EMG variables caused by this geometric movement artefact (Rainoldi, 2000). The anatomical design helps to identify immediately the landmarks and reference line for correct positioning of the electrodes, while the dark rectangle identifies the location of the IZ.

Finally each chart shows an extract of the EMG signal recorded from the muscle being tested to give the reader an idea of the quality that can be obtained, for a better understanding of the correlation between the subject's anatomical characteristics, the position of the electrodes and the signal obtained.

Bibliography

Cram J., Kasman G., Holtz J., *Introduction to Surface EMG*, Aspen Publications, Aspen (1998)

Duchateau J., Hainaut K., 'Effects of immobilization on electromyogram power spectrum changes during fatigue', *Eur. J. Appl. Physiol. Occup. Physiol.* 63(6): 458–62, (1991)

Gamet D., Duchene J., Garapon-Bar C., Goubel F. 'Surface electromyogram power spectrum in human quadriceps muscle during incremental exercise', *J. Appl. Physiol.* 74(6): 2704–2710, (1993)

Hermens H.J., Freriks B., Disselhorst-Klug C., RAU G., 'Development of recommendations for SEMG sensors and sensor placement procedures', *J. Electromyogr. Kinesiol.* 10(5): 361–374, (2000)

Hogrel J.Y., Duchene J., Marini J.F., 'Variability of some SEMG parameter estimates with electrode location', *J. Electromyogr. Kinesiol.* 8(5): 305–315, (1998)

Jensen C., Vasseljen O., Westgaard R.H. The influence of electrode position on bipolar surface electromyogram recordings of the upper trapezius muscle, Eur. J. Appl. Physiol. Occup. Physiol. 67(3): 266–273, (1993)

Merletti R., Rainoldi A., Farina D., 'Surface electromyography for noninvasive characterization of muscle', *Exerc. Sport Sci Rev.* 29(1): 20–25, (2001)

Rainoldi A., Melchiorri G., Caruso I., 'A method for positioning electrodes during surface EMG recordings in lower limb muscles', *J. Neurosci. Methods* 134(1): 37–43, (2004)

Rainoldi A., Nazzaro M., Merletti R., Farina D., Caruso I., Gaudenti S., 'Geometrical factors in surface EMG of the vastus medialis and lateralis muscles', *J. Electromyogr. Kinesiol.* 10(5): 327–336, (2000)

Roy S.H., De Luca C.J., Schneider J., 'Effects of electrode location on myoelectric conduction velocity and median frequency estimates', *J. Appl. Physiol.* 61(4): 1510–1517, (1986)

Zipp P., 'Recommendations for the Standardization of Lead Positions in Surface Electromyography', *Eur. J. Appl. Physiol. Occup. Physiol.* 50: 41–54, (1982)

ANTERIOR DELTOID (Deltoideus anterior)

Fig. 19.3

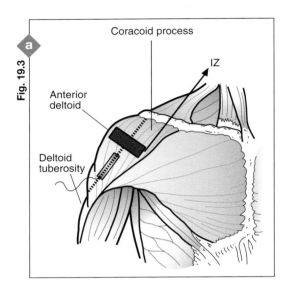

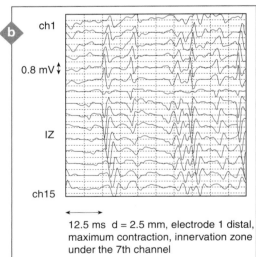

12.5 ms d = 2.5 mm, electrode 1 distal, maximum contraction, innervation zone under the 7th channel

Innervation

Circumflex or axillary nerve (C4-C6).

Anatomical characteristics

It takes origin from the anterior rim, upper surface and lateral third of the clavicle; it inserts into the deltoid tuberosity of the humerus; it flexes and rotates the glenohumeral joint medially.

Position of subject

The subject is supine, the arm along the body, the elbow flexed at 90° and the hand closed in a fist.

Direction and intensity of the movement asked of the subject

The subject is asked to flex the shoulder with the elbow flexed, with resistance against the subject's fist.

Position and orientation of probe

The probe must be positioned parallel to the line joining the deltoid tuberosity to the coracoid process.

Position of the innervation zone

The innervation zone is located 47.9% ± 5.1% (mean ± standard deviation) of the distance from the coracoid process to the deltoid tuberosity, starting from the coracoid process.

Characteristics of the electromyographic signal

The signal obtained shows clear propagation, an innervation zone of the motor units that can be readily identified, and a conduction velocity that can be estimated with physiological values.

POSTERIOR DELTOID (Deltoideus posterior)

Innervation

Circumflex or axillary nerve (C4-C6)

Anatomical characteristics

It takes origin from the inferior lip of the posterior rim of the spine of the scapula; it reinserts into the deltoid tuberosity of the humerus; its principal action is pushing the humerus back.

Position of subject

The subject is prone with the arm abducted at 90°, and the elbow flexed.

Direction and intensity of the movement asked of the subject

The subject is asked to push the arm back against resistance at the olecranon.

Position and orientation of probe

The probe should be placed on a line parallel to the spine of the scapula, perpendicular to the lower half of the line from the acromial angle to the centre of the glenoid cavity.

Position of the innervation zone

The innervation zone is located 44% ± 5.7% (mean ± standard deviation) of the distance from the acromial angle to the centre of the glenoid cavity, starting from the acromial angle.

Characteristics of the electromyographic signal

The signal obtained shows clear propagation, an innervation zone of the motor units that can be readily identified, and a conduction velocity that can be estimated with physiological values.

Fig. 19.4

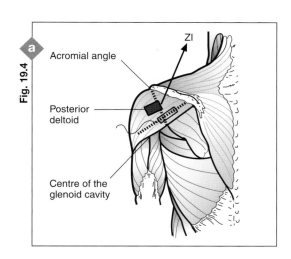

a Acromial angle — ZI — Posterior deltoid — Centre of the glenoid cavity

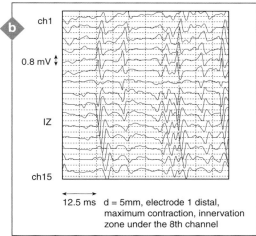

b ch1 — 0.8 mV — IZ — ch15

12.5 ms   d = 5mm, electrode 1 distal, maximum contraction, innervation zone under the 8th channel

MIDDLE DELTOID (Deltoideus lateralis)

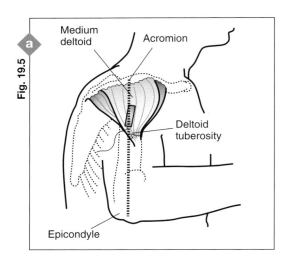

Fig. 19.5 a

Medium deltoid
Acromion
Deltoid tuberosity
Epicondyle

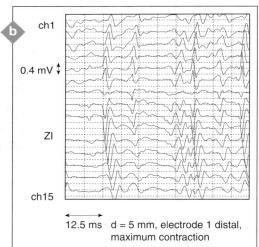

b

ch1

0.4 mV

ZI

ch15

12.5 ms   d = 5 mm, electrode 1 distal, maximum contraction

Innervation

Circumflex or axillary nerve (C4-C6).

Anatomical characteristics

It takes origin from the lateral rim and upper surface of the acromion; it inserts into the tuberosity of the humerus; its action is abduction of the shoulder.

Position of subject

The subject is seated with the spine straight, the elbow flexed at 90° and the arm abducted at 45°.

Direction and intensity of the movement asked of the subject

The subject is asked simply to abduct the shoulder against resistance applied to the lateral surface of the distal third of the humerus.

Position and orientation of probe

The probe should be placed above the deltoid tuberosity, slightly inclined towards the anterior part of the body in relation to the line joining the acromion to the epicondyle.

Position of the innervation zone

The position of the innervation zone of the motor units cannot be recognized in the majority of cases.

Characteristics of the electromyographic signal

The electromyographic signal does not show good propagation and the conduction velocity cannot be estimated.

INFRASPINATUS (Infraspinous muscle)

Innervation

Suprascapular nerve (C5, C6).

Anatomical characteristics

It takes origin from the two middle thirds of the infra-spinous fossa of the scapula; it inserts into the middle facet of the greater tubercle of the humerus and the joint capsule of the shoulder; it rotates the humerus outwards and stabilizes the head during movements of the glenoid joint.

Position of subject

The subject is seated, with the trunk upright, and the arm along the body in a neutral position as regards rotation.

Direction and intensity of the movement asked of the subject

The subject is asked to rotate the humerus outwards, with the elbow flexed at 90°, against resistance applied to the dorsal side of the wrist in the direction of internal rotation.

Position and orientation of probe

The probe should be positioned on the upper half of the line running from the centre of the medial rim of the scapula to the posterior acromial angle.

Position of the innervation zone

The innervation zone is located 28% ± 6.4% (mean ± standard deviation) of the distance from the centre of the medial rim of the scapula to the acromial angle, starting from the medial rim of the scapula.

Characteristics of the electromyographic signal

The signal obtained shows clear propagation, an innerv-ation zone of the motor units that can be readily iden-tified and a conduction velocity that can be estimated with physiological values.

Fig. 19.6

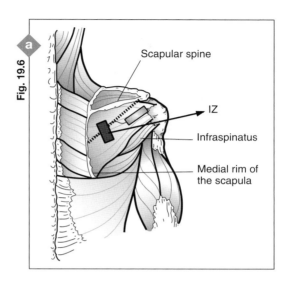

a

Scapular spine

IZ

Infraspinatus

Medial rim of the scapula

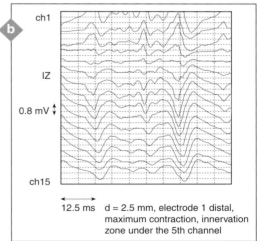

b

ch1

IZ

0.8 mV

ch15

12.5 ms   d = 2.5 mm, electrode 1 distal, maximum contraction, innervation zone under the 5th channel

TERES MAJOR (Teres major muscle)

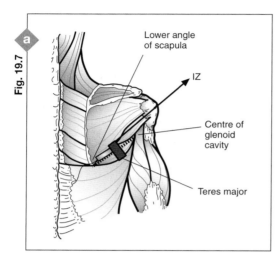

Fig. 19.7

a

Lower angle
of scapula

IZ

Centre of
glenoid
cavity

Teres major

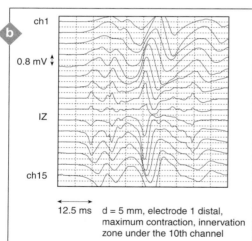

b

ch1

0.8 mV ↕

IZ

ch15

12.5 ms   d = 5 mm, electrode 1 distal,
maximum contraction, innervation
zone under the 10th channel

Innervation

Branch of the internal subscapular nerve (C5-C7).

Anatomical characteristics

It takes origin from the dorsal surfaces of the lower
angle and lower third of the lateral rim of the scapula;
it inserts into the crest of the lesser tubercle of the
humerus; it rotates medially, adducts and extends the
humerus.

Position of subject and direction and intensity of the movement asked of the subject

The subject is prone with the arm abducted at 90°
and the hand hanging over the couch supported on the
examiner's leg, on which distinct pressure is applied.

Position and orientation of probe

The probe should be positioned on the lower half of
the line joining the lower angle of the scapula to the
centre of the glenoid cavity.

Position of the innervation zone

The innervation zone is located 62.8% ± 6.2%
(mean ± standard deviation) of the distance from the
lower angle of the scapula to the centre of the glenoid
cavity, starting from the lower angle of the scapula.

Characteristics of the electromyographic signal

The signal obtained shows clear propagation, an innervation zone of the motor units that can be readily identified and a conduction velocity that can be estimated
with physiological values.

LATISSIMUS DORSI (Latissimus dorsi muscle)

Innervation

Thoracodorsal nerve (C6-C8).

Anatomical characteristics

It takes origin from the spinous processes of the last six thoracic vertebrae, the last three or four ribs and the posterior third of the external lip of the iliac crest; it inserts into the intertubercular groove of the humerus. It depresses the stump of the shoulder, elevates the homolateral hemipelvis and returns the humerus to the flexed position.

Position of subject

The subject is prone with the arm extended along the body.

Direction and intensity of the movement asked of the subject

The subject is asked to depress the shoulder while at the same time elevating the pelvis on the same side.

Position and orientation of probe

The probe should be positioned in the middle third of a line inclined at 30° to the line joining the angle of the glenoid cavity to the L5 spinous process.

Position of the innervation zone

The innervation zone is located 18.5% ± 3.9% (mean ± standard deviation) of the distance from the angle of the glenoid cavity to L5, starting from the angle of the glenoid cavity.

Characteristics of the electromyographic signal

The signal obtained shows clear propagation, an innervation zone of the motor units that can be readily identified and a conduction velocity that can be estimated with physiological values.

Fig. 19.8

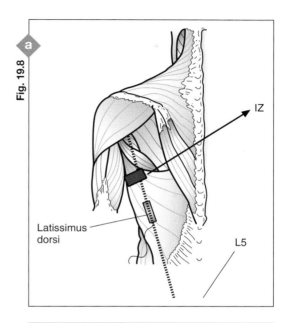

a

IZ

Latissimus dorsi

L5

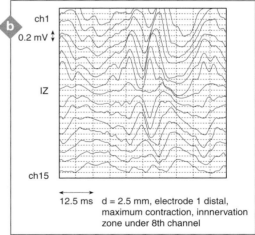

b

ch1
0.2 mV

IZ

ch15

12.5 ms   d = 2.5 mm, electrode 1 distal, maximum contraction, innervation zone under 8th channel

PECTORALIS MAJOR (Greater pectoral muscle)

Fig. 19.9

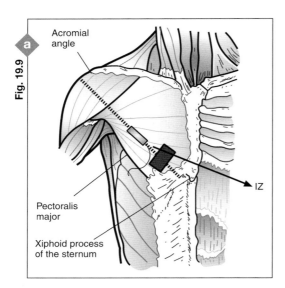

a

Acromial angle

Pectoralis major

Xiphoid process of the sternum

IZ

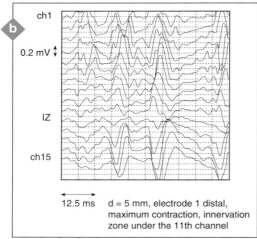

b

ch1

0.2 mV

IZ

ch15

12.5 ms

d = 5 mm, electrode 1 distal, maximum contraction, innervation zone under the 11th channel

Innervation

Long thoracic nerve and branches of the anterior thoracic nerve (C5-T1).

Anatomical characteristics

It takes origin from the anterior surface of the sternum, the cartilages of the first 6–7 ribs and the aponeurosis of the obliquus externus; it inserts into the crest of the greater tubercle of the humerus; it adducts and rotates the humerus medially.

Position of subject

The subject is erect or supine with the arm abducted at about 30° and the forearm flexed at 90°.

Direction and intensity of the movement asked of the subject

The subject is asked to adduct the arm against resistance at the elbow.

Position and orientation of probe

The EMG signal is obtained along the fibres of the lower part of the muscle, where the best propagation is obtained. The probe should be positioned along the line running from the acromial angle to the xiphoid process of the sternum.

Position of the innervation zone

The innervation zone is located $75.5\% \pm 9.4\%$ (mean $\pm$ standard deviation) of the distance from the acromial angle to the xiphoid process of the sternum, starting from the acromial angle.

Characteristics of the electromyographic signal

The signal obtained shows clear propagation, an innervation zone of the motor units that can be readily identified and a conduction velocity that can be estimated with physiological values.

SERRATUS ANTERIOR (Anterior serratus muscle)

Innervation

Long thoracic nerve (C5-C7).

Anatomical characteristics

It takes origin from the outer surfaces and upper rims of the eight or nine upper ribs; it inserts into the costal surface of the medial rim of the scapula.

Position of subject

The subject is supine, flexing the glenohumeral at 90°, with the elbow extended and the hand closed in a fist.

Direction and intensity of the movement asked of the subject

The subject is required to push the fist towards the ceiling against resistance applied by the examiner.

Position and orientation of probe

The probe should be placed along the muscle fibres of the upper digitations of the muscle.

Position of the innervation zone

The EMG signal propagates along the whole of the muscle at all the possible sampling sites (along the 5th to the 9th ribs). The innervation zone is probably located behind the accessible region, towards the scapula.

Characteristics of the electromyographic signal

The signal obtained shows clear propagation and a conduction velocity that can be estimated with physiological values.

The innervation zone of the motor units is not identified.

Fig. 19.10

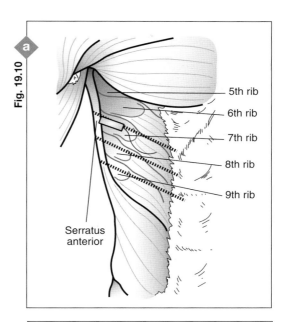

a

5th rib
6th rib
7th rib
8th rib
9th rib

Serratus anterior

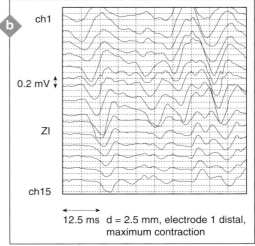

b

ch1

0.2 mV

ZI

ch15

12.5 ms   d = 2.5 mm, electrode 1 distal, maximum contraction

UPPER TRAPEZIUS (Trapezius superior)

Fig. 19.11

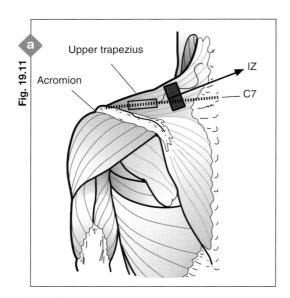

a

Upper trapezius

Acromion

IZ

C7

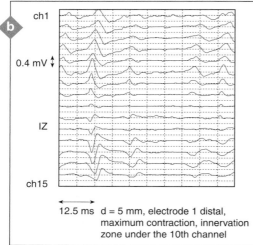

b

ch1

0.4 mV

IZ

ch15

12.5 ms d = 5 mm, electrode 1 distal,
maximum contraction, innervation
zone under the 10th channel

Innervation

Spinal accessory nerve (XI cranial nerve; C2, C3).

Anatomical characteristics

It takes origin from the transverse processes of the cervical vertebrae and from the middle third of the upper occipital line; it inserts into the lateral third of the clavicle and the acromion.

Position of subject

The subject is seated with the trunk upright.

Direction and intensity of the movement asked of the subject

The subject is asked to elevate the shoulder without any cervical movement; resistance is applied vertically to the shoulder in the direction of depression.

Position and orientation of probe

The probe is positioned in the distal half of the line joining C7 and the acromion.

Position of the innervation zone

The innervation zone is located 46% ± 4.7% (mean ± standard deviation) of the distance between C7 and the acromion, starting from C7.

Innervation

Spinal accessory nerve (XI Cranial nerve; C2, C3).

Anatomical characteristics

It takes origin from the spinous processes of the first to the fifth thoracic vertebrae; it inserts into the medial rim of the acromion and the upper part of the spine of the scapula; its principal action is adduction of the scapula.

Position of subject

The subject is prone with the shoulder abducted at 90°.

Direction and intensity of the movement asked of the subject

The subject is asked to push the arm back; resistance is applied against the olecranon in a posteroanterior direction.

Position and orientation of probe

The probe is positioned at a maximum distance of 8 cm lateral to the spinous processes of D2 on a horizontal line.

Position of the innrvation zone

The innervation zone is located 7.3 cm ± 0.5 cm (mean ± standard deviation) horizontally from D2.

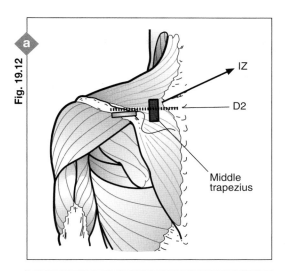

Fig. 19.12

a

IZ

D2

Middle trapezius

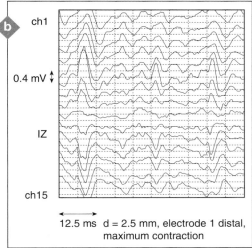

b

ch1

0.4 mV

IZ

ch15

12.5 ms   d = 2.5 mm, electrode 1 distal, maximum contraction

LOWER TRAPEZIUS (Trapezius inferior)

Fig. 19.13

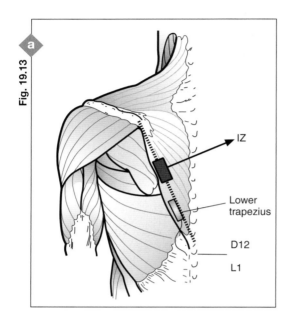

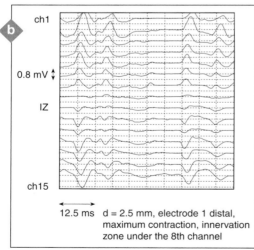

12.5 ms   d = 2.5 mm, electrode 1 distal, maximum contraction, innervation zone under the 8th channel

Innervation

Spinal accessory nerve (XI Cranial nerve; C2, C3).

Anatomical characteristics

It takes origin from the spinous processes of the sixth to the twelfth thoracic vertebrae; it inserts into the apex of the spine of the scapula; it adducts and medializes the superointernal angle and depresses the scapula.

Position of subject

The subject is prone with the arm completely elevated.

Direction and intensity of the movement asked of the subject

The subject is asked to elevate the arm against resistance applied at the elbow.

Position and orientation of probe

The probe is positioned in the lower third of the line joining the medial angle of the scapula to the spinous process of DI2.

Position of the innervation zone

The innervation zone is located 36% ± 9.5% (mean ± standard deviation) of the distance from the medial angle of the scapula to DI2, starting from the medial angle of the scapula.

GREATER RHOMBOID (Rhomboideus major)

This is not a superficial muscle since it is covered entirely by the middle trapezius; its fibres are nevertheless orientated perpendicular to those of the muscle overlying it, and if clear propagation is obtained, the EMG signal can be truly attributable to this muscle.

Innervation

Rhomboid nerve and dorsal nerve of the scapula (C4, C5).

Anatomical characteristics

It takes origin from the spinous processes of the second to the fifth thoracic vertebrae; it inserts into the medial rim of the scapula, between the spine and the lower angle; it adducts and elevates the scapula, and medializes the lower angle.

Position of subject

The subject is prone with the arm rotated inwards and the back of the hand supported on the thoracic vertebrae.

Direction and intensity of the movement asked of the subject

The subject is asked to push the elbow back against resistance applied by the examiner.

Position and orientation of probe

The probe is positioned on the lower third of a line at 45° starting from D3, towards the medial rim of the scapula.

Position of the innervation zone

The innervation zone is located 51.3% ± 4.9% (mean ± standard deviation) of the distance from D3 to the medial rim of the scapula, starting from D3 along a line inclined at 45° downwards.

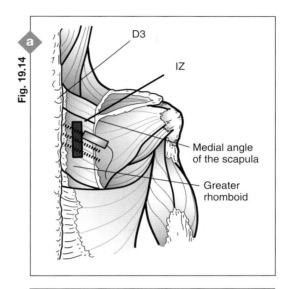

Fig. 19.14

a — D3, IZ, Medial angle of the scapula, Greater rhomboid

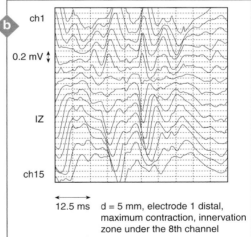

b — ch1, 0.2 mV, IZ, ch15, 12.5 ms, d = 5 mm, electrode 1 distal, maximum contraction, innervation zone under the 8th channel

LESSER RHOMBOID (Rhomboideus minor)

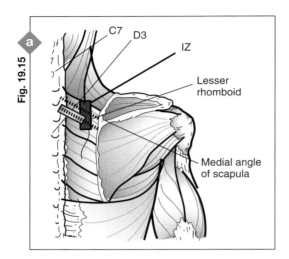

Fig. 19.15 a

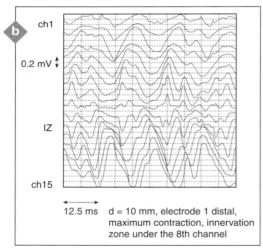

b

0.2 mV

ch1

IZ

ch15

12.5 ms   d = 10 mm, electrode 1 distal,
maximum contraction, innervation
zone under the 8th channel

This is not a superficial muscle since it is covered entirely by the middle trapezius and its fibres are orientated perpendicular to the latter. This anatomical detail means that, if clear propagation is obtained, the EMG signal is truly attributable to this muscle.

Innervation

Rhomboid nerve and dorsal nerve of the scapula (C4, C5).

Anatomical characteristics

It takes origin from the spinous processes of the seventh cervical vertebra and the first thoracic vertebra; it inserts into the medial rim, starting from the medial angle of the scapula; it adducts, elevates and rotates the scapula.

Position of subject

The subject is prone and the arm rotated inwards with the back of the hand supported on the thoracic vertebrae.

Direction and intensity of the movement asked of the subject

The subject is asked to push the elbow back against resistance applied by the examiner.

Position and orientation of probe

The probe is positioned in the upper two-thirds of a line at 45° starting from C7 towards the medial angle of the scapula.

Position of the innervation zone

The innervation zone is located 70.4% ± 4.2% (mean ± standard deviation) of the distance from C7 to the medial angle of the scapula, starting from C7 along a line at 45° inclined downwards.

BICEPS: LONG HEAD (Biceps brachii capitus longum)

Innervation

Musculocutaneous nerve (C5, C6).

Anatomical characteristics

It takes origin from the supraglenoid tubercle of the scapula; it inserts into the radial tuberosity; its principal action is flexion and supination of the forearm on the elbow. Its other function is flexion of the arm.

Position of subject

The subject is seated with the trunk upright, and with the forearm flexed at 90° and supinated.

Direction and intensity of the movement asked of the subject

The subject is asked to perform isometric flexion of the forearm against resistance applied at the wrist (palmar side).

Position of the innervation zone

The probe is positioned in the lower third of the line running from the acromion to the epicondyle.

Characteristics of the electromyographic signal

The innervation zone is located 57% ± 3.1% (mean ± standard deviation) of the distance from the acromion to the epicondyle, starting from the acromion.

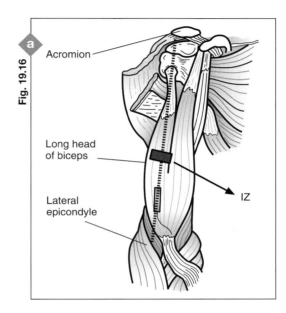

Fig. 19.16

a

Acromion

Long head of biceps

Lateral epicondyle

IZ

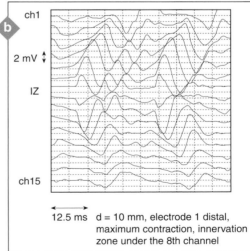

b

ch1

2 mV

IZ

ch15

12.5 ms d = 10 mm, electrode 1 distal, maximum contraction, innervation zone under the 8th channel

BICEPS: SHORT HEAD (Biceps brachii caput breve)

Fig. 19.17

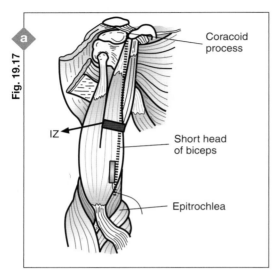

a

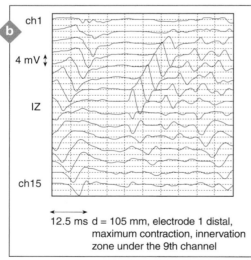

b

4 mV

ch1

IZ

ch15

12.5 ms d = 105 mm, electrode 1 distal, maximum contraction, innervation zone under the 9th channel

Innervation

Musculocutaneous muscle (C5, C6).

Anatomical characteristics

It takes origin from the apex of the coracoid process of the scapula; it inserts into the radial tuberosity; its principal actions are flexion and supination of the forearm on the arm.

Position of subject

The subject is seated with the trunk upright and with the forearm flexed at 90° and supinated.

Direction and intensity of the movement asked of the subject

The subject is asked to perform isometric flexion of the forearm against resistance applied at the wrist (palmar side).

Position of the innervation zone

The probe is positioned in the lower third of a line running from the coracoid process to the epitrochlea.

Characteristics of the electromyographic signal

The innervation zone is located $55.3\% \pm 4\%$ (mean $\pm$ standard deviation) of the distance from the coracoid process to the epitrochlea, starting from the coracoid process.

20

PRACTICAL APPLICATIONS IN SURFACE ELECTROMYOGRAPHY: LITERATURE REVIEW

V. Contardo
V. Marchione

There is a constant need in rehabilitation, as in medicine, to base clinical practice on objective data, particularly in the rehabilitation of athletes where a knowledge of the intrinsic mechanisms of muscle work and optimization of recovery times is crucial.

When evaluating athletic movements, the study of the forces acting on each joint is particularly important, both to determine the role of the muscles in achieving an optimal performance, and to evaluate the damage caused by athletic actions performed incorrectly.

Surface EMG is clearly an excellent tool for this purpose (Clarys, 1993).

Kinesiological EMG (KEMG) can be used to analyse movements and posture, and to evaluate isometric contractions with increasing tension up to maximal voluntary contraction, functional muscle activity, coordination and synchronization, the specificity and efficiency of training methods, the relation between strength and EMG, the interaction between man and machine, and the influence of materials used during training and rehabilitation (e.g. tape, braces) on muscle activity, fatigue, and load in relation to problems associated with the spine or joints (Clarys, 2000).

The limits of surface electromyography do not currently allow evaluation of muscle activity under dynamic conditions, nor detection of deeper muscles, owing to signal interference believed to derive from these recordings and from the non-detectability of some muscles which are undoubtedly key to the complex equilibrium of an athletic action. During movement, muscle fibres undergo a change in length and this inevitably alters their position in relation to the arrangement of electrodes placed on the skin. Furthermore, most muscles do not have fibres arranged longitudinally between the point of origin and the point of insertion; they are arranged obliquely (pennate muscles), and their arrangement alters further during contraction. It should be kept in mind that a solid, consistent evaluation of the forces generated by a muscle (Marchetti, 1996) cannot disregard variables that may influence athletic performance (such as ground conditions, the equipment used, the impact during the athletic movement, etc.). These factors require the investigator to reproduce conditions as close as possible to actual conditions in the study environment.

A standardization study of EMG is vital in the light of all these phenomena, and in its absence these methods do not yield objective data useful for research, nor do they contribute to the development of the practical application of the method. The European Union has just recently promoted efforts aimed at clarifying applications, making it possible to efficiently exchange data and knowledge on the analysis of movement and on the evaluation of neuromuscular disorders, owing to the combined work of experts from 16 European countries. This concerted action, named the surface electromyography for non invasive assessment of muscles project (SENIAM Project), was completed in 1999, after three years of work, and resulted in the a number of basic recommendations, such as:

— sensors and procedures for sensor positioning;
— methods of recording and acquiring the SEMG (Surface EMG) signal;
— models for the simulation and interpretation of signals; and
— a system for reporting data relating to studies based on the electromyographic signal.

Practical applications in surface electromyography: literature review

What the clinician should infer from this interdisciplinary tool is a more analytical and objective method of working, which uses data from neurophysiology, from acquiring the EMG signal, from muscle activation mechanisms, and from studies of neuromuscular coordination, compensation mechanisms of muscles adjacent to the joint studied and fatigue in relation to the application of increasing loads, as part of the rehabilitation process. It will then be possible, on this basis and in the light of a knowledge of anatomy and biomechanics and of the specific nature of the athletic action, to create a specific treatment plan for each athlete and for different lesions, based not only on the traditional association between symptom and cure, but also on an understanding of the physiological signals and mechanisms, also known as 'signal understanding'.

Physiological studies

An understanding of the real applications of surface EMG, considering what it can show and its limits, provides rehabilitation therapists with an objective evaluation tool as well as an opportunity for collaboration between bioengineering centres and research clinics, already available in countries which are more advanced in this sector.

Olympic disciplines such as swimming, cycling, running and skiing have frequently been considered in electromyographic studies; minor sports, however, feature only in isolated reports.

A detailed evaluation of basic physiological and pathophysiological studies can nevertheless provide excellent starting points for understanding some of the phenomena occurring during training, including muscle fatigue, a key factor in the damage caused by overtraining. One of the limitations of this approach is undoubtedly the fact that studies with high scientific validity are conducted in isometric contraction, which is not the case in athletic actions (Marchetti, 1996). But it does constitute a form of bench test such as that used on an engine before and after a race, to measure variables that cannot be observed during the race itself.

It is not therefore immediately obvious what benefit clinicians can gain from surface EMG studies, since the method does not currently allow measurements that can be directly related to practice. Yet the use of this method can provide a more detailed knowledge of the neurophysiological mechanisms involved under given conditions and, on this basis, and supported by the clinical rationale, can help to plan the best treatment or the best training programme.

The literature contains some useful papers in this respect; some of them will be referred to below, with the aim of providing practical starting points.

The activation of agonist and antagonist muscles during athletic actions can be mentioned as a first example. It seems that even during an athletic performance at the highest level, some, though very little, antagonist muscle activity persists simultaneously with agonist activity. This phenomenon is interpreted as a function of the central nervous system (CNS) which preserves joint congruity by activating the Golgi receptors.

Kyrolainen and Komi (1994) conducted a study of the stretch reflex with the aim of evaluating the difference in reflex response following mechanical stimulation in rapid elongation in power- and endurance-trained athletes. The muscles evaluated were the soleus, the gastrocnemii and the anterior tibial. The subjects were asked to sit with both feet supported on a platform, the axis of which was aligned with the axis of rotation of the tibiotarsal joint. Thirteen different stimuli were delivered with varying angular amplitudes, at different velocities. The movement amplitudes and latency times of the reflexes were then evaluated. The results showed that endurance athletes were more sensitive to stretch and had a faster monosynaptic response recovery time than power athletes, in other words the motor response needed a smaller interval between one stimulus and the next. The possible explanations considered by the authors were related to differences in musculotendinous properties, neural structures or properties of the neuromuscular spindles. In fact endurance athletes have a high percentage of slow twitch muscle fibres which have a lower threshold and are therefore recruited before fast twitch muscle fibres, characteristic of power athletes. The endurance fibres were, in fact, spontaneously active and were recruited more readily with stretching. The question remains to be answered, however, of how much the various training programmes used previously may have had an impact on reflex recruitment.

A further interesting aspect is how the CNS controls the intensity of activation/deactivation of the motor units of the same muscle, differentiating several anatomical segments with a variety of force vectors. This 'functional differentiation' is explained by Wickham and Brown (1998), who identified seven segments in the deltoid in a cadaver dissection study and named them D1, D2, D3, D4, D5, D6 and D7, going from the most anterior to the most posterior (Fig. 20.1). Only one of these segments, D3, inserted into the deltoid tuberosity; the insertion of the others

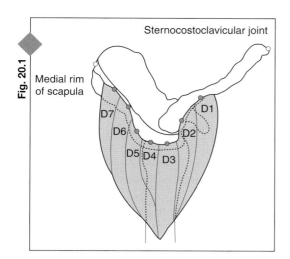

Fig. 20.1

Sternocostoclavicular joint

Medial rim of scapula

D7 D6 D5 D4 D3 D2 D1

The origin of the seven segments of the deltoid. It should be noted that segments D1 and D2 have a predominantly clavicular origin, segments D3 and D4 have an acromial origin and segments D5-D7 take origin from the spine of the scapula.

finds that some motor units carry out synergic work, others stabilization work and still others antagonistic action.

The phenomenon of functional differentiation is also analysed by a study on the upper trapezius conducted by Jensen (1997), which identified various compartments inside the muscle, each of which was activated independently of the others.

In the complex dynamics of the elevation of the humerus, the well-known scapulohumeral rhythm in which the stabilizers-rotators of the scapula have a key role should also be taken into consideration (Lear, 1998). In this respect, Bagg (1986) evaluates the behaviour of the upper, middle and lower trapezius and the anterior serratus during elevation movement in the scapular plane (Fig. 20.2).

The activity of the upper trapezius increases from the first degrees of elevation, and then reaches a constant plateau between 90° and 120°; beyond this level, the activity of the muscle increases gradually, reaching a maximum peak at the end of elevation. The important finding is obtained from the intermediate phase, in which the increase in force is reduced: Bagg noted interindividual variability in this phase.

The activity of the middle trapezius has proved to be variable in each of the phases studied; the increase in force is demonstrated after 100°; this suggests that although the middle trapezius fibres do not have a rotatory function because of their arrangement, they do have an important stabilizing function.

The lower trapezius has been found to have a low EMG signal amplitude up to about 90°, beyond which the signal shows a rapid increase in amplitude (see Fig. 20.2).

The activity of the anterior serratus increases gradually until the start of abduction, plateaus around 90° and then increases beyond this level. All four muscles examined showed a plateau phase.

The conclusions were that the activity of each muscle was closely related to the migration of the rotation centre, which moves during abduction in the direction of the AC joint. This would explain why the lower trapezius, for example, increases its own activity only beyond 90° at which point the work of its fibres becomes more advantageous.

The activity of the scapular rotators during abduction of the arm shows that the upper trapezius, the anterior serratus and the lower trapezius have an important rotatory function in the intermediate phase of elevation. The lower trapezius, whose activity undergoes a rapid increase at around halfway through the elevation, has the most important role as regards the mechanical advantage at which it finds itself,

was more proximal or more anterior, generating different force vectors depending on the position of the limb. The authors then conducted surface electromyography on eighteen healthy volunteers to evaluate activation time, duration, intensity of contraction (% MVC) and maximal force peak. The volunteers, in a seated position with the upper limb placed in a load cell at 40° abduction in the plane of the scapula, had to perform, after a period of familiarization with the task required, fifteen isometric contractions in abduction and fifteen isometric contractions in adduction, with two load cells placed over and under the arm, respectively. The results showed that, during abduction, segments D2 and D3 contributed initially to the increase in force, followed by D1, D4 and D5, while segment D6 had a stabilization function and D7 actually had an antagonist function. The authors also identified that segments D6 and D7 had an adductor function, though of brief duration. In this study, the authors have emphasized the importance of identifying the functional units inside a muscle, and thus go beyond the traditional description which attributes a single function, or in some cases a principal and accessory function, to each muscle. What the authors wanted to demonstrate is clearly described as regards the posterior deltoid, which is normally identified as producing extension, abduction and external rotation; this paper analyses it in greater detail, and

Fig. 20.2

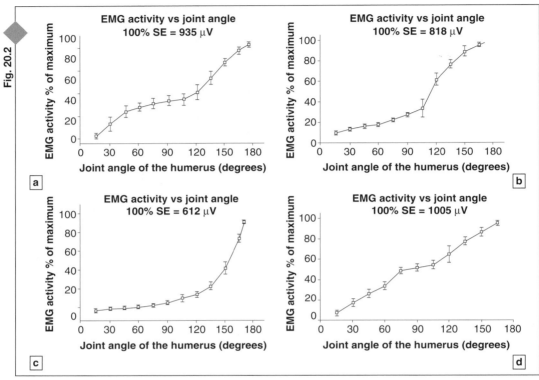

(a) Activity of the upper trapezius: the plateau phase occurs between 45° and 105° of elevation of the arm (subject no. 13);
(b) activity of the middle trapezius: the plateau phase occurs at 15° and 105° of elevation of the arm (subject no. 15); (c) activity of
the lower trapezius: the activity is minimal until the arm is elevated at 90°. A plateau phase is observed between 30° and 90°
(subject no. 18); (d) activity of the anterior serratus: a short plateau phase is evident between 75° and 105° of elevation of the arm
(subject no. 18).

increasing the rotatory forces which are already active. The fibres of the upper trapezius, on the other hand, lose their role of scapular rotators as they become progressively closer to the AC joint, principally maintaining the function of scapula elevation.

Shoulder disorder studies

Impingement

The conservative treatment of shoulder impingement often includes exercise programmes aimed at recovering a normal movement pattern. One of the aetiological factors of impingement is related to abnormal kinematics of the shoulder. EMG then becomes useful for studying the alternating kinematic pattern, although according to some authors (Ludewig, 2000), there is no scientific evidence for an alternating kinematic movement/abnormal EMG in patients with impingement.

The kinematic changes that happen in shoulder impingement include movements that bring the greater tuberosity of the humerus closer to the acromioclavicular arch (Reddy, 2000). During elevation of the shoulder, in particular, the following conditions apply:

— excessive anterior or superior translation of the humeral head on the glenoid fossa;
— inadequate external rotation of the humerus;
— decreased superior scapular rotation; and
— posterior tipping (rotation around a mediolateral axis) of the scapula on the chest.

Other kinematic modifications of the scapular movement are often related to a reduction in the muscle activity of the anterior serratus and an increase in the muscle activity of the upper part of the trapezius; these factors disturb the balance between the force of the upper and lower stabilizers of the scapula, as will be explained below.

EMG studies performed according to the scapulothoracic pattern are often not sufficiently specific

Fig. 20.3

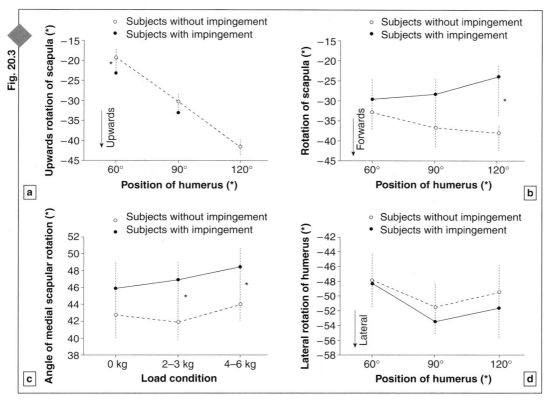

Summary of the kinematic data: **(a)** upper rotation of the scapula (phase x group interaction) (* = groups significantly different with humerus at 60°; F statistic; df = 1.50; P < 0.025; n = 52); **(b)** scapular tipping (phase x group interaction) (* = groups significantly different with humerus at 120°; F statistic; df = 1.50; n = 52); **(c)** medial scapular rotation (group × load interaction) (F statistic; df = 1.50; n = 52) (* = groups significantly different under load conditions with 2.3 kg and 4.6 kg; **(d)** external rotation of the humerus (group effects).

for diagnosis of the patient, or are limited to analysis of a specific sport (Reddy, 2000). Ludewig and Cook (2000) studied the kinematics of the shoulder and the associated muscle activity in fifty-two patients with symptoms of impingement, in comparison with an asymptomatic control group, performing an activity that required elevation movements of the upper limb. EMG analysis detected the activity of the upper and lower trapezius muscle and the anterior serratus, while electromagnetic sensors recorded the three-dimensional movements of the trunk, scapula and humerus during elevation of the limb in the scapular plane, under three conditions: without weight, with a 2.3 kg weight, and with a 4.6 kg weight (the weight was applied at the wrist). The movement phases were divided into: 31–60°, 61–90° and 91–120°.

The results showed that the group with impingement reported a decrease in upper scapular rotation in the first of the three phases, an increase in anterior tipping of the scapula at the end of the third phase and an increase in medial rotation under all three conditions with an increased load. At the same time, electromyographic activity increased for the upper and lower part of the trapezius in the group with impingement at the end of the second phase, although the increase for the upper trapezius was apparently limited to work with 4.6 kg. A reduction was noted in the activity of the anterior serratus during movements with weight in the various phases of movement (Figs. 20.3, 20.4).

Reddy (2000) concludes by emphasizing the importance of scapular tipping and the function of the anterior serratus muscle in rehabilitation of shoulder impingement.

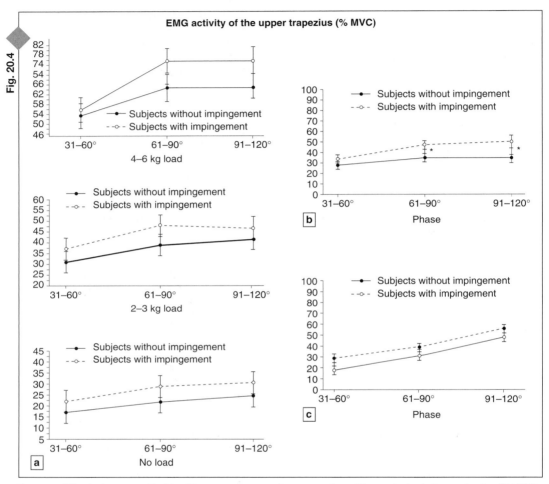

Fig. 20.4

Summary of the electromyographic data of the groups (expressed as a percentage of the maximal voluntary contraction [% MVC]): **(a)** upper trapezius, effects for each load condition (* = groups significantly different in phases 61–90° and 91–120°; F statistic; df = 1.50; n = 52); **(b)** lower trapezius muscle, phase by group interaction (* = groups significantly different in the 61–90° and 91–120° phases (F statistic; df = 1.50; n = 52); **(c)** anterior serratus (group effects). Note the variations in scale between the graphs.

Reddy (2000) analysed the needle EMG activity of the deltoid and rotator cuff muscles in fifteen patients with subacromial impingement, during scapular abduction movement between 30° and 120° in the scapular plane, in comparison with healthy volunteers. The study demonstrated less electromyographic activity for the deltoid and rotator cuff than in the healthy volunteers, in particular during the first phase of elevation.

According to the author, normal muscle activation of the shoulder in the muscles described is characterized by synchronous action. The gradual increase in

the EMG activity of the deltoid may indicate that this muscle uses progressive force to elevate the arm, while the consistently high levels of activity of the supraspinatus maintain glenohumeral stability throughout the arc of movement.

Shoulder instability

EMG is often used in shoulder instability as a tool for the specific study of muscle activity in this disorder, owing to the importance of certain muscles in the rehabilitation phase. The muscles considered responsible for glenohumeral stability are the rotator cuff and the stabilizing muscles of the scapula.

There are various electromyographic techniques for taking these measurements; many studies use needle EMG in particular since it allows signals to be obtained without movement artefacts caused by other muscles or interference, as with the subscapularis which cannot be reached by surface EMG.

The aim of these studies was to identify the mode of activation of the muscles located around the shoulder and the humerus, during different movements chosen by the authors, in patients considered to have reduced shoulder stability.

Kronberg (1991) reported that muscle activity in healthy individuals happened simultaneously, in both agonist and antagonist muscles, emphasizing that coordinated muscle contraction is fundamental to shoulder stability during its movement. According to the author, alternating muscle activity in patients with shoulder instability also helps to understand the mechanism of instability and to devise an appropriate rehabilitation programme for these patients. In a comparison of the results of muscle activation in throwers with shoulder instability with those of healthy volunteers, Glousman (1988) similarly maintains that rehabilitation programmes can help to reduce instability. McMahon (1996) showed that the EMG activity of the anterior serratus was reduced in patients with shoulder instability during elevation in the scapular plane and flexion, compared to healthy volunteers. According to the study, this aspect indicates an abnormality in the coordinated rotation of the scapula on the thorax, and therefore impairment of the scapulothoracic rhythm, since the muscle is also an important rotator of the scapula and contributes to its rotation in the initial phase of elevation in the scapular plane and flexion. The study by Glousman (1988) also showed a reduction in EMG activity in the anterior serratus in throwers with shoulder instability in the three phases of throwing, compared to normal individuals. Kronberg (1991) found a reduction (in a study admittedly consisting of only six subjects) in EMG activity in the anterior and middle parts of the deltoid muscle, whereas the activity of the subscapularis was significantly increased in internal rotation at 45° with the arm abducted. This increase in activity could be explained, according to the author, by an increased muscle fibre length at rest in patients with generalized shoulder laxity, or by a reduction in muscle strength. The studies conclude that muscle strengthening, proprioception and coordination, in the rehabilitation of the muscles named, are crucial to the prevention

of shoulder instability (Kronberg, 1991; Glousman, 1988).

Applications in physiotherapy

A complete knowledge of the kinematics of the normal and pathological shoulder forms the basis for developing training and rehabilitation strategies (Glousman, 1993).

Various studies (Fujisawa, 1998; McCann, 1993) have used needle EMG to obtain more specific information, particularly on the deeper muscles; others have used surface EMG and still others dynamic EMG.

Dynamic EMG, along with movement analysis, has improved understanding of biomechanics during athletic activities and rehabilitation protocols (Bradley, 1991). Surface EMG is an excellent aid during rehabilitation, since it is a non-invasive tool for the evaluation of improvements and of normal and abnormal activation patterns. A better knowledge of studies conducted with EMG has helped to increase the basic knowledge of physiotherapists, and to support the clinical evaluation and consequently the evaluation of treatment efficacy (Bradley, 1991). EMG has been used, in the various studies of shoulder physiotherapy conducted, to analyse the following:

— the scapular muscles in a shoulder rehabilitation programme (Moseley, 1992; Decker, 1999);
— electromyographic activity, with weight applied during rehabilitation exercises, using elastic resistance in six exercises. The exercises were: internal rotation, external rotation, straight fist, and rowing with arms wide, intermediate and together. The maximum load peaks for all the exercises were between 21 and 54 N; the authors conclude that these exercises are indicated in post-traumatic lesions and in postoperative patients (Hintermeister, 1998);
— the electromyographic activity of the rotator cuff during passive shoulder exercises after surgery. The results of the study suggest that passive and physiotherapist-assisted movements, and Codman's (pendulum) exercise did not differ significantly from those obtained with CPM (Continuous Passive Movement), and that both CPM and passive physiotherapist-assisted movements increase passive articular function, without damaging cuff reconstruction (Dockery, 1998);
— electromyographic activity during isometric shoulder exercises in and out of water. The muscles considered were the supraspinatus, the

infraspinatus, the subscapularis, the pectoralis major (clavicular part and costal part), the deltoid (anterior, middle and posterior) and the latissimus dorsi. The electrodes used were intramuscular wires 0.05 mm in diameter for the supraspinatus and infraspinatus; needle electrodes were used for the deeper subscapularis muscle, inserted from the medial rim of the scapula; AG-AgCI surface electrodes were used for the pectoralis major, the deltoid and the latissimus dorsi. During this study, a protective water-repellent film was placed over the electrodes to prevent them coming into contact with the water. The exercises used were: flexion and abduction of the shoulder at 30°, 60° and 90°, and three rotation positions with the arm at the side, at 0°. Electromyographic activity was significantly reduced for the supraspinatus with the arm abducted at 90° in water (3.9%, manual muscle test (MMT)) and out of water (22.3% MMT). These results provide valuable information on the safety of exercises in water during rehabilitation after shoulder surgery, such as rotator cuff reconstruction. External rotation exercises are not recommended after reconstruction of the infraspinatus, either in or out of water (Fujisawa, 1998); and

— electromyographic activity during rehabilitation exercises in three phases as described by Neer (McCann, 1993). This study demonstrated that EMG may be clinically useful to confirm the gradual nature of exercises during rehabilitation. Passive exercises cause minimal EMG activity and can thus be introduced early postoperatively. Active exercises and exercises against resistance have shown a higher level of electromyographic activity for the rotator cuff and for the deltoid muscle, and are thus indicated at a later stage.

A further example of the use of EMG in physiotherapy has been described by Palmerud (1995), who analysed the distribution of muscle activity in four shoulder muscles (supraspinatus, infraspinatus, anterior and middle parts of the deltoid and upper trapezius). The aim of the study was to evaluate:

— the ability of a subject to reduce voluntarily the activity of certain muscles using EMG feedback, maintaining given positions;
— whether the reduction in the activity of a muscle coincided with an increase in the activity of other muscles;
— whether there was interindividual variability; and
— whether trapezius activity could be determined objectively as a means of describing the total load applied to the shoulder.

The study was conducted in six right-handed women without shoulder pain, using a needle electromyography technique. The subjects were asked to sit comfortably on a chair, with a monitor positioned in front providing visual feedback which the subject had to minimize as much as possible, without altering the position of the arm which was kept in abduction in the scapular plane; they were asked to perform the task at different joint angles. There was a recovery period of two minutes between tests. The study was divided into two parts: the first measured the activity of the supraspinatus, the middle deltoid and the upper trapezius at 30°, 60° and 90° abduction in the scapular plane with the elbow extended; the second part monitored the supraspinatus, the infraspinatus, the anterior deltoid, the middle deltoid and the upper trapezius at 30° abduction in the scapular plane with the elbow flexed at 90°. The results showed that:

— it is possible to reduce EMG activity voluntarily without altering the load or position of the arm, but only in the upper trapezius. This result was found in all the positions and in all the tests. The opposite effect was found in the infraspinatus and the deltoid, which actually demonstrated increased activity. The results for the supraspinatus showed no significant variations in activity;
— there is no significant evidence of a transfer of loads to other shoulder muscles;
— the results were not conclusive as regards identifying interindividual variability, since all the subjects had the ability to reduce the activity of the trapezius, but at different levels; and
— the activity of the trapezius cannot be directly related to the total load on the shoulder.

Studies in specific sports

The mechanics of the shoulder during athletic actions have been evaluated dynamically using needle EMG so that an optimal rehabilitation programme can be devised (Glousman, 1993; Pink, 1991).

Dynamic EMG and analysis on high-speed film are used to evaluate the shoulder during throwing sports and swimming, tennis and golf, to identify the damaging mechanism and to plan the correct treatment and prevention programme. Evaluation of the shoulder function in these sports has shown that the rotator cuff is the structure which must be considered particularly in all sports, although the emphasis and role of individual muscles differ (Clarys, 1993). The clinical observation of common shoulder injuries in athletes has revealed selective muscle weakness of the rotator cuff rather than impairment of the muscles. Let us look at a few examples.

Swimming

Pink M (1991) has described the pattern of activation in 12 muscles of the normal shoulder in 12 freestyle swimmers, using needle EMG. The freestyle movement was divided into 4 phases:
— early recovery;
— late recovery;
— early push; and
— late push.

The muscle pattern during freestyle swimming was similar during the entry and exit phases of the hand in the water. The upper trapezius and rhomboids performed a complementary action: the trapezius caused the scapula to rotate upwards, while the rhomboids pulled it back. The three parts of the deltoid and the supraspinatus worked in synchrony to position the arm in the entry and exit phases of the hand in the water. The pectoralis major together with the latissimus dorsi, the anterior serratus and the teres minor were activated in the propulsive phase of the stroke. An interesting finding was that both the subscapularis and the anterior serratus were activated throughout the arc of the stroke (approximately 20% of MMT) and were more exposed to muscle fatigue. Pink (1993a) evaluated the normal shoulder during butterfly stroke. The movement was divided into the same four phases, with results similar to those reported in the previous study.

Pink (1993b) conducted a study in swimmers with shoulder pain (10% of whom had a diagnosis of impingement), demonstrating that during the entry of the hand in the water in butterfly, the posterior deltoid, upper trapezius and anterior serratus muscles act simultaneously to position the humerus and the scapula for a wider entry of the arm in the water. This reduces the impingement between the supraspinatus and the coracoacromial arch. It has also been demonstrated that the anterior serratus and the teres minor do not intervene, in individuals with shoulder pain, to preserve the stability of the scapula and the balance of humeral rotation.

Tennis

Turning to tennis, many players suffer injuries caused by repetitive high forces generated around the shoulder, during the basic strokes of the game. Service, forehand and backhand were evaluated using dynamic

EMG and high-speed film in the supraspinatus, infraspinatus, subscapularis, middle deltoid, pectoralis major, latissimus dorsi, biceps brachii and anterior serratus muscles. The greatest activity during the service and forehand was recorded in the subscapularis, pectoralis major and anterior serratus. A high level of activity was recorded in the anterior serratus which helped to provide a stable platform for the humeral head and assisted glenohumeral and scapulothoracic synchrony. Greater activity was recorded during the acceleration and follow-through phases of the backhand in the middle deltoid, supraspinatus and infraspinatus muscles (Ryu, 1988).

Golf

The most studied movement in golf is the swing. Golf does not require an intensive arm movement, but the swing is a rapid movement in which the rotator cuff has to work in synchrony in order to be able to protect the glenohumeral complex (Pink, 1990). The swing, studied using needle EMG in 13 professional golfers, has been divided into 5 phases:
— take away;
— forward swing;
— acceleration;
— early follow through; and
— late follow through.

Of the eight muscles studied, the infraspinatus and the supraspinatus were more active at the extreme limits of the movement of the shoulder, with 27% and 25% of the MMT, respectively, while the figures were 68% and 93% of the MMT for the subscapularis and the pectoralis major during the acceleration phase. The greatest activity for the latissimus dorsi was recorded during the forward swing (50% MMT), while this happened for the anterior deltoid during the forward swing and the follow through (differences not significant). These results agree with those of Jobe's study (1986).

Bibliography

Bagg S.D., Forrest W., 'Electromyographic study of the scapular rotators during arm abduction in the scapular plane', *Am. J. Phys. Med.* 65(3): 111–124, (1986)

Bradley J.P., Tibone J.E., 'Electromyographic analysis of muscle action about the shoulder', *Clin. Sports Med.* 10(4): 789–805, (1991)

Clarys J.P., Cabri J., 'Electromyography and the study of sport movements', *A review. J. Sport. Sci.* 11: 379–448, (1993)

Clarys JP., 'Electromyography in sports and occupational settings: an update of its limits and possibilities', *Ergonomics* 43(10): 1750–1762, (2000)

Practical applications in surface electromyography: literature review

Decker M.J., Hintermeister R.A., Faber K.J., Hawkins R.J., 'Serratus anterior muscle activity during selected rehabilitation exercise', *Am. J. Sports Med.* 27(6): 784–791, (1999)

Dockery M.L., Wright T.W., Lastayo P.C., 'Electromyography of the shoulder: an analysis of passive modes of exercise', *Orthopedics* 21(11): 1181–1184, (1998)

Fujisawa H., Suenaga N., Minami, 'A. Electromyographic study during isometric exercise of the shoulder in head-out water immersion', *J. Shoulder Elbow Surg.* 5(7): 491–494, (1998)

Glousman R., Jobe F., Tibone J. et al., 'Dynamic electromyographic analysis of the throwing shoulder with glenohumeral instability', *Jour. Bone Joint Surg.* 2(70-A): 220–226, (1988)

Glousman R., 'Electromyographic analysis and its role in the athletic shoulder', *Clin. Orthop.* (288): 27–34, (1993)

Hermens H.J., Freriks B., Merletti R. et al., 'Raccomandazioni Europee per l'Elettromiografia di Superficie – I risultati del progetto SENIAM', Ed. Clut, Turin, (2000)

Hintermeister R.A., Lange G.W., Schultheis J.M., 'Electromyographic activity and applied load during shoulder rehabilitation exercises using elastic resistance', *Am. J. Sports. Med.* 26(2): 210–212, (1998)

Jensen C., Westgaard R.H., 'Functional subdivision of the upper trapezius muscle during low-level activation', *Eur. J. Appl. Physiol.* 76: 335–339

Jobe F.W., Moynes D.R., Antonelli D.J., 'Rotator cuff function during a golf swing', *Am. J. Sports Med.* 14(5): 388–392, (1986)

Kronberg M., Broström L.Å., Németh G., 'Differences in shoulder muscle activity between patients with generalized joint laxity and normal controls', *Clin. Orthop. Related Res.* 269: 181–192, (1991)

Kyrolainen H., Komi P.V., 'Stretch reflex responses following mechanical stimulation in power- and endurance-trained athletes', *Int. J. Sports. Med.* 15: 290–294, (1994)

Lear L.J., Gross M.T., 'An electromyographical analysis of the scapular stabilizing synergists during a push-up progression', *JOSPT* 28(3): 146–157, (1998)

Ludewig P.M., Cook T.M., 'Alternations in shoulder kinematics and associated muscle activity in people with symptoms of shoulder impingement', *Phys. Ther.* 3(80): 276–290, (2000)

Marchetti M., Felici F., 'Surface electromyography and sport. European activities on surface electromyography, Proceedings of the first general SENIAM workshop', Turin (1996)

McCann P.D., Wotten M.E., Kadaba M.P. et al., 'A kinematic and electromyographic study of shoulder rehabilitation exercises', *Clin. Orthop.* 288: 179–188, (1993)

McMahon P.J., Jobe F.W., Pink M. et al., 'Comparative electromyographic analysis of shoulder muscles during planar motions: anterior glenohumeral instability versus normal', *J. Shoulder Elbow Surg* 2(5): 118–123, (1996)

Moseley J.B. JR, Jobe F.W., Pink M. et al., 'EMG analysis of the scapular muscles during a shoulder rehabilitation program', *Am. J. Sports. Med.* 20(2): 128–134, (1992)

Palmerud G., Kadefors R., Sporrong H. et al., 'Voluntary redistribution of muscle activity in human shoulder muscles', *Ergonomics* 4(38): 806–815, (1995)

Pink M., Jobe F.W., Perry J., 'Electromyographic analysis of the shoulder during the golf swing', *Am. J. Sports Med.* 18(2): 137–140, (1990)

Pink M., Perry J., Browne A. et al., 'The normal shoulder during freestyle swimming. An electromyographic and cinematographic analysis of twelve muscles', *Am. Jour. Sport Med.* 6(19): 569–576, (1991)

Pink M., Jobe F.W., Perry J., 'The normal shoulder during the butterfly swim stroke. An electromyographic and cinematographic analysis of twelve muscles', *Clin Orthop. Mar.* (288): 48–59, (1993a)

Pink M., Jobe F.W., Perry J., 'The painful shoulder during the butterfly stroke: an electromyographic and cinematographic analysis of twelve muscles', *Clin. Orth. Rel. Re.* 288: 60–72, (1993b)

Reddy A.S., Mohr K.J., Pink M.M., Jobe F.W., 'Electromyographic analysis of the deltoid and rotator cuff muscles in persons with subacromial impingement', *J. Shoulder Elbow Surg.* 6(9): 519–523, (2000)

Ryu R.K., McCormick J., Jobe F.W., 'An electromyographic analysis of shoulder function in tennis players', *Am. J. Sports. Med.* 5(16): 481–485, (1988)

Wickham J.B., Brown J.M.M., 'Muscles within muscles: the neuromotor control of intra-muscular segments', *Eur. J. Appl. Physiol.* 78: 219–225, (1998)

Glossary

Acceleration phase
Central phase of throwing; for the upper limb this consists of extension, passing from external to internal rotation; the structures involved follow a proximal to distal recruitment pattern: pelvis, trunk, shoulder, forearm, hand.

Agonist
Muscle which exerts the action specific to it, i.e. the action which in functional anatomy is its specific function.

Antagonist
Muscle which acts in opposition to the movement of the agonist. It has a dual action: it regulates the intensity and velocity of the agonist movement and then slows the same movement; the functionally most important roles are coordination of movement and prevention of excessive width of joint movement which may result in damage to the joint or soft tissues (muscles, tendons, ligaments, connective tissue and skin).

Arousal
Activation – or increased activation – of the central nervous system; defined as specific or non-specific. Specific arousal is when the stimulus is consistent with the response, whereas non-specific arousal is when the response is not proportional to or consistent with the stimulus, as in the case of chronic pain.

As regards intentional movement, a distinction can be drawn between slow (tonic) and fast (phasic) activation. Specific activation allows the motor task to be performed, whereas everything that is not contributing to this is inhibited. Non-specific activation may correspond to excess activation, resulting in lack of motor coordination (e.g. in fatigue).

Arthrokinematics
Study of the movement of body segments from the point of view of trajectories, and relative positions and variations of these, regardless of the causes.

Arthrokinetics
Study of the movement of body segments from the point of view of the forces that cause or limit it.

Ballistic
This refers to throwing sports involving rapid, relatively stereotyped movement, characterized by large amplitude and considerable potential energy (throwing the javelin, discus or hammer, volleyball, water polo, etc.).

CKC (closed kinetic chain)
Combination of several joints in succession, forming a complex motor unit, in which the distal segment meets an obstruction of considerable resistance which limits the movement of the whole kinetic chain.

Closed skill
Describes sports characterized by repeating as precisely as possible a known, automatic movement (e.g. archery).

Cocking phase
A phase of throwing, consisting of extension and posterior rotation of the trunk and upper limb, to achieve the space and energy accumulation (see Compliance) for the acceleration phase. For the upper limb in particular, the shoulder is abducted, extended and externally rotated, the scapula adducted and rotated, and the thoracic and cervical spine undergoes extension and rotation. Biomechanical studies identify the last part of this phase as Late-cocking, which is particularly significant because of the intensity of the forces working on the glenohumeral joint.

Co-contraction
Simultaneous (synergic) contraction of agonist and antagonist muscles mainly to stabilize a body segment.

Compliance
Characteristic of the myotendinous unit being sufficiently elastic to store and return a large quantity of elastic energy.

Concentric – muscle contraction (types of)
Contraction that shortens muscle fibres (agonists). This contraction is incorrectly called isotonic (with constant muscle tone), since there are actually variations in tone (heterotonia); when an increase in tone occurs, this is called auxotonic contraction.

Coordination
Ability to achieve, in a harmonious and measured manner, complex movements that involve the simultaneous and synchronous contraction of several muscle groups with agonist, antagonist and synergic action.

Degrees of freedom
All movements permitted by each specific joint, i.e. two for each body plane in which movement is possible.

DOMS
Delayed Onset Muscular Soreness.

Eccentric – Muscle contraction (types of)
Muscle contraction during which the agonist muscle fibres are lengthened. It often corresponds to a braking

Glossary

action on a load, which may be submaximal, maximal (corresponding to maximum isometric force) or supramaximal; the corresponding movement is also known as yielding.

Factors predisposing to disease or risk factors

Combination of elements that can cause a disease to occur; they may be intrinsic or extrinsic, related to the individual or to the context. The presence of a single risk factor in an athlete is rarely sufficient to cause a disease to occur.

Feedback

The return of some of the responses of a system acting as a stimulus; it may be negative (inhibitory) or positive (inductive). In a motor or functional context, it can be applied to a single movement or to a chain of movements, made following a motor action or a particular previous sense and sensory stimulus, to allow the motor action itself to take place and any corrections necessary to be made following modifications of the external and internal environment.

Feedforward

In a motor or functional context, it can be applied to a motor programme, acquired with experience by the CNS, which is sufficient to decide on and perform an action, without peripheral information.

Follow-through phase

Last phase of throwing, in which the whole movement arc is completed. For the upper limb this involves concluding the extension, adduction and internal rotation carried out from the cocking position; this is the phase of antagonist action by the muscle chains.

Grinding

Joint noise perceptible during assessment.

Impairment

According to the ICF concept, this comprises various aspects connected to the disorder; examples of impairment are change in ROM, change in coordination, instability, pain, changes in balance, anxiety and depression.

Impingement

Typical disorder of the shoulder. Three main types of impingement are recognized: subacromial, subcoracoid and posterosuperior or internal.

Isometric – muscle contraction (types of)

Muscle contraction characteristic of static exercise, in which the muscle or muscle chain, owing to a condition of constant length or minimal shortening, opposes resistance not superior to its maximum strength.

Late-cocking

See Cocking phase

Load/carriability

Concept proposed by the multidimensional load/carriability model, included in the ICF; it considers the general response (of the individual) and local response (of a body structure) to environmental stresses. Evaluating load (e.g. quality and quantity of training) can provide crucial information for proposing diagnoses and prognoses and for the therapeutic approach.

Mid-range

Intermediate joint position in relation to the total amplitude of movement possible.

Motor end plate

Nerve ending in the innervated nerve fibre.

Motor reaction time

Start of neuromuscular activity detectable on the EMG but not yet visible as the start of movement.

Motor unit (MU)

Functional unit of the neuromuscular system. It consists of a complex of structures formed by the alpha motor neuron, its axon, the motor end plate and the innervated muscle fibres.

Muscle tone

Active tension of a reflex nature which depends largely on the myotactic stretching reflex.

Muscle stiffness

Level of resistance of muscle fibres following the lengthening of muscle as a result of its intrinsic viscoelastic properties, independent of nerve activity. The adjective stiff may be used with a negative meaning in current usage in medical literature, corresponding to 'not stretchable'.

Neuromotor

Relating to neurological aspects (afference and efference) of motricity; these can include the ideomotor aspect, i.e. the ability of the CNS to devise a motor programme.

Neuromuscular

Relating to the nervous and muscular systems, i.e. the connection between the CNS and the effector muscle (concept of coordination) and vice versa (concepts of kinesthesia, bathyesthesia and proprioception).

OKC (open kinetic chain)

Combination of several joints which work together functionally, forming a complex unit in which the distal segment moves freely without external resistance (no obstruction).

Open skill
Sports in which the quantity and origin of information to be processed vary and the action is not repetitive (e.g. team games).

Outcome
Result, i.e. objective of treatment, to be identified during evaluation, in relation to the prognostic health profile (PHP). It is a form of mediation between the need to use an objective indicator for the therapist and the patient's expectations; one or more measurable outcomes are advisable as indicators of the efficacy of the therapy.

Overstrain
Excessive strain in terms of intensity or quality, including a single strain, beyond the carriability of the structure, since it is not physiologically anticipated (e.g. excessive traction); particularly with reference to the joint (e.g. throwing at increased acceleration or with increased loads).

Overuse
Excessive strain in terms of quantity, repeated to a point beyond the carriability of the joint in question; it is usually caused by a repetitive action tending to be stereotyped (e.g. freestyle swimming).

Pattern of activation
Recruitment or modality of activation in sequence of several motor units.

Periodization (of training)
Division in time of work rates necessary for the physical and athletic preparation of an athlete to achieve a performance or series of performances for a planned deadline; the most frequent periodizations are yearly or four-yearly.

Plyometric
(From the Greek pleion = more and metron = measure) muscle exercise which uses the stretch-shortening cycle, consisting of eccentric pretensioning of the first agonist muscle (or muscle group), followed immediately by the explosive concentric contraction of the same muscle.

Popping or clicking
Joint noise perceptible during evaluation.

Premotor or cognitive reaction time
Precedes reaction time.

Programming (of training)
Organization and tailoring of objectives and methods necessary for the physical and athletic preparation of an athlete.

Range of motion (ROM)
Of a joint usually expressed in degrees; the internal ROM is understood to be an arc of movement less than the resting length of the principal agonist muscles of the same movement; external ROM is understood to be an arc of movement greater than the resting length of the principal agonist muscles of the same movement.

Rapidity
See Velocity.

Reaction time
Interval between the nerve stimulus and the start of the motor response.

Scaption
Scapular plane, i.e. the plane tangential to the scapula.

Scapulohumeral rhythm
Functional characteristic of the shoulder joint, in which movements of the humerus are accompanied, in a fixed sequence, by movements of the scapula and clavicle.

Slack
Resting state of soft tissues, capable of being subjected to mechanical stress; capsular slack is eliminated during the evaluation of joint structures by passive mobilization, providing information on joint function.

Staleness syndrome – Overtraining syndrome
The result of prolonging a state of overreaching which alters the body's neuroimmunoendocrine response.

Strain
Excessive or inappropriate strain on a functional structure (see Overstrain)

Velocity
Ratio between the movement of a body in space and the time taken to travel the distance.

Viscosity
Passive resistance intrinsic to the muscle, it is dependent on velocity and temperature.

Bibliography

Various authors, *Dizionario Oxford della Medicina*, I. Gremese, Rome (1996)

Angel R.W., 'Muscular contractions elicited by passive shortening', In: Desmedt J.E. (eds), *Motor Control Mechanism in Health and Disease*, Raven Press, New York (1983)

Benaglia PG., Sartorio F., Piralla F., *Il concetto pliometrico*, Sport&Medicina, March–April, (1996)

Berkinblit M.B., Feldman A.G., Fukson O.I., 'Adaptability of innate motor patterns and motor control mechanisms', *Behav Brain Sci* 9: 585–638, (1986)

Boccardi S., 'Le strutture propriocettive nella patologia ortopedico traumatologica', *Le Scienze Motorie*, III, n. 2, (1994)

Boccardi S., Lissoni A., *Cinesiologia*, vol. I–III, Soc. Ed. Universo, Rome (1980)

DIETZ V., 'Human neuronal control of automatic functional movements: interaction between central programs and afferent input', *Phys. Rev.*, 72(1): 33–69, (1992)

Donskoj D.D., Zatziorskij V.M., *Biomeccanica*, Soc. Stampa Sportiva, Rome (1983)

Erikson E., 'Finalità della biomeccanica applicata allo sport', In: Proceedings of the congress 'Biomeccanica e gesto sportivo', Ed. Delta, Terni (1991)

Fazio C., Loeb C. *Neurologia*, vol. I, III ed., Soc. Ed. Universo, Rome (1998)

Gowitzke B.A., Milner M., *Le basi scientifiche del movimento umano*, EMSI, Rome (1984)

GRAZIATI G., *Compendio di bioingegneria dell'apparato locomotore*, Ed. Ciba, Milan (1993)

Hewitt RM, Miller EC, Sanford AH., *The American illustrated Medical Dictionary*, 22. Saunders, Philadelphia (1956)

Huijing P.A., 'Parameter interdependence and success of skeletal muscle modelling', *Human Movement Sci* 14: 573–608, (1995)

Kandel E.R., Schwartz J.H., Jessell T.M., *Principi di neuroscienze*, Ed. Ambrosia, Milan

Kapandji I..A. Fisiologia Articolare, vol. I–III., Soc. Ed. Demi, Rome (1974)

Katz R., Rondot P., 'Muscle reaction to passive shortening in normal man', *Electroenceph. Clin. Neuroph.*, 45: 90–99, (1978)

Kelso J.A.S., Schoner G., 'Toward a physical (synergetic) theory of biological coordination', In: R. Graham E A. Wunderlin (eds). *Springer Proceedings in Physics* 19, pp. 224–237, (1987)

Latash M.L., *Control of human movement*, Human Kinetics Publisher, (1993)

Le Veau B.F., *Biomeccanica del movimento umano*, Verduci Ed., Rome (1993)

Nicoletti R., *Il controllo motorio*, Il Mulino, Bologna (1992)

Pirola V., *Cinesiologia – Il movimento umano applicato alla rieducazione e alle attivitàsportive*, Edi. Ermes, V ed., Milan (2002)

Rothwell J.C., *Il controllo del movimento volontario nell'uomo*, Masson, Milan (1991)

Rumolo R., Vitolo E. et al. *Dizionario medico Dompè*, Masson, Milan (1992)

Saltzman E.I., Kelso J.A.S. *Toward a dynamic account of motor memory and control*, Haskins Laboratories: Status Report on Speech Research, SR 71-72: 199–218, (1982)

Tittel K., *Anatomia Funzionale dell'uomo*, Edi. Ermes, Milan (1991)

Van Ingen Schenau G.J., Van Soest A.J., Gabreels F.J.M., Horstink M.W.I.M., 'The control of multijoint movements relies on detailed internal representations', *Human Movement Sci*, 14: 511–538, (1995)

Wells K.E., Luttgens K., *Kinesiologia: basi scientifiche del movimento umano*, Verduci Ed., Rome (1990)

Colour Plates

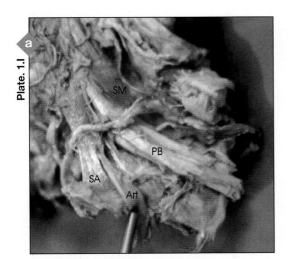

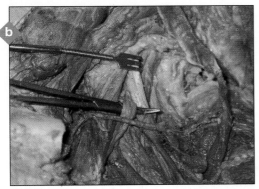

Variants of the shoulder muscles: (a) small scalene muscle (b) accessory scalene muscle, consisting of a duplication of the anterior scalene.
PB: brachial plexus; Art: subclavian artery; SA: anterior scalene muscle; SM: middle scalene muscle.

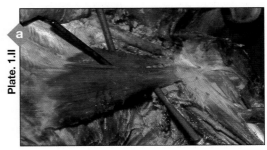

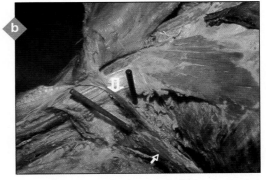

Supernumerary pectoralis minor muscle, (b) dorsopectoral muscle (axillary or Langer's arch).
Langer's arch   Latissimus dorsi m.

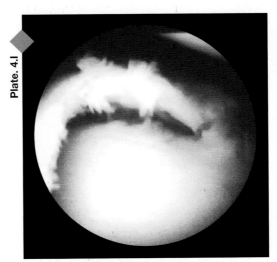

Type II SLAP lesion. Arthroscopic image.

Plate. 9.I

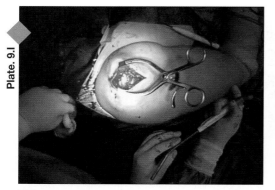

Mini-open surgery.

Plate. 10.II

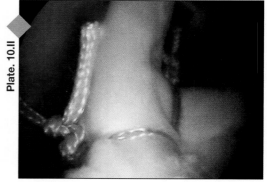

Debridement and fixation of the labrum and LHB for type II.

Plate. 9.II

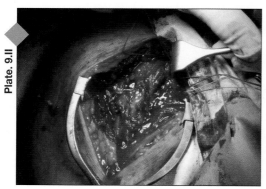

Open surgery.

Plate. 10.III

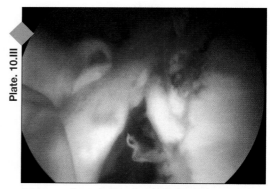

Arthroscopy for evaluation of unstable shoulder.

Plate. 10.I

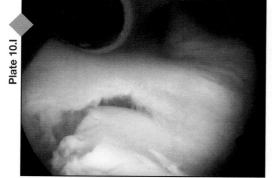

Type II SLAP lesion.

Plate. 10.IV

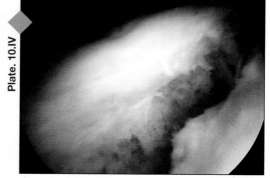

Lesions of the glenoid rim.

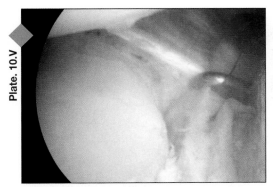

Arthroscopy demonstrates the posterior structures of the shoulder joint.

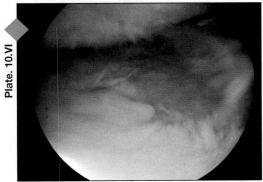

Surgical arthroscopy to remove inflamed synovial membrane and cartilage debris in a patient with premature osteoarthritis.

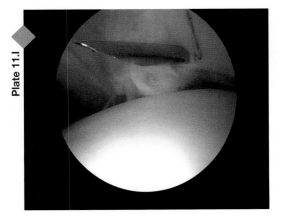

Arthroscopic image of an early lesion of the glenohumeral joint (view through the posterior portal, left shoulder).

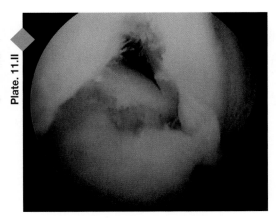

Arthroscopic image of a late lesion of the subacromial space (view through the lateral portal, right shoulder).

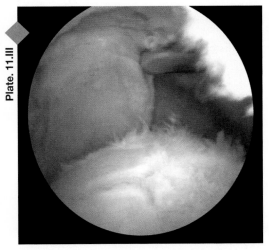

Arthroscopic image of a glenohumeral joint lesion that is too late (view through the posterolateral portal, right shoulder).

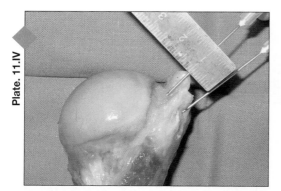

Insertion of the supraspinatus tendon in a cadaveric shoulder. Note the extension of the insertion over an area of at least 10 mm.

Plate 11.V

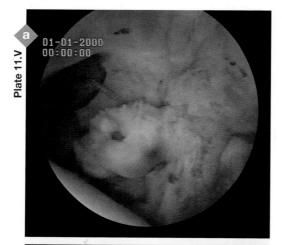

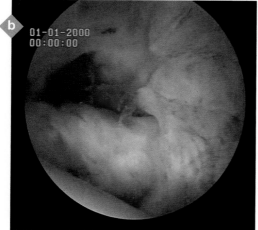

Complete upper lesion of the subscapularis tendon and repair (view through the posterior portal, left shoulder).

Plate 11.VI

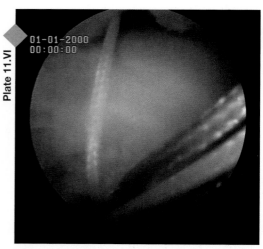

Medial anchor with double thread. Note the proximity of the joint cartilage of the humerus (view through the lateral portal, right shoulder).

Index

Index

Index

Index

Index

Index

Index

S

sacpulohumeral rhythm 31
sacpulothoracic osteokinematics 32
sacroiliac joint, stability 226
scalene muscles 19–20; fig.1.14; pl.1.1
scapula
  anomalies 63
  anterior tilt 116, 225
  cranial rotation 225
  dyskinesia 221, 223
  glenohumeral (sacpulohumeral) rhythm 31
  inferior angle 116; fig.8.6
  lateral view fig.1.3
  mobility 48, 64
  muscles 224, 225, 230
  position in relation to trunk 116
  posture 48
  proprioceptive neuromuscular facilitation (PNF) 188–9, 248
  rehabilitation exercises 182, 183, 187–8; figs.13.1–4
  resting position 116
  retraction strength 120
  rhythmic stabilization 188–9; fig.13.7
  stability 227
  throwing movements 227
  winged 80, 116
scapular sliding 46
scapular dyskinesia 49
scapular fracture 104
scapular protraction 116
scapular spine 9
  angle 11
  coracoid process, and 11
  prominence on 80
  root 116; fig.8.4
scapulohumeral complex 225
  anterior view fig.1.3
  dislocation 90, 147
  frontal section fig.1.3
  instability 146–7
  osteoarthritis 90
  surgical treatment 146–8
scapulohumeral periarthritis 57, 102
scapulohumeral rhythm
  alteration 153
scapulothoracic dyskinesis 116
scapulothoracic joint
  crepitation 211
  examination 120–1
  gliding 211–12; fig.14.32
  manipulation 211; fig.14.30
  mobilization techniques 210–12; figs.14.30–3
  movements 210; fig.14.29
  proprioceptive training 212; fig.14.33

  stabilization 230
  traction 211; fig.14.31
scapulothoracic muscles
  examination 119
  shortening 46
  weakness 45
scar tissue 62, 183–4
scleroderma 104
self-assessment questionnaires 111–14
sensory afferences 48; fig.8.2
septic arthritis 104
shock wave treatment 146
shot put 52
shoulder pain and disability index (SPADI) 174
shoulder severity index (SSI) 174
shoulder surgery perception (SSP) scale 177
sickness impact profile (SIP) 174
simple shoulder test (SST) 174
soft tissue neoplasia 104
softball 71, 74–5; fig.5.4
Speed's manoeuvre 128
Speed's test 65, 84; fig.6.11
spine
  cervical 48
  compensatory movement 80
  dorsal kyphosis, effect 46
  lumbar 48
  scapular see scapular spine
  stability 225
  thoracic 48
spinoappendicular muscles 250
stability 45–55, 224–5
  active stabilization 29–31
  aetiopathogenesis 45–6
  agonist-antagonist muscle imbalance 45–6, 48–9, 50, 53
  at rest 31
  capsuloligamentous stabilization 46–7
  compensation actions 47
  conceptual model 224; fig.15.5
  dislocation and 45
  effective force 49
  functional 47–50, 183
  glenohumeral joint 25–31
  global (secondary or movement) stabilizers 49
  gravity 31
  local (primary or deep) stabilizers 49
  lumbar spine 48, 227, 230
  mobility, and 45
  overhead sports 50–2
  pelvic 50, 226, 230
  proximal stability for distal mobility 182
  quantifying 119–20
  rotation strength, internal and external 225–6
  rotator cuff and 49, 225, 233
  sacroiliac joint 226

Index